December 2012

Donated by Randy Fuller RN
Educator for Obstetrical Services
Beverly Hospital

D1256859

EVIDENCE-BASED HANDBOOK OF NEONATOLOGY

EVIDENCE-BASED HANDBOOK OF NEONATOLOGY

editor

William Oh

The Warren Alpert Medical School
of Brown University, USA

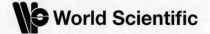 **World Scientific**

NEW JERSEY · LONDON · SINGAPORE · BEIJING · SHANGHAI · HONG KONG · TAIPEI · CHENNAI

Published by

World Scientific Publishing Co. Pte. Ltd.

5 Toh Tuck Link, Singapore 596224

USA office: 27 Warren Street, Suite 401-402, Hackensack, NJ 07601

UK office: 57 Shelton Street, Covent Garden, London WC2H 9HE

British Library Cataloguing-in-Publication Data
A catalogue record for this book is available from the British Library.

ISBN-13 978-981-4313-46-9
ISBN-10 981-4313-46-7

Typeset by Stallion Press
Email: enquiries@stallionpress.com

Printed in Singapore by Mainland Press Pte Ltd.

*This book is dedicated to
my wife, Mary,
who enthusiastically supported my career over the years;
and, to
my children and grandchildren, Ken, Amy, Laurie, Travis,
Katie, Kristen, Matthew, Thomas, Malia, and Tyler.*

Foreword

expertise from a large number of colleagues to outline current evidence-based practice. By choosing topics that are important, contemporary and yet even controversial, and outlining the rationale for care, they are helping us to move our discipline forward. We look forward to exciting future developments. In additional contfoversies, to continuing opportunities to interact with the trainees and the students who have given us so much inspiration and to improving .... the lives of our patients and families.

James F. Padbury, MD
Oh-way Professor of Pediatrics for Perinatal Research
The Women Alpert Medical School of Brown University

In 1975, the American Board of Pediatrics established the first sub-board certification for neonatology. Prior to that, our field was largely the purview of boutique clinical services in prestigious universities where pediatric, obstetric and related disciplines had a special interest in the care of high-risk and critically ill newborns. Our discipline has grown substantially in both its academic impact and the scope of research conducted. We have witnessed extraordinary advances in the care of our patients and families. There may be four epochs or four major "sea of changes" in our discipline. The first would surely be the creation of the subspecialty certification itself, while the second, I would argue was the licencing and clinical use of surfactant. The third is the widespread use of antenatal steroids, motivated by the NIH Consensus Conference. The final "sea of change" may well be the widespread adoption of the single-family model of newborn intensive care. While we have all experienced extraordinary improvements in the survival of ever-smaller and more delicate infants, their neurodevelopmental outcomes leave room for improvement. This new model of care may in fact be the next "sea of change" to have the greatest impact.

As our specialty has grown, it has also matured academically. We have come to pride ourselves on the widespread use of evidence-based practice. In our clinical and teaching roles, we strive to guide current care into new and better approaches of caring for our patients and their families using an evidence basis for decision making. In this handbook, Dr. William Oh, one of the pioneers of our discipline, has brought together expertise from a large number of colleagues to outline current evidence-based practice. By choosing topics that are important, contemporary and yes, even controversial, and outlining the rationale for care, they are helping us to move our discipline forward. We look forward to exciting future developments, to additional controversies, to continuing opportunities to interact with the trainees and the students who have given us so much inspiration and to improving the care and the lives of our patients and families.

James F. Padbury, MD
Oh–Zopfi Professor of Pediatrics for Perinatal Research
The Warren Alpert Medical School of Brown University

Preface

For the past six decades, neonatology has emerged as a vibrant subspecialty of pediatrics. Basic science and translational research in Perinatal Biology, and their application to clinical trials have generated a large amount of data that allow for implementation of evidence-based interventions for various neonatal ailments. The result is a significant improvement in survival rates among high-risk infants, particularly the very low birth weight infants. In fact, during this time period, the neonatal mortality rates in the United States have declined from approximately 20/1000 in the 1950s to the current estimate of 7/1000 in live births. Similar declines in neonatal mortality rate have also occurred in many developed and developing countries around the world.

The downside of this phenomenon is that while survival rates have improved markedly among the very low birth weight infants, their late morbidities and neurodevelopmental outcomes have not been as favorably affected. This is in part due to the application of interventions that have not been thoroughly tested for their efficacy and the adverse effects resulting in the lack of improvement of the illness; in the worse scenarios they produced injuries to various organ systems including the lung and central nervous systems. The delay in recovery accounts for the prolonged hospital stay associated with inadequate nutrition and, in the absence of family-centered care, deprivation of parental bonding. Injury to central nervous systems, inadequate nutrition, and lack of parentral bonding result in neurodevelopmental impairment among survivors. This observation clearly illustrates the importance of practicing evidence-based medicine, using intervention and management that have been tested in appropriately designed clinical trials. The purpose of this handbook is to present evidence-based management strategies for various common clinical problems in the newborn infants.

By nature of being a handbook, this publication is not meant to be all-inclusive as in a textbook of neonatology. There are several well-respected textbooks of neonatal and perinatal medicine that the readers can use. The main goal of this handbook is to present pathophysiology and management of common ailments affecting the newborn. I selected topics based on three guiding principles: (1) the ailments affect a large number of newborn infants; (2) the topics have new developments; and (3) the subject is somewhat controversial, particularly with reference to management. I have assembled a group of authors who were former fellows or close colleagues at Brown Medical School and in other major academic institutions to write the 21 chapters in this handbook. Each of the authors is expert in his/her field who can provide specific and authoritative comments on the subject. They thrive to use as much available evidence in the literature as possible which in part accounts for the lengthy reference list.

I hope that this handbook will provide useful information to the clinicians and other care providers in the field of neonatology in our quest to continue the trends of improving outcomes both in terms of survival and quality of survivors.

William Oh, MD

Editor

2010

Contents

Contributors

Ira Adams-Chapman, MD
Assistant Professor of Pediatrics
Emory University
Atlanta, GA
USA
iadamsc@emory.edu

Eduardo Bancalari, MD
Department of Pediatrics
University of Miami
Miami, FL
USA
ebancalari@miami.edu

Stephen Baumgart, MD
Professor of Pediatrics
George Washington University
School of Medicine & Health
   Sciences
Washington, D.C.
USA
STbaumga@cnmc.org

Joseph M. Bliss, MD, PhD
Assistant Professor of Pediatrics
The Warren Alpert Medical
   School of Brown University
Providence, RI
USA
jbliss@wihri.org

Waldemar A. Carlo, MD
Professor of Pediatrics
University of Alabama at
   Birmingham
Birmingham, AL
USA

Ronald I. Clyman, MD
Professor of Pediatrics
University of California,
   San Francisco
San Francisco, CA
USA
clymanr@peds.ucsf.edu

Donald R. Coustan, MD
Professor of Obstetrics and
  Gynecology
The Warren Alpert Medical
  School of Brown University
Providence, RI
USA
dcoustan@wihri.org

Mara G. Coyle, MD
Associate Professor of Pediatrics
  (Clinical)
The Warren Alpert Medical
  School of Brown University
Providence, RI
USA
coylem@southcoast.org

Lloyd R. Feit, MD
Associate Professor of
  Pediatrics
The Warren Alpert Medical
  School of Brown University
Providence, RI
USA
lfeit@lifespan.org

Sara R. Ford, MD
Clinical Assistant Professor of
  Pediatrics
The Warren Alpert Medical
  School of Brown University
Providence, RI
USA
sford@lifespan.org

**Thor Willy Ruud Hansen,
  MD, PhD**
Professor of Pediatrics
University of Oslo
Oslo, Norway
t.w.r.hansen@medisin.uio.no

John Kelleher, MD
Department of Pediatrics
University of Alabama at
  Birmingham
Birmingham, AL
USA

Jae H. Kim, MD, PhD
Assistant Professor of Pediatrics
University of California,
  San Diego
San Diego, CA
USA
neojae@ucsd.edu

Yuh-Jyh Lin, MD
Associate Professor of Pediatrics
Director, Pediatric Pulmonology
National Cheng Kung University
  Hospital
Tainan, Taiwan
Lin.yuhjyh@gmail.com

François I. Luks, MD, PhD
Professor of Surgery, Pediatrics,
  Obstetrics & Gynecology
The Warren Alpert Medical
  School of Brown University
Providence, RI
USA
Francois_luks @brown.edu

Leslie T. McKinley, RD
Neonatal Nutritionist
Women and Infants Hospital
Providence, RI
USA
lmckinley@wihri.org

Ran Namgung, MD
Professor of Pediatrics
Yonsei University College of
    Medicine
Seoul, Korea
ranng@yuhs.ac

Barbara M. O'Brien, MD
Assistant Professor of Obstetric
    and Gynecology
The Warren Alpert Medical
    School of Brown University
Providence, RI
USA
bobrien@wihri.org

William Oh, MD
Professor of Pediatrics
The Warren Alpert Medical
    School of Brown University
Providence, RI
USA
woh@wihri.org

James F. Padbury, MD
Oh–Zopfi Professor of Pediatrics
    for Perinatal Research
The Warren Alpert Medical
    School of Brown University
Providence, RI

USA
jpadbury@wihri.org

Ted Rosenkrantz, MD
Professor of Pediatrics
University of Connecticut
Hartford, CT
USA
TedR1@aol.com

Richard J. Schanler, MD
Professor of Pediatrics
Albert Einstein College of
    Medicine
Bronx, New York
USA
RSchanle@NSHS.edu

Seetha Shankaran, MD
Professor of Pediatrics
Wayne State University
Detroit, Michigan
USA
sshankar@med.wayne.edu

Ilene R. S. Sosenko, MD
Department of Pediatrics
University of Miami
Miami, FL
USA
isosenko@miami.edu

Roman Starikov, MD
Teaching Fellow in Obstetrics and
    Gynecology
The Warren Alpert Medical
    School of Brown University

Providence, RI
USA
Rstarikov@wihri.org

Bonnie E. Stephens, MD
Assistant Professor of Pediatrics
The Warren Alpert Medical
    School of Brown University
Providence, RI
USA
Bstephens@wihri.org

Barbara J. Stoll, MD
Professor and Chair of Pediatrics
Emory University
Atlanta, GA
USA
Barbara_Stoll@oz.ped.emory.edu

Reginald C. Tsang, MBBS
Professor Emeritus of Pediatrics
University of Cincinnati
Cincinnati, OH
USA
rctsang@gmail.com

Maximo Vento, MD
Associate Professor of Pediatrics
University of Valencia
Valencia, Spain
maximo.vento@uv.es

Betty R. Vohr, MD
Professor of Pediatrics
The Warren Alpert Medical
    School of Brown University

Providence, RI
USA
Bvohr@wihri.org

**Rajan Wadhawan, MBBS,
    MD**
Assistant Professor of Pediatrics
University of South Florida
Tampa, FL
USA
wadhawar@allkids.org

Katharine D. Wenstrom, MD
Professor of Obstetrics and
    Gynecology
The Warren Alpert Medical
    School of Brown University
Providence, RI
USA
kwenstrom@wihri.org

Tsu-Fuh Yeh, MD, PhD
Distinguished Professor of
    Pediatrics
College of Medicine
China Medical University
Taichung, Taiwan

Senior Neonatologist
John Stroger Hospital of Cook
    County
Chicago, Illinois
USA
tsufuhy@yahoo.com

PART

I

The Fetus

Chapter

Prenatal Diagnosis

Barbara M. O'Brien and Katharine D. Wenstrom

Introduction

During the last few decades, options for prenatal diagnosis have significantly expanded due to improvements in genetic technology and prenatal imaging modalities. The term prenatal diagnosis is an inclusive term involving genetic counseling, fetal risk assessment, noninvasive and invasive fetal testing, as well as population screening.[1]

Patients seek prenatal diagnosis for a variety of reasons, including advanced maternal age, family history of a birth defect or genetic disorder, abnormal maternal serum screen, exposure to a potential teratogen, or a maternal medical disorder that can affect the fetus. Pregnant women are routinely offered screening for a list of autosomal recessive diseases; those who are determined to be carriers also seek prenatal diagnostic services.

This chapter will discuss the different options available for prenatal diagnosis of congenital disorders, as well as the approach to screening ongoing pregnancies for genetic disease.

The Impact and Etiology of Birth Defects

The medical impact of birth defects is considerable. In 2006, the most recent year for which final statistics are available, the infant mortality rate was 6.69 per 1000 live births.[2] The leading causes of infant deaths were congenital malformations, deformations and chromosomal abnormalities. Eight percent (1/13) of conceptuses are chromosomally abnormal, accounting for 50% of all first-trimester abortions and 6 to 11% of all still-births and neonatal deaths. By grade school, a major or minor structural birth defect will be recognized in 8% of all children, and another 8% will have developmental delay.[3]

Dysmorphologists divide birth defects into three major categories: malformations, deformations and disruptions. Malformations are the result of intrinsic abnormalities in one or more genetic processes directing fetal development, regardless of whether the precise genetic etiology is known.[4] A common malformation is a neural tube defect.

In contrast to malformations, deformations occur when genetically normal tissues are exposed to extrinsic factors that physically impinge on the fetus, resulting in abnormal development of that tissue or structure. An example of a deformation is a contracture of an extremity resulting from fetal compression during prolonged oligohydramnios. The third major category of birth defect is a disruption. Disruptions occur when normal tissue is damaged by a vascular accident, trauma, or exposure to a terato-gen. A common disruption is a limb amputation resulting from an amniotic band that wraps around the limb, cutting off the blood supply to and eventually destroying the tissues distal to the band.

Screening Versus Diagnosis of Genetic Disorders

A key concept in the field of prenatal diagnosis is the distinction between screening tests and diagnostic tests. The goal of a screening test is to determine the risk of disease in an asymptomatic individual who is other-wise believed to be at low risk. Genetic screening tests seek to identify individuals who are at increased risk of having a child with a specific dis-order, for whom prenatal diagnostic testing may be warranted. In contrast to screening tests, diagnostic tests confirm or rule out a specific disease in an individual who is suspected of having or is at high risk of developing that disease.

An ideal perinatal genetic screening test should fulfill the criteria for a general medical screening test with one important addition: it should be possible to do the screening test and get the results early enough in gestation to permit the patient to consider her options, and to undergo safe and legal pregnancy termination if desired.[1] The other five criteria are: it should identify a common or important fetal disorder, be cost effective and easy to perform, have a high detection rate and low false positive rate, be reliable and reproducible, and screen for a disorder for which there is an accurate diagnostic test.

Chromosomal Abnormalities

Although the majority of aneuploid pregnancies end in miscarriage, a variety of chromosome abnormalities can occur in live births. Most trisomies result from maternal meiotic nondisjunction, a phenomenon that occurs more frequently as women (and their gametes) age. Numeric sex chromosome abnormalities can result from either maternal or paternal nondisjunction; inversions and translocations may be sporadic or familial.

Autosomal trisomy

Although any woman at any age can have a trisomic fetus, the frequency of meiotic errors and resulting fetal aneuploidy steadily increases with each year of maternal age. Traditionally, women who would be age 35 or older at the time of delivery were thought to be at sufficient risk to warrant the routine offering of fetal karyotype analysis by chorionic villus sampling (CVS) or genetic amniocentesis. Age 35 was an arbitrary cutoff chosen because, from that age onwards, the risk of fetal Down syndrome begins to increase sharply with each year. Additionally, the midtrimester risk of Down syndrome or the term risk of any aneuploidy roughly equaled the risk of pregnancy loss after amniocentesis at that time (approximately 1:200). However, over the last 20 years, improvements in amniocentesis technique have resulted in post-amniocentesis pregnancy loss rates ≤ 1:300 at most centers. Accordingly, the maternal age at which age alone increases the risk of fetal aneuploidy sufficiently to warrant an invasive diagnostic test has become blurred, with many younger women requesting genetic amniocentesis or CVS. Conversely, because the sensitivity of Down syndrome screening tests has increased to 85–95%

over the same time period, many older women prefer to undergo serum screening before deciding about invasive testing. According to the American College of Obstetricians and Gynecologists (ACOG),[5] both fetal aneuploidy screening and invasive diagnostic testing should now be made available to all women regardless of age, and all pregnant women should be counseled accordingly. Women whose obstetric history, family history, or ultrasound findings suggest an increased risk, whose serum screening test indicates increased risk, and who have had a previous pregnancy complicated by trisomy 21, 18, or 13, or any other trisomy in which the fetus survived at least to the second trimester should be offered the opportunity to proceed directly to diagnostic testing. After having a trisomic pregnancy, the risk of having another pregnancy complicated by the same or a different trisomy is estimated to be 1% until the age-related risk exceeds this figure, after which the risk is determined by the maternal age. Invasive diagnostic testing should be performed only after a full discussion of the risks of the procedure relative to the patient's estimated risk of fetal aneuploidy.

Sex chromosome abnormalities

Sex chromosome abnormalities occur in 1 of every 1,000 births. The most common are 45, X; 47, XXY; 47, XXX; 47, XYY; and mosaicism (the presence of two or more cell populations with different karyotypes). Because a fetal XXX or XXY karyotype can result from maternal meiotic nondysjunction of the X chromosome, this history increases the recurrence risk of another fetal trisomy to 1%; women with this history should be offered prenatal testing in subsequent pregnancies. Because monosomy X (Turner syndrome) and 47, XYY arise by a different mechanism, these aneuploidies are not associated with a significant recurrence risk. However, a woman whose fetus had either of these karyotypes may request genetic testing for reassurance.

Translocations and inversions

A translocation usually involves the reciprocal exchange of genetic material between two different (nonhomologous) chromosomes. A break occurs in one arm of each chromosome, and all the genetic material distal to each break point is exchanged.

In a balanced translocation, no genetic material is gained or lost, and the individual carrying the rearrangement usually is phenotypically normal. However, a carrier of a balanced translocation may make unbalanced gametes, resulting in infertility, early pregnancy loss, or structurally or developmentally abnormal offspring. The translocation carrier's risk of having an affected child with an abnormal amount of chromosomal material should be estimated individually, taking into account the chromosomes involved, the amount of genetic material exchanged, the gender of the transmitting parent, and the method of ascertainment. In general, translocation carriers identified after the birth of an abnormal infant are at increased risk (5 to 30%) of having another abnormal child. Those identified during an infertility workup are at low risk (0 to 5%) of having an abnormal child, but are at increased risk of continued infertility, most likely because their translocation leads to nonviable gametes or conceptuses.

A Robertsonian translocation results from the centromeric fusion of two acrocentric chromosomes. Acrocentric chromosomes (chromosomes 13, 14, 15, 21, and 22) are those with the centromere located very near one end. Although the carrier of a Robertsonian translocation is usually phenotypically normal, he or she is at risk of producing unbalanced gametes. Whether the unbalanced gametes will result in abnormal offspring depends on the type of translocation, the chromosomes involved, and the gender of the carrier parent. The most clinically important Robertsonian translocations are those involving chromosome 21 and another acrocentric chromosome, most commonly chromosome 14 (t[14;21]). Carriers of these translocations have the potential to have a liveborn child with trisomy 21. The risk of trisomy 21 is 15% if the translocation is maternal and 2% or less if it is paternal.

Inversions arise when two breaks occur in the same chromosome and the segment between the break points is inverted before the breaks are repaired. No genetic material is lost, but the gene sequence is altered. Most carriers of inversions are phenotypically normal. However, because inversion carriers usually produce both balanced and unbalanced gametes, fertility may be affected. When both break points occur in the same arm of the chromosome (paracentric inversion), the centromere is not involved.

The unbalanced gametes therefore contain either no centromere or two centromeres, and are thus so abnormal as to preclude fertilization. For this reason, the carrier of a paracentric inversion has virtually no risk of having abnormal offspring. However, if the break points occur in the opposite arms of the chromosome (pericentric inversion), then the centromere is involved. The unbalanced gametes produced in this case may contain duplications or deletions, but still be capable of fertilization. As a result, the carrier of a pericentric inversion has a 5 to 10% risk of having abnormal children if the carrier status was ascertained after the birth of an abnormal child and 1 to 3% if not. All carriers of chromosome rearrangements should be counseled and offered prenatal diagnosis based on their history and estimated risk.

Triploidy

A triploid conception is one in which three complete haploid ($n = 23$) chromosome complements are present, resulting in 69 total chromosomes. This abnormality occurs in 1 to 2% of recognized pregnancies, accounting for 15% of chromosomally abnormal abortuses. Most commonly, triploidy results from double fertilization of a normal haploid egg (dispermy) or from fertilization with a diploid sperm. Such conceptions usually are partial hydatidiform moles and end spontaneously in the first trimester; the recurrence risk is minimal, and genetic testing in future pregnancies is unnecessary. A fetus rarely develops in association with triploidy. Fetuses resulting from the fertilization of a diploid ovum (digynic) are severely growth restricted and have small, noncystic placentas. Fetuses resulting from dispermy (diandric) are relatively normal in size but have large, cystic placentas. This form of triploidy is frequently associated with the midtrimester onset of severe preeclampsia. Women who experienced triploidy in association with a fetus surviving past the first trimester have a 1 to 2% risk of recurrence of any numerical aneuploidy and should be offered genetic testing in subsequent pregnancies.

Parental aneuploidy

Women with trisomy 21 or 47, XXX and men with 47, XYY usually are fertile and have a 30% risk of trisomic offspring. Men with trisomy 21 or 47, XXY and women with 45X usually are sterile.

Maternal Serum Screening

Maternal serum screening for Down syndrome

Down syndrome, which occurs at a rate of one per 660 live births, is the most common form of mental retardation with a confirmed genetic cause. The majority of Down syndrome cases (97%) are caused by trisomy 21, with the remainder caused by other cytogenetic abnormalities such as translocations and mosaicism. The Down syndrome phenotype includes moderate to severe mental retardation, with an average intelligence quotient (IQ) of 40, and characteristic facial features. Patients typically have short stature and can have a variety of birth defects: 50% have a congenital heart defect, most frequently complete atrioventricular canal; 10% have gastrointestinal abnormalities; and approximately 50% have visual and hearing deficits.[6]

Down syndrome screening is available in both the first and second trimesters, depending on when the woman presents for prenatal care, and can be performed in a variety of ways. Although most current screening protocols achieve high detection rates with low screen-positive rates, none of the screening options is perfectly sensitive or specific. Current invasive fetal diagnostic methods achieve near 100% diagnostic accuracy, but are complicated by low but real risks of procedure-related pregnancy loss.

Genetic amniocentesis to identify aneuploidy such as trisomy 21 (Down syndrome) in the fetuses of women at high risk has been available for almost 50 years. As noted earlier, the definition of "high risk" in a singleton pregnancy traditionally, if arbitrarily, included being 35 years or older at the time of delivery. However, because women aged 35 or more have <12% of all pregnancies, the majority (80%) of Down syndrome infants actually are born to women younger than age 35. Thus, even if all women age 35 or more elected to have genetic amniocentesis, only 20% of affected fetuses would be identified. With the development of several multiple-marker screening tests, the majority of women of all ages who are at increased risk to have a child with Down syndrome can now be identified in the first or second trimesters.[7]

The second trimester "quad screen," consisting of maternal serum AFP, estriol, hCG, and inhibin, identifies approximately 81% of all Down syndrome cases and 75% of all cases of trisomy 18 at a screen positive rate of 5%.[8] For women who present for prenatal care in the first few months of pregnancy, first-trimester Down syndrome screening is also possible, using maternal serum analytes either alone or in combination with a sonographic marker. First-trimester screening is typically performed between 10 and 13 weeks' gestation. The first-trimester screening test with the best detection rate at the lowest screen-positive rate includes both maternal serum analyte levels and sonographic measurement of the fetal nuchal translucency. Free β-human chorionic gonadotropin (hCg) and pregnancy-associated plasma protein A (PAPP-A) are the most discriminatory first-trimester analytes studied to date; free β-hCg levels are higher than expected and PAPP-A levels are lower in pregnancies complicated by fetal Down syndrome.[9,10] The most predictive ultrasound marker is measurement of the nuchal translucency (NT), an echolucent area seen in longitudinal midsagittal views of the back of the fetal neck between 10 and 14 weeks' gestation. Because the NT increases in size as the fetus grows, using a specific size cut off to define an abnormal result leads to decreased test sensitivity. Expressing the NT as a multiple of the median (MoM) accounts for gestational, age-related size changes and also allows it to be used in the algorithm along with maternal serum analyte levels to calculate a composite risk. Because the NT is a very small area, measurements are difficult to obtain accurately and reproducibly, and minor measurement inaccuracies can lead to major changes in risk estimation. Specific training in standardized measurement techniques is required, and adherence to specific guidelines for measuring the NT is imperative. In addition, because NT medians vary not only from center to center but also from operator to operator, and the medians gradually change or "drift" over time, each center's or operator's medians should be monitored carefully and adjusted as necessary.[11]

Four large trials of combined first-trimester ultrasonographic and serum screening, including 103,856 patients and 328 cases of Down syndrome, have been completed and yielded similar results. The BUN, FASTER, SURUSS, and OSCAR trials enrolled women who underwent screening between 10 weeks 4 days and 13 weeks 6 days of gestation and determined the risks of Down syndrome and trisomy 18 based on maternal age, free beta hCG, PAPP-A, and NT measurement. When the false positive rates were held at 5%, these four trials averaged a detection rate of 84%.[12–15]

The sensitivity of Down syndrome screening can be further improved by combining first and second trimester screening tests. In the integrated screening test, both first trimester analytes and NT and second trimester analytes are measured, and one composite screening test result is provided after completion of the second trimester portion of the test. The advantage of this strategy is that the detection rates increase to 94–96%, at a false positive rate of ≤5%.[16] The disadvantage is that no result is provided until the second trimester. All analytes must be assayed in the same lab and the patient must complete the entire two-part test or else does not receive a result. An alternative is the sequential screening test, in which the first trimester screening test is performed, the woman is informed of the result and then may or may not go on to second trimester screening. In the sequential step wise approach, the likelihood ratio derived from the first trimester screen is used to modify the likelihood ratio determined by the second trimester screen, and only women with a final screen positive result are offered invasive testing. This strategy results in a 95% detection rate at a = 5% false positive rate.[17] In contingent sequential screening, the first trimester result is placed in one of three categories; those at highest risk are offered diagnostic testing, those at lowest risk need no further screening, and those at intermediate risk go on to the second trimester screening test. This strategy has an 88 to 94% detection rate at a 5% false positive rate.[18]

Advantages of both forms of sequential screening include that the woman can choose to act on the result of the first trimester test; the woman whose risk is very low may decide not to proceed to the second trimester test, while the woman whose risk is very high may choose to have a CVS procedure rather than wait for the second part of the test. Down syndrome detection rates are still high — 88 to 95% — but a reduced number of second trimester tests need to be done and fewer women need to undergo invasive testing, thus making the screening process less expensive and losing fewer normal fetuses as the result of an invasive diagnostic procedure. Disadvantages include the necessity of doing both tests in the same lab, and the need to provide test results and counseling twice. One important rule to remember: when either form of sequential screening is chosen, it is essential that both tests be done in the same lab. The lab will then be able to use the risk estimate determined by the first trimester test as the *a priori* risk for the second trimester test, yielding the most accurate ultimate risk estimate at the lowest screen positive rate. If the tests are done separately, the final screen positive rate will be the sum of the rates of the first and second trimester tests, and thus too high.

Current ACOG guidelines regarding screening for fetal Down syndrome recommend that screening and invasive testing for fetal aneuploidy should be made available to all women who present for prenatal care before 20 weeks' gestation, regardless of maternal age. Although the ability to choose from among a variety of screening strategies may be attractive to some patients, others may find it confusing. It is therefore reasonable for practitioners to choose a limited number of strategies to routinely offer patients, such as sequential screening for women who present early enough to undergo first trimester screening, and the quad screen for women who present later. In areas where NT measurement is not available, both first trimester screening and combined first and second trimester screening can be done using only maternal serum analytes; the detection rates are somewhat lower than when NT is included, but still acceptable.

Maternal serum screening for neural tube defects

Neural tube defects (NTDs) are the most common birth defect world wide, affecting 1 to 2 per 1,000 live births. All variations of the multiple marker screening test include maternal serum alpha-fetoprotein (AFP), because this marker also screens for fetal NTDs. Because 95% of all NTDs occur in families with no previously affected children or relatives, all pregnant women should be offered NTD screening, regardless of their family history. Maternal serum AFP screening identifies 90% of fetuses with open spina bifida or anencephaly and at least half of all fetuses with a ventral wall defect.[19]

All pregnancies characterized by confirmed elevated maternal serum AFP should be evaluated ultrasonographically. In the second trimester fetus, 90 to 99% of open NTDs can be diagnosed by ultrasound examination. Not only can open spine defects be directly visualized, but

99% of fetuses with an open spina bifida have at least one of five ultra-sonographic cranial signs: lemon sign (frontal scalloping or notching), obliteration of the posterior fossa, banana sign (chiari deformation), ventriculomegaly, and small biparietal diameter.[20] As the resolution of ultrasound imaging has improved, controversy has arisen regarding the value of amniocentesis to measure amniotic fluid AFP levels when a woman with an elevated maternal serum AFP has an ultrasound exam that is reassuring. Although many sonographers report nearly 100% diagnostic accuracy with ultrasonography alone, this detection rate is influenced by the skill and experience of the person evaluating the images, the quality of the ultrasound equipment, the patient's habitus, and the position of the fetus.[21] The maternal serum AFP level is another important factor to consider, since levels ≤3.5 MOM are unlikely to be false positive. Amniotic fluid AFP analysis and confirmation of the presence of acetylcholinesterase — which indicates direct exposure of neural tissue to amniotic fluid — identifies all NTDs except the 3 to 5% of fetuses whose spine defect is covered by skin. The decision of whether to perform amniocentesis should be on an individual basis, considering both the quality of the ultrasound evaluation and the patient's desires. If an amniocentesis is performed, a fetal karyotype should be obtained; in the setting of elevated maternal serum AFP, 16% of abnormal fetuses and 0.61% of normal-appearing fetuses will have chromosome abnormalities.[19]

Fetus with Major Structural Defects Identified by Ultrasonography

The discovery of a structural malformation of a major fetal organ or structure or the finding of two or more minor malformations or dysmorphisms (i.e. choroid plexus cyst, extra digit, single umbilical artery), increases the risk of aneuploidy sufficiently to warrant genetic testing of the fetus, regardless of maternal age or parental karyotypes. An exception to this rule is a fetal defect known to be familial and not associated with aneuploidy (e.g. fetal cleft lip discovered during an ultrasound examination ordered because the mother has a cleft lip).

Single-Gene Disorders

Patient or family history

Single-gene or "Mendelian" disorders are generally transmitted as auto-somal dominant, autosomal recessive, or X-linked recessive traits. An exception is any new single-gene disorder that results in infertility or death before reproduction; these occur as the result of a spontaneous new mutation. For example, gene deletions on the Y chromosome are fre-quently not transmissible because they result in infertility.

The number of single-gene disorders that can be diagnosed prenatally is rapidly increasing. The list of diagnosable diseases currently includes auto-somal dominant diseases such as neurofibromatosis, myotonic dystrophy, adult polycystic kidney disease, Huntington's disease, and osteogenesis imperfecta; autosomal recessive conditions such as cystic fibrosis, phenyl-ketonuria, congenital adrenal hyperplasia, and Tay-Sachs and other enzyme deficiency diseases; and X-linked diseases, including hemophilia A, Duchenne's muscular dystrophy, and Fragile X syndrome. Any patient with a personal or family history of a monogenic disorder should be referred for genetic counseling and consideration of carrier testing or prenatal diagnosis before conception or early in pregnancy.

Ethnic groups at high risk

Although single-gene disorders are generally rare, some ethnic groups are at a higher risk of having certain diseases than the general population and should be counseled and offered genetic screening accordingly. If only one person in a couple is a member of a high-risk group, that person can be tested first; if he or she is not determined to be a carrier, the partner may not need to be screened.

African Americans have an increased risk of having sickle-cell disease, the most common hemoglobin disorder in the United States. Approximately 8% of African Americans carry the sickle hemoglobin gene, which also is found with increased frequency in those of Mediterranean, Caribbean, Latin American, or Middle Eastern descent.[4]

Individuals of Southeast Asian origin are at an increased risk of car-rying hemoglobin E, the second most common abnormal hemoglobin in the world, and those of Mediterranean or Asian origin are at increased risk of having α-thalassemia or β-thalassemia. Hemoglobin E has an abnormal beta chain in which lysine is substituted for glutamic acid, resulting in susceptibility to oxidative stress. The thalassemias occur as the result of a functional deletion of one or more of the two β genes or two or more of the four α genes. The loss of these genes leads to decreased production of the hemoglobin chain in question, reduced production of normal hemoglobin A, the production of an alternate hemoglobin (hemoglobin A2) in the case of beta thalassemia, hemolysis and anemia which can be severe.

Cystic fibrosis (CF) is an autosomal recessive condition that results in chronic pulmonary and exocrine pancreatic disease, as well as infertility in affected males due to congenital absence of the vas deferens. It is the most common monogenic disorder in the Caucasian population, with a carrier frequency of 1 in 22 in Caucasians of North European heritage; it also occurs frequently in those of Ashkenazi Jewish descent (carrier frequency 1: 24) and Native American heritage (carrier frequency unknown). Ethnic groups at low risk of CF include African Americans (carrier rate 1:65), Hispanic Americans (1:46), and Asian Americans (1:94). Although the National Institutes of Health and the ACOG have recommended that cystic fibrosis screening be offered to all pregnant Caucasians of North European descent or Ashkenazi Jewish heritage, they also recommend that it be made available to pregnant women of other ethnic groups because of this disparity in mutation frequency.

More than 1,300 different gene mutations that cause cystic fibrosis have been identified. The most common cystic fibrosis mutation in Caucasians, ΔF508, accounts for 75% of CF cases in this group.[4] If a specific gene mutation has been identified in an affected family, individuals at risk can be tested for that particular mutation. When there is no family history of cystic fibrosis, since it is not possible to screen for all 1300 known mutations during carrier testing, most laboratories now screen for a panel of 23 mutations that each have a frequency of at least 0.1% in American CF patients. If certain specific mutations are identified in the first mutation panel, the lab will screen for one or more of seven second-tier mutations, to help clarify the results and predict the prognosis.

Because the current screening test identifies only 23 of the 1,300 known CF mutations, an individual who has a negative cystic fibrosis screening test cannot be told that she does not carry the cystic fibrosis gene. However, because the 23 mutations evaluated account for the majority of CF cases in this country, she can be informed that the negative test significantly reduces her risk of carrying a CF mutation, from one in 22 (the *a priori* risk based solely on ethnic origin) to one in 246.[22] If both members of the couple test negative, their risk of having a child with cystic fibrosis is reduced to one in 242,100.

In addition to cystic fibrosis, ACOG recommends that counseling and carrier screening for Tay-Sachs disease, familial dysautonomia, and Canavan disease be offered to all patients of Jewish heritage.[23] Carrier screening for other disorders for which this group is at risk such as mucolipidosis IV, Niemann-Pick disease type A, Fanconi anemia group C, Bloom syndrome and Gaucher disease, should also be made available.

Nonmendelian inheritance

Certain single-gene disorders are transmitted in nonclassical (non-mendelian) ways. For example, some inherited diseases occur as a result of a mutation in mitochondrial DNA (i.e. Leber's hereditary optic atrophy, Kearns-Sayre syndrome, and myoclonic epilepsy with ragged red fibers). Because mitochondria are passed to the ovum exclusively by the mother, mitochondrial disorders are characterized by maternal inheritance.

Another nonclassical inheritance pattern involves germline mosaicism. Although it was previously believed that conditions caused by new autosomal dominant mutations (i.e. osteogenesis imperfecta type II or achondroplasia) occurred sporadically in the single ovum or sperm involved in fertilization, and thus had no recurrence risk, there is evidence that some individuals actually carry two or more populations of germ cells, one of which contains the new mutation. Because the autosomal dominant mutation is carried by many germ cells, not just one, it is therefore possible to have another affected child. As a result, the risk of having another child with the same condition caused by a new autosomal dominant mutation is generally quoted as being somewhere between 1% and 7%, not zero.[4]

Hereditary Unstable DNA

Hereditary unstable DNA is the name for certain genes that can change in size and become inactivated, thus changing the phenotype, as they are passed from parent to child. Most of these genes contain a series of trinucleotide repeats — for example, 100 copies of CGG — that can increase or decrease in size as the gene is transmitted. Once a region of repeats reaches a critical size, the gene is usually turned off and the protein it encodes is no longer produced. Fragile X, the most common inherited form of mental retardation, is caused by a region of CGG repeats in the FMR1 gene on the X chromosome. When the region expands to more than 200 repeats, it is methylated, thus turning the FMR1 gene off; the Fragile X phenotype is caused by the lack of FMR1 protein. Prenatal testing for Fragile X syndrome should be offered to known carriers of the premutation or mutation. Testing for Fragile X syndrome should be considered for any child with developmental delay of uncertain etiology, autism, or autistic behavior, or for any individual with mental retardation of uncertain etiology. Because Fragile X premutation carriers can have ovarian failure or an elevated follicle-stimulating hormone level before 40 years of age, women with premature ovarian failure without a known cause should be screened to determine whether they have the Fragile X premutation.[24] Although such women will not need this information to inform their own reproductive choices, it would be valuable to potentially affected family members.

Multifactorial Disorders

Multifactorial disorders are caused by a combination of factors, some genetic and some nongenetic (i.e. environmental). Multifactorial disorders tend to recur in families but are not transmitted in any distinctive pattern. Many congenital structural abnormalities involving a single organ system are multifactorial, having an incidence in the general population of approximately one per 1,000. Examples of multifactorial traits are:

* Cleft lip, with or without cleft palate
* Congenital cardiac defects

- Diaphragmatic hernia
- Hydrocephalus
- Müllerian fusion defects
- Neural tube defects (NTDs)
- Posterior urethral valves
- Pyloric stenosis
- Renal agenesis
- Talipes equinovarus.

Because most of the defects on the above list also may occur as a result of a genetic syndrome, a single-gene disorder, or a chromosome abnormality, a thorough evaluation by a geneticist or fetal pathologist (in the case of pregnancy loss) may be necessary before multifactorial inheritance can be assumed. Counseling about multifactorial inheritance should include the following points[25]:

- The risk to first-degree relatives of the affected individual (mother, father, brother, sister) is higher than in the general population. The most commonly quoted risk is an empirical risk based on experience with similar families (recurrence rate of 1 to 5% in most cases).
- The risk is sharply lower (<1%) for second-degree and more distant relatives.
- The recurrence risk is higher when more than one family member is affected and when the defect is more severe (indicating the presence of more abnormal genes or environmental influences).
- If the trait is more common in one gender than in the other, the risk is higher if the affected individual is of the less susceptible gender (again, indicating the presence of more abnormal genes).

Invasive Fetal Testing

Pre-procedure counseling

Prenatal genetic screening and testing is voluntary. Counseling by a genetic counselor, geneticist, or physician with special expertise in prenatal diagnosis can assist patients in making an informed decision about prenatal diagnosis, and should be considered for all but the most straight-forward counseling issues. Among the factors that the patient may consider are the likelihood of fetal aneuploidy as determined by a screening test result or the family history, the severity of the disease in question, treatment options, personal and family values regarding reproductive choices, and the risks of the diagnostic test.

Amniocentesis

Traditional amniocentesis for prenatal diagnosis of aneuploidy or genetic disease usually is offered between 14 and 20 weeks' gestation. Recent large multicenter trials have reported post-procedure pregnancy loss rates of 1:300 to 1:500 after traditional amniocentesis; in the FASTER trial, the loss rate was closer to 1:1600.[26] Early amniocentesis, performed between 11 and 13 6/7 weeks, results in significantly higher pregnancy loss and complication rates than does traditional amniocentesis. In one multicenter randomized trial, the rate of spontaneous pregnancy loss after early amniocentesis was 2.5%, compared to 0.7% after traditional amniocentesis. There were more failures of amniotic fluid cultures after the early procedure, necessitating an additional invasive diagnostic procedure in these patients.[27] Early amniocentesis also was associated with significantly more cases of talipes than was traditional amniocentesis. For all these reasons, many centers no longer offer amniocentesis before 14 weeks of gestation.

Chorionic villus sampling

The primary advantage of chorionic villus sampling (CVS) is that results are available earlier in pregnancy. Early reports of an association between CVS and limb reduction and oromandibular defects virtually all involved cases in which the procedure was performed before 10 weeks' gestation. Subsequently, several large studies showed that CVS does not increase the risk of these anomalies above the background risk when the procedure is performed at or beyond 10 weeks' gestation. CVS at this gestational age is believed to be as safe as second trimester amniocentesis.[28]

Pre-implantation Genetic Diagnosis (Embryo Biopsy)

Preimplantation diagnosis is now available in many urban centers. After *in vitro* fertilization, a biopsy of the blastomere (at the 8 to 16 cell stage) or the polar body is performed, followed by genetic testing using PCR and/or FISH, and intrauterine transfer of the embryo once it is confirmed that the embryo is unaffected. The benefits of preimplantation diagnosis are obvious. The drawbacks include having to conceive by using reproductive technology, the fact that only a limited number of FISH probes can be applied to a single cell, and the possibility of misdiagnosis due to "allele dropout," or failure to correctly identify an abnormal allele because one of the parental alleles in a heterozygous cell fails to amplify.[29] In addition, many authorities strongly recommend that the preimplantation diagnosis be confirmed by CVS or amniocentesis, thus incurring the risk and expense of an invasive diagnostic procedure.

Future Direction and New Therapies Under Investigation

Cell-free fetal DNA circulates in maternal blood during pregnancy and has many potential applications in obstetric care.[30] Although not yet widely available, cell-free fetal DNA (and RNA) found in maternal blood during pregnancy could be used for noninvasive prenatal diagnosis to determine fetal sex, diagnose certain single gene disorders, to determine fetal blood genotyping, and to diagnose fetal Down syndrome or another aneuploidy. Specialist centers already offer noninvasive determination of fetal sex and RHD typing for high risk pregnancies, and other test options will probably become widely available in the near future.[31]

Array-based comparative genome hybridization (aCGH) is a molecular technique that detects very small DNA deletions and duplications — an increase or decrease in the number of base pairs, or "copy number variation" (CNV) — that would not be recognized with standard high resolution karyotyping. It utilizes a microarray constructed of small segments of DNA (oligonucleotides), representing thousands of discrete genomic locations, fixed to a slide. A microarray could be designed to represent a complete normal genome, or could be composed of selected DNA sequences that correspond to a single chromosome or chromosome region, known genes, or multiple loci of interest. The patient's DNA and a sample of normal reference DNA are fragmented and labeled differentially using two different color fluorophores, and allowed to hybridize to the oligonucleotides on the microarray slide. A fluorescent scanner determines the relative amounts of the two fluorophores bound to each oligonucleotide; equal binding of the two fluorophores indicates that the patient's DNA is identical to the reference DNA, while unequal binding indicates copy number variation, or a very small duplication or deletion in that region. Computer software converts the scanner information into data showing the size and location of the copy number changes within the tested DNA.

aCGH could be used to complement a high resolution karyotype. For example, aCGH has been used to evaluate apparently balanced chromosome translocations, and microdeletions have been identified that were not detected with a standard high resolution karyotype. In small series of neonates with specific structural anomalies, dysmorphisms, or developmental delay who have been evaluated by aCGH, approximately 11 to 12% have been found to have previously unrecognized copy number abnormalities. In a series of 300 cases, array technology used in the prenatal setting identified many additional molecular abnormalities beyond what was detected by routine karyotype. Although 13% of the abnormalities detected were benign inherited variants, this did not present major counseling difficulties.[32]

The utility of aCGH for the prenatal evaluation of anomalous fetuses is being explored. ACOG states that targeted array CGH, in concert with genetic counseling, can be offered as an adjunct tool in prenatal cases with abnormal anatomic findings and a normal conventional karyotype, as well as in cases of fetal demise with congenital anomalies when a conventional karyotype cannot be obtained.[33]

It is possible that aCGH might eventually obviate the need for a standard karyotype; because aCGH identifies copy number abnormalities, it could identify trisomies such as Down syndrome and other numerical aneuploidies, marker chromosomes, unbalanced translocations, and of course, deletions and duplications.

References

1. *Creasky and Resnik's Maternal-Fetal Medicine*, 6th ed. Saunders Elsevier, 2009, p. 221 Apr 17.

2. Heron M, Hoyert DL, Murphy SL *et al*. (2009) Deaths: Final data for 2006, *Natl Vital Stat Rep* **57**(14): 1–134.

3. Milunsky A (ed.) (1992) *Genetic disorders and the fetus: Diagnosis, prevention and treatment*. 3rd ed. Johns Hopkins University Press, Baltimore, Maryland.

4. *Thompson and Thompson: Genetics in Medicine* (2007) 7th ed. Saunders Elsevier, pp. 420–421.

5. ACOG Practice Bulletin #77, Screening for Fetal Chromosomal Abnormalities, (2007) *Obstetrics Gynecol* **109**(1): 217–227.

6. California Birth Defects Monitoring Program (2004). Available at: www.cbdmp.org/bd_down_syn.htm

7. Hook EB *et al*. (1981) Rates of chromosome abnormalities at different maternal ages, *Obstet Gynecol* **58**: 282.

8. Wald NJ, Kennard A, Hackshaw A *et al*. (1997) Antenatal screening for Down's syndrome, *J Med Screen* **4**: 181–246.

9. Cuckle H. (2000) Biochemical screening for Down syndrome, *Eur J Obstet Gynecol Reprod Biol* **92**: 97–101.

10. Spencer K, Souter V, Tul N *et al*. (1999) A screening program for trisomy 21 at 10–14 weeks using fetal nuchal translucency, maternal serum free beta-human chorionic gonadotropin and pregnancy-associated plasma protein-A. *Ultrasound Obstet Gynecol* **13**: 231–237.

11. D'Alton ME, Malone FD, Lambert-Messerlian G *et al*. (2003) Maintaining quality assurance for nuchal translucency sonography in a prospective multicenter study: Results from the FASTER Trial. *Am J Obstet Gynecol* **187**: S79.

12. Wapner RJ. (2005) First Trimester Screening: The BUN Study. *Seminar Perinatol* **29**(4): 1236–1239.

13. Malone FD, Canick JA, Ball RH *et al*. (2005) First trimester or second trimester screening or both for Down's syndrome, *N Engl J Med* **353**: 2001–2011.

14. Wald NJ, Rodeck C, Hackshaw AK *et al*. (2003) First and second trimester antenatal screening for Down syndrome: The results of the Serum, urine and ultrasound Screening Study (SuRRuS), Health Technol Assess, **7**: 1.

15. Dhaifalah I, Vrbicka D, Santavy J. (2006) OSCAR (One-Step Clinic for Assessment of Fetal-Risk): Our experience with first trimester screening for chromosomal abnormalities, *Ceska Gynekol* Sept **71**(5): 363–369.
16. Wald NJ, Watt HC, Hackshaw AK. (1999) Integrated screening for Down's syndrome on the basis of tests performed during the first and second trimesters, *N Engl J Med* **341**: 461–467.
17. Wapner R, Thom E, Simpson J *et al.* (2003) First-trimester screening for trisomies 21 and 18, *N Engl J Med* **349**: 1405–1413.
18. Wright D, Bradbury I, Benn P *et al.* (2004) Contingent screening for Down syndrome is an efficient alternative to non-disclosure sequential screening, *Prenat Diagn* **24**: 762–766.
19. Watson WJ, Chescheir NC, Katz VL *et al.* (1991) The role of ultrasound in evaluation of patients with elevated maternal serum alpha-fetoprotein: A review. *Obstet Gynecol* **78**: 123–128.
20. Campbell J, Gilbert WM, Nicolaides KH *et al.* (1987) Ultrasound screening for spina bifida: Cranial and cerebellar signs in a high-risk population. *Obstetrics & Gynecology* **70**(2): 247–250.
21. Sepulveda W, Donaldson A, Johnson RD *et al.* (1995) Are routine alpha-fetoprotein and acetylcholinesterase determinations still necessary at second-trimester amniocentesis? Impact of high-resolution ultrasonography. *Obstet Gynecol* **85**: 107–112.
22. ACOG Committee Opinion #325, Update on Carrier Screening for Cystic Fibrosis. (2005) *Obstet Gynecol* **106**: 1465–1468.
23. ACOG Committee Opinion #442, Preconception and Prenatal Carrier Screening for Genetic Diseases in Individuals if Eastern European Jewish Descent. (2009) *Obstet Gynecol* **114**: 950–953.
24. ACOG Committee Opinion #338, Screening for Fragile X Syndrome. (2006) *Obstet Gynecol* **107**: 1483–1485.
25. Thompson and Thompson: Genetics in Medicine, 2007. 7th ed. Saunders Elsevier, p. 173.
26. Malone FD, Wald NJ, Canick JA *et al.* (2003) First and second trimester evaluation of risk (FASTER) Trial: Principal results of the NICHD multicenter Down syndrome screening study. *Am J Obstet Gynecol* **187**: S56.
27. Tredwell SJ, Wilson D, Wilmink MA. (2001) Canadian Early and Mid-Trimester Amniocentesis Trial Group (CEMAT), and the Canadian Pediatric Orthopedic Review Group. Review of the effect of early amniocentesis on

foot deformity in the neonate. *Journal of Pediatric Orthopedics* **21**(5): 636–641.

28. Caughey AB, Hopkins LM, Norton ME. (2006) Chorionic villus sampling compared with amniocentesis and the difference in the rate of pregnancy loss. *Obstet Gynecol* Sep **108**(3 Pt 1): 612–616.

29. Swanson A, Strawn E, Lau E *et al.* (2007) Preimplantation genetic diagnosis. *Wisc Med J* **106**: 145.

30. Lo YMD, Corbetta N, Chamberlain PF *et al.* (1997) Presence of fetal DNA in maternal plasma and serum. *Lancet* **350**: 485–487.

31. Wright CF, Chitty LS. (2009) Cell-free fetal DNA and RNA in maternal blood: Implications for safer antenatal testing. BMJ; **339**: b2451.

32. Van den Veyver IB, Patel A, Shaw CA *et al.* (2009) Clinical use of array comparative genomic hybridization (aCGH) for prenatal diagnosis in 300 cases. *Prenatal Diagnosis* **29**: 29–39.

33. Array Comparative Genomic Hybridization in Prenatal Diagnosis. (2009) ACOG Committee Opinion No. 446. American College of Obstetricians and Gynecologists. *Obstet Gynecol* **114**: 1161–1163.

Chapter 2

Effects of Maternal Medication on the Fetus and Newborn

Donald R. Coustan and Roman Starikov

Introduction

Prior to the early 1960s, the placenta was widely regarded as an effective barrier, protecting the fetus from any substances, including medications, ingested by the mother. Thalidomide, an effective tranquilizer, analgesic and sleeping medication, which also ameliorated nausea in pregnancy, was marketed in the late 1950s, although not in the United States. The discovery that thalidomide could cause birth defects such as phocomelia, and that thousands of infants around the world had been impacted, led to its removal from the market in 1961. In 1962, Congress passed laws requiring that new drugs be tested for safety in pregnancy before approval for sale in the US. This event also changed the prevailing view of the placenta, from that of a barrier to that of a "sieve," allowing anything ingested by the mother to pass to the developing fetus. Strictly speaking, the truth lies somewhere in between; some substances pass the placenta more readily than others.

In this chapter, we shall discuss the level of available evidence regarding medication use in pregnancy and effects on the fetus, describe possible pitfalls in interpreting the available evidence, and then cover what is known about some of the more commonly prescribed drugs. In the space available, it will be impossible to include all possible prescription and over the counter medications, and the reader is referred to Refs. 1 and 2 for broader coverage of this topic.

The Evidence: Pitfalls in Assigning Teratogenicity

One of the biggest concerns in prescribing medications for pregnant women is the possibility of unintended adverse effects on the fetus. Teratogenicity is often considered to be a phenomenon confined to the first trimester, when major organ systems are forming. However, growth, differentiation and development continue throughout pregnancy and even into neonatal life; and these may be impacted at any time along the way. Tetracyclines, for example, can cause staining of the deciduous teeth and inhibit growth of long bones when the fetus is exposed in the second and/or third trimesters, but not the first trimester. For that reason, it is important to have as much information as possible regarding risks of medications throughout pregnancy. However, risk is not the only consideration. If medications provided no benefit to our patients, the risk/benefit equation would be simple: any risk at all would not be worth taking. We prescribe medications because we believe they will be beneficial to our patients, mother and/or fetus. The greater the benefit, the greater the acceptability of the theoretical risk. An example of such a calculation would be the case of a pregnant woman with a Starr–Edwards heart valve prosthesis. Heparin is the anticoagulant of choice in pregnancy because it does not cross the placenta and because coumarin derivatives can cause fetal hemorrhage in any trimester, in addition to specific problems in the first trimester. However, coumarin derivatives are more effective than heparin in preventing clots on non-biologic prosthetic heart valves, so a frank risk/benefit discussion needs to be held with such a patient. Either option would be acceptable as long as the patient demonstrates an understanding of the issues.

Our current emphasis on evidence-based medicine provides increasing discomfort with treatment that is based on less than level I evidence. With a few exceptions, it is difficult to design and to perform double-blind, randomized placebo-controlled trials of medication administration to healthy pregnant women who do not otherwise need treatment. Ethical considerations preclude such studies if more than negligible risk to mother or fetus is present. While some randomized trials have been performed comparing different treatment regimens in patients with a particular condition, the condition itself may confound our understanding of the effects of the drug on the fetus. A good deal of the information available to us comes from case reports, descriptive association studies from large databases, or case-control studies. The following paragraphs describe some of the pitfalls in assigning teratogenicity based on this type of data.

1. *The illness, rather than the drug, may be teratogenic.* As an example of this phenomenon, it is possible to demonstrate that fetuses exposed to prednisone *in utero* are at greater risk for congenital heart block than are non-exposed pregnancies. However, this does not necessarily imply that prednisone causes heart block. Patients with systemic lupus are likely to receive prednisone as part of the treatment of their disease. Some patients with lupus have circulating anti-R_o antibodies, which may be associated with heart block in the fetus and neonatal lupus. It is the anti-R_o antibodies that cause the heart block, and the association with prednisone is a confounder.

2. *A fetal malformation may cause a maternal symptom, which is then treated with a medication.* An example of this phenomenon might be found historically when hydramnios was treated with diuretic medications in order to reverse the excessive amniotic fluid volume. It should be noted that this treatment was not effective. Nevertheless, it should be possible to demonstrate an increased likelihood of esophageal atresia among infants exposed to diuretics during pregnancy. While an understanding of the embryology would tell us that the esophageal atresia occurred long before the diuretics were administered, the association would nonetheless be present and the birth defect could be mistakenly attributed to the medication.

3. *A drug might inhibit the spontaneous abortion of an already malformed fetus.* While no medication has been demonstrated to reliably inhibit spontaneous first trimester abortion, in which a high proportion of abortuses are chromosomally and/or structurally abnormal, if such a treatment were successful, we might mistakenly attribute the malformations to the drug and consider the drug to be teratogenic.

A potential example of this phenomenon might have been progesterone, which was once widely used to prevent threatened abortion.
Although it was subsequently demonstrated to be ineffective in
randomized trials, if progesterone worked at preventing early miscarriage, we might have been confronted with an epidemic of
abnormal fetuses, whose abnormalities were not caused by the drug,
but whose survival was due to the treatment.

4. *A drug might frequently be used in combination with a second drug
   which is teratogenic.* An example of this pitfall would be the standard
   use, some years ago, of phenobarbital and phenytoin to treat epilepsy.
   The well-characterized fetal hydantoin syndrome could easily have
   been ascribed to phenobarbital.

5. *A common factor might predispose both to the use of a particular
   medication and to congenital malformations.* Infertility is generally
   considered to be present when a couple has been unsuccessful in
   attempting to conceive over a predetermined period of time, often a
   year. On average, then, infertile couples are older than couples not
   requiring infertility treatment. It would stand to reason that any treatment or diagnostic procedure typically used for infertility, such as
   clomiphene, would be associated with a greater risk of age related
   occurrences, such as Down syndrome, if data are not corrected for
   maternal age.

6. *The association might be confounded by study design issues such as
   recall bias or multiple comparisons.* **Recall bias** may be introduced
   when a retrospective study design requires individuals who have
   undergone an adverse outcome (i.e. the birth of an infant with a major
   abnormality) to recall events during early pregnancy (i.e. taking specific over the counter medications). If such individuals are compared
   with controls who have experienced a normal outcome in their pregnancies, the affected subjects are much more likely to recall the
   details of early pregnancy than are unaffected controls. **Multiple
   comparisons** may provide random associations that do not pan out on
   further examination. For example, when a large database is queried
   regarding associations between any of multiple medications and any of
   multiple congenital malformations, one statistically significant association will emerge by chance, on average, for every 20 comparisons

(i.e. the 5% level of significance). Such associations should be considered hypothesis generating, and should be validated in a separate population.

As described above, assigning a teratogenic role or other adverse consequence for a given medication is fraught with difficulty in the absence of well-controlled studies, and much of what we believe we know about interactions between medications and pregnancy is based on less than level I evidence. The remainder of this chapter will describe the apparent effect of a number of medications, chosen for their particular interest to the neonatologist, on the fetus. Though space limitations preclude a complete listing of medications, the reader is referred to standard sources for further information about these and other medications.[1,2]

Medications Specific to Pregnancy

Tocolytic agents

A number of medications are used to inhibit uterine activity in patients with preterm labor. Although a number have been shown to prolong pregnancy for 2–7 days, long enough for the mother to receive corticosteroids to enhance fetal pulmonic maturation and to enable transfer to a tertiary perinatal center, none have been demonstrated to delay delivery long enough to impact perinatal mortality nor perinatal morbidity such as RDS or NEC, with the possible exception of calcium channel blockers. **Betamimetics** such as terbutaline are associated with a number of maternal side effects, including chest pain, dyspnea, tachycardia, tremor, headaches, nausea, and hyperglycemia. **Cyclooxygenase (COX) inhibitors** such as indomethacin have been demonstrated to be more effective than betamimetics in prolonging pregnancy for 48 hours,[3] and are much less likely to cause maternal side effects. However, COX inhibitors have also been associated with the constriction or the closure of the ductus arteriosus *in utero*, a generally transient effect which is much more likely after 32 weeks (50%) than before (5–10%).[4] Prolonged use is also associated with oligohydraminos, so COX inhibitors are generally used prior to 32 weeks, for no longer than 48 hours. **Calcium channel blockers**, primarily nifedipine, are associated with few maternal side effects, are effective in prolonging pregnancy for seven days, and in a Cochrane review of 12 trials were associated with a significant reduction in RDS, NEC and IVH.[5] **Magnesium sulfate** is not a particularly effective tocolytic and is associated with maternal side effects such as pulmonary edema;[6] this drug is primarily used to treat pre-eclampsia and as a fetal neuroprotective agent, both of which uses are discussed below.

Corticosteroids to enhance pulmonic maturation

A 1994 NICHD Consensus Panel report recommended that a single course of corticosteroids be given to all pregnant women between 24 and 34 weeks, who are considered to be at risk for delivery within seven days, to enhance fetal pulmonic maturation. This recommendation was confirmed in a second panel report in 2000.[7] Because it is not always possible to predict with accuracy when a premature birth is going to occur, and because a course of corticosteroids has its maximal effect between 48 hours and seven days after initiation, many caregivers opted to administer weekly courses of steroids as long as the patient had not yet delivered. Because the scientific evidence was insufficient, that second panel[7] recommended that repeat corticosteroid doses not be given except in the context of clinical trials. They noted that there are animal and human data that suggest deleterious effects on the fetus regarding cerebral myelination, lung growth and the functioning of the hypothalamic-pituitary-adrenal axis. A number of subsequent randomized trials suggested that weekly doses of steroids may be associated with lower birth weight and reduced head circumference.[8,9] whereas other studies did not find such disadvantages.[10] Most studies that found decreased head circumference or lower birth weight reported the effect only after at least three courses of steroids. A randomized trial in 2009 evaluated the use of a single "rescue course" of steroids in patients remote from their initial course, who were expected to deliver within a week and had intact membranes.[11] Exposed infants were less likely to experience a composite adverse outcome (RDS, BPD, IVH, PVL, sepsis, NEC or perinatal death) if delivered before 34 weeks than placebo-exposed controls. Birth weights and head circumferences were similar in both groups. Currently many centers are using "rescue courses" of steroids under circumstances similar to those of the randomized trial.

Neuroprotective drugs

Preterm birth is a strong risk factor for the development of cerebral palsy. After case-control studies suggested that maternal treatment with magnesium sulfate prior to preterm delivery was associated with protection against cerebral palsy, the NICHD MFMU Network conducted a randomized placebo-controlled, double blind trial of intravenous magnesium sulfate in women at imminent risk of preterm delivery between 24 weeks and 31-weeks-and-6-days gestation.[12] In this study of over 2200 gravidas, moderate or severe cerebral palsy occurred in 1.9% of the treated group versus 3.5% of the control group (RR 0.55, CI 0.32 to 0.95). Neonatal death rates were not different between the two groups. The use of magnesium sulfate for this purpose was not tested after 32 weeks, so there is no evidence regarding a neuroprotective effect at later gestational ages. Details of the protocol may be found in the original reference. A subsequent Cochrane Review[13] of this and other randomized trials concluded that "the neuroprotective role for antenatal magnesium sulphate therapy given to women at risk of preterm birth is established," with a number needed to treat to avoid one case of CP of 63. While future studies will undoubtedly explore various aspects of this therapy, and while ACOG has not yet made a recommendation regarding its use, neonatologists can anticipate that more and more babies will be born after maternal magnesium sulfate treatment. While adverse effects such as diminished FHR variability, neonatal depression and hypotension have been attributed to magnesium sulfate, the randomized trial cited above found no difference between treated and control babies with respect to Apgar scores, need for resuscitation, hypotension, or hypotonicity.

Medications used to treat pre-eclampsia

Although antihypertensive medications are frequently needed to treat severe pre-eclampsia, the only medication specific to this disorder is magnesium sulfate. While magnesium sulfate is discussed above in the context of its use as a neuroprotective agent in pregnancies at risk of imminent delivery before 32 weeks and in the context of its poor tocolytic properties, its use in pre-eclampsia merits further consideration. While it has been used over many years to prevent eclamptic convulsions, its efficacy was not tested in randomized trials until relatively recently. In the largest randomized trial, women with pre-eclampsia receiving magnesium sulfate had a 58% lower risk of eclampsia than those receiving a placebo.[14] A Cochrane analysis of six randomized trials concluded that the number needed to treat to prevent one case of eclampsia was 100.[15] When toxic levels of magnesium sulfate are reached, respiratory and cardiac arrest may occur, so it is not an entirely benign drug.

Other Medications

Psychotropics

It is estimated that approximately one-third of all pregnant women are exposed to a psychotrophic medication at some time during gestation.[16] Untreated depression can result in maternal complications such as alcohol abuse, suicide attempt and neglect of nutrition and prenatal care. Potential neonatal complications include low birth weight, decreased fetal growth and smaller head circumference.[17] Psychotropic medications are divided into the following categories:

1) anxiolytics,
2) anticonvulsants and mood stabilizing agents,
3) selective serotonin inhibitors (SSRIs),
4) tricyclic antidepressants (TCAs),
5) atypical antidepressants, and
6) antipsychotics.

Anxiolytic agents such as benzodiazepines have not been associated with a significant risk of teratogenicity, although CNS symptoms such as depression, hypotonia, apneic spells and neonatal withdrawal have been observed in infants with prolonged antenatal exposure to benzodiazepines.[18] The teratogenic effect of anticonvulsants has already been mentioned. Lithium carbonate is a common **mood stabilizing agent** that is used for treatment of bipolar disorder. Older literature suggested that first-trimeter exposure to lithium carbonate was associated with increased risk of congenital heart disease, particularly Ebstein's anomaly.[19] These reports resulted from retrospective and possibly biased reports, and more recent epidemiologic data indicate that the teratogenic risk of first-trimester exposure to lithium is lower than previously suggested.[20] Late-gestation neonatal exposure to lithium has been associated with floppy infant syndrome, flaccidity, lethargy and poor suck reflexes. Lithium has been also associated with neonatal cardiac arrhythmia, nephrogenic diabetes insipidus, changes in neonatal thyroid function and hypoglycemia.[21] **SSRIs** such as fluoxetine are commonly used to treat depression. Despite conflicting data, SSRIs have been reported to be associated with omphalocele and atrial and ventricular septum defects, especially when used early in pregnancy.[22] Paroxetine has specifically been found to increase the risk of congenital cardiac malformation by 1.5–2.0 fold and therefore should be avoided during pregnancy.[23]

SSRIs have also been associated with persistent pulmonary hypertension in the newborn.[24] **Tricyclic Antidepressants (TCAs)** were initially associated with limb anomalies; subsequent studies failed to confirm this association. **Atypical antidepressants** such as bupropion, nefazodone, venlafaxine have not been well-studied in pregnancy. Limited data do not suggest increased risk of fetal malformations. **Antipsychotics** whether typical or atypical have not been associated with teratogenic or toxic effects on the fetus. There are no long-term neurobehavioral studies of exposed children to atypical antipsychotics currently available.

Anticonvulsants

Intrauterine exposure to anti-epileptic drugs (AEDs) has been associated with increased risk of major congenital malformations. However, it has been reported that tonic-clonic seizures in pregnancy can cause fetal heart rate depression, fetal hypoxia and fetal intracranial hemorrhage.[25,26] There are no randomized controlled trials of AEDs in pregnancy, but many are known to interfere with folic acid metabolism, so folate supplements are generally prescribed and prospective pregnancy registries provide some information about the risk of exposure *in utero*. Increased risk of neural tube defects has long been recognized in fetuses exposed to AEDs. Older AEDs such as phenytoin, valproic acid and carbamazepine have been associated with major congenital malformations. **Valproic acid** has been associated with the "valproate syndrome" that includes distinct facial features, musculoskeletal abnormalities and congenital heart defects. Antenatal exposure to valproic acid increases the risk of neural tube defects by 1.0–3.8% and the effect appears to be dose dependent.[16] Valproic acid has been found to impair cognitive function by three years of age for infants exposed to *in utero*.[27] **Carbamazepine** syndrome includes facial dysmorphism, spina bifida, hypoplastic nails, cardiac malformations and developmental delays. **Phenytoin** exposure is associated with fetal hydantoin syndrome which includes craniofacial dysmorphology, microcephaly, growth and mental retardation, distal phalangeal and nail hypoplasia, neonatal coagulopathy congenital heart defects and cleft palate. Most newer AEDs have not been sufficiently studied with the possible exception of lamotrigine. Several large AED pregnancy registries report a rate of major congenital malformations following first-trimester exposure, with monotherapy exposures of 2–3%.[28] In one report, lamotrigine was associated with a 10-fold increase of oral clefts as compared to unexposed infants.[29] Other new AEDs such as levetiracetam, oxcarbazepine and topiramate are not well studied in pregnancy and various registries in North America are currently collecting data.

Antidiabetic medications

The goal of antidiabetic drugs is to maintain maternal blood glucose levels as close to euglycemia as possible, to prevent fetal hyperinsulinemia and its adverse ramifications. Insulin, the standard therapy, has the advantage of not crossing the placenta to any measurable extent because of its large molecular size. It has the disadvantages of being administered by injection, and of having the potential to cause maternal hypoglycemia. Two oral antidiabetic medications have also been used in pregnancy. **Sulfonylureas**, which work by stimulating pancreatic insulin production and release, have been demonstrated to have similar efficacy to insulin in controlling maternal glycemia in patients with gestational diabetes.[30] No glyburide was measurable in the cord bloods of infants whose mothers were treated with the medication during the cited study, and an earlier investigation of isolated perfused placental cotyledons had not demonstrated transplacental passage[31]; glyburide was not considered to be able to cross to the fetus. Using state-of-the-art measurement techniques, the NICHD Obstetric-Fetal Pharmacology Research Unit Network recently reported that fetal glyburide levels are 70% of maternal levels.[32] Appropriate studies in either animal models or in humans have not evaluated the potential effect of an insulin secretogogue on the fetal insulin dynamics, either short-term or later in life. **Metformin**, an insulin sensitizer, has also been compared to insulin in a randomized trial in women with gestational diabetes.[33] Perinatal outcomes were similar in the two groups, and patient satisfaction was predictably higher with metformin. However, 46% of the patients receiving metformin required the addition of insulin in order to achieve satisfactory glycemic control. Metformin has also been demonstrated to cross the placenta, with fetal levels approximately twice of those in the maternal circulation.[34] As with glyburide, little is known about fetal effects of exposure to this insulin sensitizer *in utero*, although adverse effects in the offspring have not been reported to date. There is currently no evidence regarding any specific precautions to be taken for neonates exposed to either of these antidiabetic drugs, other than the usual management of infants of diabetic mothers. There is little information available regarding other antidiabetic drugs such as thiadolazinediones, alpha-glucosidase inhibitors and GLP agonists as they are not generally used in pregnancy.[35]

Medications used to treat thyroid disease

Hypothyroidism, which may be associated with a greater likelihood of spontaneous abortion, pre-eclampsia, abruption, IUGR and stillbirth, is generally treated with levothyroxine. This drug crosses the placenta poorly, although it is likely that some transfer occurs. Neonates with congenital absence of the thyroid, for example, are normal at birth suggesting that maternal thyroid hormone reached the fetus in amounts adequate to support normal development. There is evidence that mild asymptomatic untreated hypothyroidism in the mother, as evidenced by elevated TSH levels with low T_4 concentrations, is associated with decreased IQ in the offspring.[36] It has not yet been established whether treatment of this condition will improve outcomes; this hypothesis is currently the subject of a randomized double blind trial being carried out by the NICHD Maternal-Fetal Medicine Units Network. Maternal **hyperthyroidism** is commonly treated with propylthiouracil (PTU), a thioamide which inhibits thyroglobulin production in the thyroid gland and also inhibits conversion of T_4 to T_3 peripherally. PTU crosses the placenta and may suppress the fetal thyroid gland, with the resultant increase in fetal TSH possibly leading to fetal goiter. If the mother has thyroid-stimulating immunoglobulins, which can cross the placenta and cause transient fetal and neonatal hyperthyroidism, treatment with PTU may temporarily suppress the fetal response. Neonatal thyrotoxicosis shows up when the PTU effect has worn off, typically after the baby has been discharged from the hospital.

References

1. Briggs GG. (2008) *Drugs in Pregnancy and Lactation*, 8th ed. Lippincott Williams and Wilkins, Philadelphia.
2. http://www.reprotox.org/Default.aspx
3. King JF, Flenady V, Cole S *et al.* (2005) Cyclo-oxygenase (COX) inhibitors for treating preterm labour. *Cochrane Database of Systematic Reviews*, Issue 2. Art. No.: CD001992. DOI: 10.1002/14651858.CD001992.pub2.
4. Moise KJ Jr. (1993) Effect of advancing gestational age on the frequency of fetal ductal constriction in association with maternal indomethacin use. *AJOG* **168**: 1350–1353.
5. King JF, Flenady V, Papatsonis D *et al.* (2003) Calcium channel blockers for inhibiting preterm labour. *Cochrane Database of Systematic Reviews*, Issue 1. Art. No.: CD002255. DOI: 10.1002/14651858.CD002255.
6. Mercer BM, Merlino AA, For the Society for Maternal-Fetal Medicine. (2009) Magnesium sulfate for preterm labor and preterm birth. *Obstetrics & Gynecology* **114**: 650–668.
7. 2001 NIH Consensus Development Panel: Antenatal corticosteroids revisited. *Obstetrics and Gynecology* **98**: 144–150.

8. Guinn DA, Atkinson MW, Sullivan L *et al*. (2001) Single vs weekly courses of antenatal corticosteroids for women at risk for preterm delivery: a randomized controlled trial. *JAMA* **286**: 1581–1587.

9. Wapner RJ, Sorokin Y, Thom EA *et al*. (2006) Single vs weekly courses of antenatal corticosteroids: Evaluation of safety and efficacy. *AJOG* **195**: 633–642.

10. Crowther CA, Haslam RR, Hiller JE *et al*. (2006) Neonatal respiratory distress syndrome after repeat exposure to antenatal steroids: A randomized controlled trial. *Lancet* **367**: 1913–1919.

11. Garite TJ, Kurtzman J, Manuel K *et al*. (2009) Impact of a "rescue course" of antenatal corticosteroids: A multicenter randomized placebo-controlled trial. *AJOG* **200**: 248.e1–248.e9.

12. Rouse DJ, Hirtz DG, Thom E *et al*. (2008) A randomized, controlled trial of magnesium sulfate for the prevention of cerebral palsy. *NEJM* **359**: 895–905.

13. Doyle LW, Crowther CA, Middleton P *et al*. (2009) Magnesium sulphate for women at risk of preterm birth for neuroprotection of the fetus. *Cochrane Database Systematic Reviews* **21**: CD004661.

14. Altman D, Carroli G, Duley L *et al*. (2002) Do women with pre-eclampsia, and their babies, benefit from magnesium sulphate? The Magpie Trial: A randomised placebo-controlled trial. *Lancet* **359**: 1877–1890.

15. Duley L, Gulmezoglu AM, Henderson-Smart DJ. (2003). Magnesium sulphate and other anticonvulsants for women with pre-eclampsia. *Cochrane Database of Systematic Reviews*. 2003; *Issue 2, Art. No. CD000025, DOI 10.1002/145651858.CD00025*.

16. American College of Obstetricians and Gynecologists: Use of psychiatric medications during pregnancy and lactation. (2000) *ACOG Practice Bulletin*, Number 87, Nov 2007.

17. Hoffman S, Hatch MC. (2000) Depressive symptomatology during pregnancy: Evidence for an association with decreased fetal growth in pregnancies of lower social class women. *Health Psychol* **19**: 535–543.

18. McElhatton PR. (1994) The effects of benzodiazepine use during pregnancy and lactation. *Reprod Toxicol* **8**: 461–475.

19. Weinstein MR, Goldfield M. (1975) Cardiovascular malformations with lithium use during pregnancy. *Am J Psychiatry* **132**: 529–531.

20. Jacobson SJ, Jones K, Johnson K *et al*. (1992) Prospective multicentre study of pregnancy outcome after lithium exposure during first trimester. *Lancet* **339**: 530–533.

21. Woody JN, London WL, Wilbanks GD Jr. (1971) Lithium toxicity in a newborn. *Pediatrics*, **47**: 94–96.
22. Wogelius, Pia, Nørgaard, Mette; Gislum, Mette. (2006) Maternal use of selective serotonin reuptake inhibitors and risk of congenital malformations. *Epidemiology* **17**: 701–704.
23. Bar-Oz B, Einarson T, Einarson A *et al.* (2007) Paroxetine and congenital malformations: Meta-Analysis and consideration of potential confounding factors. *Clin Ther* **29**: 918–926.
24. Chambers CD, Hernandez-Diaz S, Van Marter LJ *et al.* (2006) Selective serotonin-reuptake inhibitors and risk of persistent pulmonary hypertension of the newborn. *N Engl J Med* **354**: 579–587.
25. Minkoff H, Sheffer RM, Delke I *et al.* (1985) Diagnosis of intracranial hemorrhage in utero after a maternal seizure. *Obstet. Gynecol* **65**: S22–S24.
26. Teramo K, Hiilesmaa V, Bardy A *et al.* (1979) Fetal heart rate during a maternal grand mal epileptic seizure. *J Perinat Med* **7**: 2–6.
27. Meador KJ, Baker GA, Browning N *et al.* (2009) Cognitive function at three years of age after fetal exposure to antiepileptic drugs. *N Engl J Med* **360**: 1597–1605.
28. The Lamotrigine Pregnancy Registry, Interim Report 1 September 1992 through 31 March 2007, July 2007.
29. Holmes LB, Wyszynski DF, Baldwin EJ *et al.* (2008) Increased frequency for isolated cleft palate among infants exposed to lamotrigine during pregnancy. *Neurology* **70**: 2152–2158.
30. Langer O, Conway DL, Berkus MD *et al.* (2000) A comparison of glyburide and insulin in women with gestational diabetes mellitus. *NEJM* **343**: 1134–1138.
31. Elliott BD, Langer O, Schenker S *et al.* (1991) Insignificant transfer of glyburide occurs across the human placenta. *Amer J Obstet Gynecol* **165**: 807–812.
32. Hebert MF, Ma X, Naraharisetti SB *et al.* (2009) Are we optimizing gestational diabetes treatment with glyburide? *Clinical Pharmacology & Therapeutics* **85**: 607–614.
33. Rowan JA, Hague WM, Gao W *et al.* (2008) Metformin versus Insulin for the Treatment of Gestational Diabetes. *NEJM* **358**: 2003–2015.
34. Vanky E, Zahlsen K, Spigset O *et al.* (2005) Placental passage of metformin in women with polycystic ovary syndrome. *Fertil Steril* **83**: 1575–1578.

35. Coustan DR. (2007) Pharmacological management of gestational diabetes. *Diabetes Care* **30**(Suppl 2): S206–S208.

36. Haddow JE, Palomaki GE, Allan WC *et al.* (1999) Maternal thyroid function during pregnancy and subsequent neuropsychological development of the child. *N Engl J Med* **341**: 549–555.

PART

II

Transitional Period

Chapter

3

Delivery Room Management of the Newborn Infant

Maximo Vento

Definition/Concept

According to World Health Organization estimates, between 0.5–3% of approximately 120 million infants born every year suffer birth asphyxia requiring resuscitation; some 900,000 of these newborns die each year, and a similar number of infants will develop motor and/or neurocognitive dysfunctions.[1,2] The incidence of birth asphyxia is higher in developing countries because of a higher prevalence of risk factors, namely: women who are in poor health when they become pregnant; high incidence of pregnancy and delivery complications in these women; often inadequate or nonexistent care during labor and delivery.[3,4] Resuscitation of a newborn is the most frequent intervention in the neonatal period; however, many newborns do not receive adequate care in the delivery room (DR) because birth attendants have not been adequately trained, necessary equipment is lacking, international guidelines are not put into practice and certain traditional practices are not only ineffective, but may be also harmful.[5]

In this chapter, the pathophysiology of asphyxia and resuscitation procedures will be described based on the International Consensus on Cardiopulmonary Resuscitation (ILCOR) 2005 guidelines[6] and evidence-based information published in recent years.

43

Pathophysiology of Asphyxia

Cardio-circulatory changes during fetal to neonatal transition

Life *in utero* occurs in a low oxygen atmosphere. The fetus is persistently hypoxic compared to the adult, whereas human maternal arterial and venous pO_2 is ~12 kPa (90 mmHg) and 9.3 kPa (70 mmHg), respectively; the highest arterial or venous pO_2 in the late gestation fetus rarely exceeds 4 kPa (30 mmHg).[7] Concomitantly, pulmonary circulation is excluded from the cardio-vascular circuit through the extra cardiac (*ductus arteriosus*) and intracardiac shunting (*foramen ovale*). The pCO_2 of the fetus is slightly higher than adult levels with an umbilical venous pCO_2 from 35–45 mmHg (4.6–6 kPa). Elimination of CO_2 from the fetus is enhanced by maternal hyperventilation during pregnancy. Maternal oxygenated blood coming from the placenta through the umbilical vein will bypass pulmonary circulation and flow directly into the aorta and get distributed throughout the body; fetal venous return will be delivered by both umbilical arteries to the placenta where CO_2 will be eliminated.[8]

During labor, the fetus experiences brief periods of ischemia and hypoxia because with each uterine contraction, flow to the fetus decreases transiently, impairing placental gas exchange. However, the fetus is allowed to recover between each contraction and blood gases performed in the umbilical cord immediately after birth are within a "normal" range.[9]

In the first few minutes after cord clamping, with the initiation of breathing, lungs are fully expanded and fluid inside the alveoli and respiratory airways is rapidly absorbed. In addition, pulmonary blood flow increases dramatically, and intracardiac and extracardiac shunts reverse direction and subsequently close. The first breaths of normal-term neonates exert negative pressures that may reach up to about −80 cmH_2O when they start to expand their lungs.[10] To aid initial lung expansion,[10] the fluid-filled alveoli may require higher peak inspiratory and end-expiratory pressures than what is commonly used in resuscitation later in infancy.[11,12] Expansion of the lungs and the increase in alveolar oxygen tension both mediate the fall in pulmonary vascular resistance and increase in pulmonary blood flow after birth. The effect of gestational age on the development of the lung and pulmonary circulation influences how newborn infants at different gestational ages are resuscitated. Surfactant deficiency in the premature infant reduces lung compliance.[13] Premature infants and infants born by cesarean section, without the effect of labor, may not clear the lung fluid and expand their alveoli as easily as term babies born by vaginal delivery.[14] If meconium is passed into the amniotic fluid, it may be inhaled before or during delivery and lead to inflammation of the lung and airway obstruction. Complications of meconium aspiration are more likely in infants small for their gestational age, such as those born after term or with significant perinatal compromise.[15]

Pathophysiologic changes during asphyxia

Dawes *et al.*[16] performed experiments with rhesus monkeys asphyxiated by sealing their heads in a bag containing saline immediately after delivered by cesarean section (Fig. 1). Respiratory rate increased for a few breaths and then stopped (primary apnea). However, after one or two minutes, gasping re-initiated with vigor and higher frequency, and was accompanied by thrashing movements of the extremities. In this period, spontaneous ventilation could still be induced by appropriate sensory stimuli. Simultaneously, heart rate (HR) dropped from 200 bpm to 100 bpm. Respiratory efforts gradually decreased and completely ceased at around 8 min. Cardiac activity continued until approximately 10 min. The period between the last gasp and cardiac arrest is known as secondary or terminal apnea.[16] The time gap between secondary apnea and initiation of resuscitation directly correlates with success of resuscitation.

Metabolic changes in asphyxia

Asphyxia is characterized by intermittent periods of hypoxia and ischemia. During hypoxia, limited oxygen availability decreases oxidative phosphorylation, resulting in a failure to resynthesize energy-rich phosphates, especially ATP leading to alterations in cellular ion flux leading to cell cytotoxic edema. During re-oxygenation, if an excess of oxygen is given, a burst of oxygen free radicals will be formed, further increasing cellular damage and especially inducing cell apoptosis, thus amplifying the initial damage caused by hypoxia/ischemia. Thus, the oxygen amount given during resuscitation of the asphyxiated neonate is essential to prevent a further increase in damage upon resuscitation.[7,17,18]

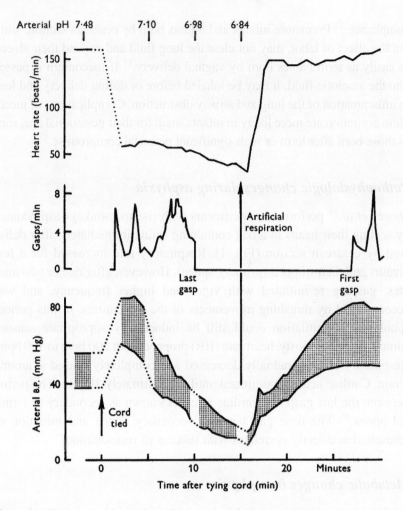

Figure 1. Heart rate, gasps and arterial pressure of rhesus monkeys asphyxiated immediately after birth.[16] Reprinted with permission from Wiley Interscience.

Action Plan for Delivery Resuscitation

Anticipating the need for resuscitation

Personnel

Caregivers responsible for attending births in the DR should have adequate training in basic neonatal resuscitation skills which include evaluation of clinical status of the newborn bag and mask ventilation and cardiac compressions. One person should be available round the clock for the care of each infant. In addition, a skilled caregiver trained in advanced neonatal resuscitation (intubation, ventilation, IV cannulation, use of drugs and fluids) should be available for second call for low-risk deliveries and present for all high-risk deliveries where he/she should take the leadership of the procedure.

Equipment

Ideally, basic DR installations should be based on the DRICU concept (Delivery Room Intensive Care Unit) which means that technology used in the intensive care unit should be available in the delivery room to adequately provide care immediately after birth.[25] Equipment should be applicable to any gestational age (23–44 weeks of gestation) and should be inventoried regularly to ensure its operational completeness (Table 1)

Communication with the obstetric team and identification of newborn at risk

Caregivers in charge of the neonate should request information from the obstetric team regarding maternal medical condition, medication and fetal status (Table 2).

Environment

Temperature

Neonates, and especially preterm infants, have a tendency towards hypothermia because of their diminished capability to generate heat (inability to shiver) and an increased ability to lose it due to an increased surface-area-to-body-weight ratio and extremely thin insulator subcutaneous tissue. Therefore, if measures are not promptly initiated to counteract this negative thermal balance, body temperature will fall, independently of the environment temperature, during the first 12 hours of life.[26] For the full-term newborn, both standard thermal care (promptly drying, and wrapping the infant in a warm blanket after birth) and placing the dried infant under a radiant heater in a draft-free room at minimum

Table 1. Equipment and drugs in the delivery room.

Equipment
— Resuscitator with overhead warmer and light, and firm, padded and heated mattress
— 2 sources of medical oxygen
— 2 sources of medical air
— 2 blenders (air/oxygen)
— Clock with timer in seconds
— Warmed towels or other covering
— Polyethylene bag, or wrap, big enough for a baby less than 1500g birthweight.
— Stethoscope, neonatal size
— Suction catheters (6F, 8F, 10F, 12F)
— Oxygen/Air admixture supply (flow rate up to 10 L) with flow meter and tubing
— Face masks (various sizes)
— Oropharyngeal airways (sizes 0 and 00)
— Positive-pressure ventilation (two in case of twin deliveries):
  • T-piece device
  • Self-inflating bag with an oxygen reservoir and a manometer if available
  • Flow-inflating bag with a pressure safety valve and manometer
— Laryngoscopes with straight blade (00, 0, 1), spare bulbs, and batteries
— Endotracheal tubes (sizes 2.5, 3, 3.5, and 4 mm ID)
— Endotracheal stylet or introducer
— Magill forceps, neonatal size
— Supplies for fixing endotracheal tubes and IVs (e.g. scissors, tape)
— End-tidal carbon dioxide detector (to confirm intubation)
  • Chemical detector (e.g. Pedicap®)
  • End tidal CO_2 monitor
— Meconium suction device (to apply suction directly to endotracheal tube)
— Feeding tubes for gastric decompression
— Umbilical vein catheterisation set and umbilical catheters (5F) with suitable skin prep solution
— Syringes with needles (assorted sizes)
— Intravenous cannulae (assorted sizes)
— Pulse oximeter with sensors adequate for different gestational ages

Drugs
— Adrenaline: 1:10 000 concentration (0.1 mg/mL)
— Volume expanders: Normal saline, O Rh -ve blood needs to be readily available for a profoundly anaemic baby
— Sodium bicarbonate: 0.5 mmol/mL solution (4.2% concentration, or diluted 8.4%)
— Naloxone hydrochloride: 400 micrograms/mL solution
— Sterile water for injection

Table 2.   Identification of the newborn at risk.

Maternal risk factors

- Prolonged rupture of membranes (>24 hours)
- Bleeding in second or third trimester
- Severe pregnancy-induced hypertension
- Chronic hypertension
- Substance abuse
- Drug therapy (e.g. lithium, magnesium, adrenergic blocking agents, narcotics)
- Diabetes mellitus
- Chronic illness (e.g. anaemia, cyanotic congenital heart disease)
- Maternal infection
- Chorioamnionitis
- Heavy sedation
- Previous fetal or neonatal death
- No prenatal care

Fetal risk factors

- Twins or triplets
- Preterm gestation (especially <35 weeks)
- Post-term gestation (>41 weeks)
- Large for dates
- Fetal growth restriction
- Rhesus, or other types of isoimmunisation especially those causing hydrops fetalis
- Polyhydramnios and oligohydramnios
- Reduced fetal movement before onset of labor
- Congenital abnormalities which may affect breathing
- Intrauterine infection

Intrapartum risk factors

- Non-reassuring fetal heart rate patterns on CTG
- Abnormal presentation
- Prolapsed cord
- Prolonged labor (or prolonged second stage of labor)
- Precipitate labor
- Antepartum hemorrhage
- Thick meconium in the amniotic fluid
- Narcotic administration to mother within 4 hours of delivery
- Forceps delivery
- Cesarean section under general anesthesia

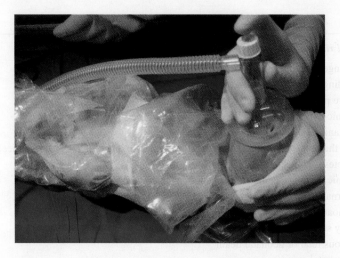

Figure 2. Premature infant completely wrapped in a polyethylene bag except for head which is covered with a cap. This method allows keeping the body temperature and performing profound resuscitation maneuvers. The baby should not be dried before wrapping.

25°C are effective in maintaining normal body temperature. For preterm infants <28 weeks gestation, randomized controlled trials have shown that covering infants up to the neck in a transparent heat-resistant plastic (poly-ethylene/poly-urethane wrapping) without previous drying, results in a higher body temperature at admission (Fig. 2). Only the head is dried and covered with a cap. All resuscitation interventions can be performed with the plastic cover in place. Currently, there is no evidence that this procedure improves mortality or long-term outcome.[27] Monitoring of body temperature should be considered, especially when resuscitation is prolonged, to avoid the small risk for inducing hyperthermia.[26] When resuscitation is not required, the mother's body can keep the infant warm by using her as a heat source by placing the infant skin-to-skin on the mother's chest or abdomen and putting a blanket or warm wrap on top.

Induced hypothermia

Hypoxic-ischemic encephalopathy (HIE) is not a single and acute event, but an evolving process that may occur for hours, days or months. Some neurons will die as a consequence of an acute asphyxial event (primary cell death) while others will initially recover from the primary insult, only to die several hours, days or even months thereafter (secondary delayed cell death). Magnetic resonance spectroscopy (MRS) has shown that asphyxiated infants whose oxidative metabolism transiently recovers after birth but who thereafter develop delayed energy failure 6–15 hours later, have a neurodevelopmental prognosis that closely correlates with the degree of energy failure at 24–48 hours postnatal. The effectiveness of any treatment is highly dependent on the timing of initiation and continuation, and its ability to interrupt active events that trigger the secondary phase of delayed cell death. Several randomized trials have been performed using selective head cooling or moderate whole-body hypothermia (33.5–34.0°C) for 72 hours in patients of ≥36 weeks gestation and <6 hours of life who fulfilled specific clinical, biochemical and neurological criteria. Follow-up was performed at 18–24 months of postnatal age using standard neurode-velopmental scales. All studies concluded that moderate hypothermia for 72 hours did not significantly reduce the combined rate of death or severe disability, but resulted in improved neurologic outcomes in survivors. There are still many unanswered questions and further trials are needed to identify those who will benefit most. Until then, cooling babies with HIE should only occur in the context of controlled trials.[28–30]

Avoidance of hyperthermia

Note that babies born to febrile mothers (>38°C) have an increased risk of death, perinatal respiratory depression, neonatal seizures and cerebral palsy.[31] Therefore the body temperature should be between 36.5°C and 37.2°C (normothermia) for newly born infants and iatrogenic hyperther-mia must be avoided.

Evaluation of the newly born infant

The assessment of the newborn's postnatal adaptation in the DR is usually done using the Apgar score[32] which evaluates five clinical signs: heart rate, respiratory effort, color, tone and response to stimuli at one and five minutes, although it can be further performed at ten minutes (Table 3). To

Table 3.   The Apgar score for evaluation of adaptation of the newborn infant after birth.[32]

Sign	0	1	2
Heart rate	Absent	<100 bpm	>100 bpm
Respiratory effort	Absent	Slow, irregular	Good, crying
Muscle tone	Flaccid	Some flexion extremities	Active motion
Reflex irritability	No respond	Grimace	Vigorous cry
Color	Pale	Cyanotic	Completely pink

avoid inter-observer variability[33] caregivers should be trained in assessing the different parameters of the Apgar score in a uniform manner; an objective means of evaluation should be pursued (e.g. pulse oximetry). Thus, an apneic infant should score "0," even if the infant is ventilated and abnormal respiratory efforts should score "1," also if the infant is ventilated. The premature infant that is hypotonic scores "1" for muscle tone, although this may be physiologic for the gestational age.

Heart rate (HR) is the most relevant clinical sign indicating adequate postnatal adaptation and/or response to resuscitation. In addition, HR in the first minutes of life has prognostic value regarding mortality in the early neonatal period.[34] HR may be assessed by palpation of umbilical cord pulsations or direct auscultation of the *praecordium*; however, randomized studies have shown that both of these methods could delay or underestimate the heart rate compared to electrocardiography.[35] Therefore, it is advised to use pulse oximetry for monitoring HR especially in case of an extended resuscitation. Healthy newborns achieve a HR around 130 bpm (110–160 bpm) within the first seconds of life; importantly, it should be consistently above 100 bpm within a minute after birth. Hence, if HR is persistently below 100 bpm, resuscitation should be initiated.

Assessment of the newborn's color also shows high inter-observer variability, especially in preterm. This can be avoided with the use of pulse oximetry.[36] Remarkably, healthy term newborns do not reach preductal oxygen saturations (with sensor located in the right wrist) between 79% and 91% until 5 min and preterm infants until 10–15 min after birth.

After initial breathing efforts, the newborn establishes a regular pattern of respiration sufficient to maintain the HR >100 bpm. If a newborn exhibits an irregular respiratory pattern but is able to maintain an adequate HR, he/she should be closely observed but not given respiratory aid. However, if irregular breathing movements are unable to sustain a HR >100 bpm, positive pressure ventilation (PPV) should be immediately applied. Importantly, in the presence of suprasternal, intercostal and subcostal retractions, PPV should be immediately applied. Finally, the absence of respiratory movements with persistent apnea generally associated with hypotonia unresponsive to stimuli, and bradycardia (HR < 100 bpm) requires immediate PPV.

Newborn moving their extremities soon after birth do not require any assistance. However, if these responses are absent, stimulus with a dry soft towel should suffice. Other methods such as slapping, foot flicking, shaking, spanking, or holding the baby upside down are potentially dangerous and should not be used. If the infant does not respond, PPV should be started.

An infant with good tone (moving the limbs and with a flexed posture) is unlikely to be severely compromised whereas a floppy infant (not moving and extended posture) is likely to need active resuscitation. However, as indicated before, special attention should be paid especially to very premature infants for whom a hypotonic state is physiologic.

Airway and Breathing

Positioning

The newborn that needs PPV should be positioned on his/her back with the head in a neutral or slightly extended position (sniffing position) (Fig. 3).

Airway suctioning

Routine oropharyngeal suction is not recommended, as a normal newborn clear its airways effectively. However, if secretions are obstructing the airway, it should be suctioned with a special catheter with an adequate size (French gauge 10–12) and pressure not surpassing 133 cmH₂O (13 kPa;

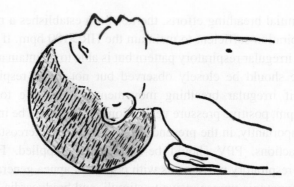

Figure 3.   Sniffing position opens the airway and facilitates air entrance.

1.9 Psi). Suction should be brief (10 seconds) and performed carefully (not further than 5 cm from the lips) because it may cause laryngeal spasm, bradycardia and/or delay the onset of spontaneous respiration.

Meconium stained liquor

In the case of meconium-stained amniotic fluid, 2–9% of the neonates will develop a meconium aspiration syndrome (MAS). Intrapartum oronasopharyngeal suctioning of meconium before the delivery of the shoulders is no longer recommended.[37] However, if meconium is thick, the baby is hypotonic and respiration is shallow or absent, mouth, pharynx and trachea should be suctioned under direct vision with the laryngoscope. If the infant is vigorous, endotracheal suction is not recommended because it may cause harm and does not improve the outcome.[37]

Ventilation strategies: initial breaths

The establishment of an adequate gas exchange by effective PPV at a rate of 30–60 bpm is, without any doubt, the single most effective maneuver to overcome bradycardia and hypoxemia. However, if HR does not improve and no thoracic expansion is observed, positioning the face mask should be corrected to avoid leakage which causes ventilation to be ineffective. In term infants, initial inflations, either spontaneous or assisted, create a functional residual capacity (FRC). The optimum pressure, inflation time, and flow required to establish an effective FRC have not been determined. However, peak inflating pressures of 30–40 cmH_2O have been shown to be effective to ventilate unresponsive term infants. Importantly, sustained inflation pressure of 30 cmH_2O for five seconds for the first breath seems to be more effective in achieving FRC than lower pressures for shorter periods of time. Once the newborn has achieved an adequate FRC, lower pressures in the range of 15–25 cmH_2O and a pace of 30–60 bpm seem to be adequate. However, the ILCOR 2005 guidelines state that optimal ventilation rates and pressures should be individualized according to each infant's response.[6]

Assisted positive pressure ventilation devices

Three different devices have been successfully employed to ventilate newborn infants: self-inflating bag, flow-inflating (anesthesia bag) and T-piece mechanical device designed to regulate pressure.

Self-inflating bags (Fig. 4a) are devices that consist of a rubber bag that re-expands due to its elastic recoil and does not depend on a gas source for inflation (it may be attached for administering gas admixture). It is simple and portable, allowing its use outside the hospital. It has a pressure-limited pop-off valve that usually triggers at 40 cmH_2O, although these valves activate at a wide range of pressures which makes it difficult to adjust to desired target values. Self-inflating bags do not administer PEEP (although certain models allow fitting of a PEEP valve), and do not permit adjusting inspiratory times. Inspiratory fraction of oxygen cannot be precisely adjusted and an additional reservoir is necessary for the administration of 100% oxygen. The preferred size in neonatology is of 240 mL because it covers the tidal volume needs of newborn infants (5–10 mL/kg).

Flow-inflating (anesthesia) bag (Fig. 4b) is connected to a compressed gas source which provides the gas admixture to inflate the bag when in use. If the face mask is not perfectly adjusted (leaks) or if the flow is too low, the bag will collapse and ventilation will be impossible. One should pay special attention on the inspiratory pressure, since these devices can reach very high pressures which could cause pulmonary air leaks. To avoid this potential problem, a pressure gauge and a blow-off valve in the circuit is mandatory. An expiratory pressure (CPAP or PEEP)

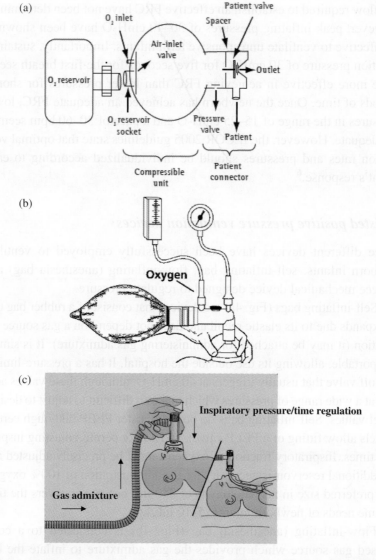

Figure 4. (a) Self-inflating bag with an additional reservoir for oxygen to allow administering higher oxygen concentrations. In addition, a pop-off valve avoids excessive pressure into the airways. (b) Flow-inflating bag receives compressed gas from the wall outlet or gas tanks. Expiratory pressure can be adjusted by regulating the flow and the outlet valve of the bag. (c) The inlet arm provides with a gas admixture. Flow can be interrupted by closing or opening a hole in the T-piece and thus positive inspiratory pressure and time can be regulated. Expiratory pressure can be regulated adjusting the outlet valve.

can be provided by controlling the pressure in the bag, by adjusting the flow of gas into the bag and the rate of gas escape at the outlet valve from the bag. Flow-inflating bags can be used to deliver sustained inflations.

The T-piece device (Fig. 4c) consists of an inlet arm attached to the patient through which the gas flows into a facemask or endotracheal tube (ETT). Positive inspiratory pressure (PIP) is achieved by interrupting the escape of gas through an outlet hole using a thumb or finger so that the pressure rises and is displayed by a manometer. PIP is adjusted varying the release valve. The inflation time is voluntarily regulated by the caregiver by varying the duration of occlusion of the outlet hole. CPAP or PEEP is delivered automatically and the pressure varied by adjusting the outlet valve. This controls the rate of escape of gas when the outlet is not occluded (i.e. in expiration) and generates a set level PEEP or CPAP. The level of PEEP or CPAP can also be adjusted by altering the flow into the system. The preferred system should always be that with which the caregivers are most acquainted and self-confident.[6]

Interfaces for gas administration

Noninvasive ventilation is generally performed with a face mask (FM), although nasal prongs may also be used, and invasive intubation is performed using an endotracheal tube (ETT). Indications, advantages and disadvantages of each interface will depend on the severity, gestational age and/or experience of the caregiver. As a rule, FM is the first choice for moderately depressed neonates while endotracheal intubation (ETI) is preferred for more severe conditions or as the second choice when FM fails to adequately recover newborn's HR.

FM is gentler to the airway, easier to use and expertise can be maintained because it is frequently used in the DR. An appropriately sized FM should be used according to the infant's birth weight and preferably with cushioned rims to avoid leakage. Available masks have diameters ranging from 35 to 72 mm that will provide adequate sealing to newborn from 24 to 40 weeks gestation (Fig. 5). Note that an adequate holding of the mask is essential and adequate training significantly reduces air leaking[38] (Fig. 6). Controlled studies comparing FM versus intubation have shown that, although inflation pressures were similar, inflation volumes, especially expiratory volumes,

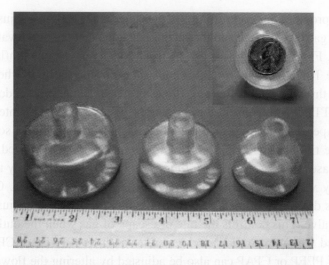

Figure 5. Different cushion-rimmed mask sizes for extreme preterm infants (Courtesy of Fischer & Paykel Healthcare Corporation Limited).

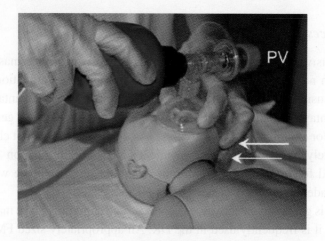

Figure 6. Adequate face mask holding technique is essential to avoid leaks.

were difficult to assess with mask ventilation because of frequent leakage even with higher inflation pressures. FM ventilation seems to induce breathing by Head's paradoxical reflex and therefore successful resuscitation is dependent on the baby's spontaneous respiration.[39] In severely asphyxiated babies, a brief trial with FM should be performed, but if no improvement is seen after 30 seconds (HR persistently <100 bpm, lack of effective breathing or is profoundly apneic and/or bradycardic with HR <60 bpm), intubation should be performed. Intubation is potentially the most injurious invasive procedure performed during neonatal resuscitation. Every effort should be made to stabilize an infant before attempting intubation to avoid the occurrence of bradycardia/hypoxia. In addition, surfactant administration can be delayed until the baby is recovered without losing its effectiveness. It is important to be gentle during intubation to avoid damaging the anatomical structures. An oral route is easier for the inexperienced resuscitator. It is also important to use an appropriately sized laryngoscope blade (0/00 [7.5 cm] for preterm babies; 1 [10 cm] for term infants) and ETT size, as well as depth of insertion (Table 4). The tip of the laryngoscope should be advanced over the tongue to the vallecula or on top of the epiglottis and elevated gently to reveal the vocal cords (Fig. 7a). Cricoid pressure may be helpful (Fig. 7b). ETT should be inserted through the vocal cords to a depth indicated by marks on the annotated tube and safely secured to avoid extubation or bronchial intubation (Fig. 7c). Common problems experienced during neonatal intubation:

- If the laryngoscope is advanced too far, the larynx will not be seen (Fig. 7d).
- If the blade does not support the tongue, it will obscure the view of the larynx.
- If the laryngoscope is not held slightly towards the left side, the larynx will not be seen.
- If the neck is flexed or over-extended, the larynx may not be seen.

Table 4. Endotracheal tube sizes and depth of insertion from the lips.

Weight (g)	Gestation (wks)	Tube size (mm)	Depth of insertion from lip (cm)
<1000	<28	2.5	6.5–7
1000–2000	28–34	3.0	7–8
2000–3000	34–38	3.0/3.5	8–9
>3000	>38	3.5/4.0	>9

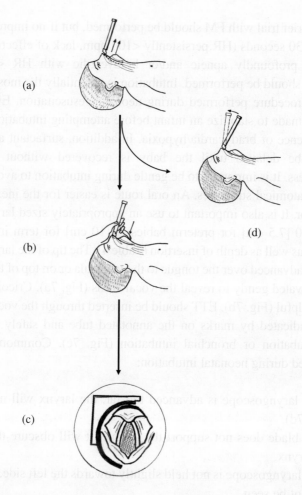

(a)

(b)

(c)

(d)

Figure 7. (a) Correct position slightly hyper-extended. The laryngoscope blade tip is advanced over the tongue to the vallecula or on top of the epiglottis. (b) Pressure on the cricoid may help visualize vocal cords. (c) The endotracheal tube is inserted in the space left between the vocal cords. (d) If the blade is advanced too far, the larynx will not be seen.

The use of a stylet inside the ETT should be done with care to prevent damaging the trachea.

Most caregivers are successful in intubating in 30 seconds; saturation and HR will not differ from those intubated in <20 seconds.[40] Once the tube is secured, the position of the tip should be verified as soon as possible to avoid hypoxia/hypercapnia. Air entering in both lungs and the absence of sounds in the stomach can be detected by auscultation; however, in preterm infants and in special situations such as diaphragmatic hernia, or pneumothorax, this may be difficult. End-tidal carbon dioxide (CO_2) detectors or colorimetric CO_2-detectors may be used to rapidly verify if the ETT tip is in a correct position. Colorimetric CO_2-detectors have been shown to be effective in confirming ETI or detecting a misplaced ETT within six inflations even in babies of less than 400 g. When CO_2 is detected, the color changes from purple to yellow. If there is no color change, the likely causes are: the ETT is not in the trachea; the PIP is inadequate; or no CO_2 is produced because of absent lung perfusion due to cardiac arrest. If a colorimetric detector indicates the presence of CO_2 the operator can be certain that the airway is patent and fresh gas is being delivered into the lungs. Interestingly, the CO_2-detector has been shown to indicate the return of circulating rhythm during chest compressions, an observation recently confirmed in an animal model of neonatal resuscitation.[40]

Special circumstances: The very preterm neonate

Postnatal adaptation of preterm <29 weeks frequently requires respiratory support to establish functional residual capacity (FRC). The controversial issue of early intubation and surfactant administration vs noninvasive CPAP is still under intense debate. However, the tendency is towards the use of noninvasive ventilation in the DR.[25,27] Observational studies have suggested that using early CPAP in very preterm infants may reduce intubation rate, need for oxygen and incidence of BPD without increasing morbidity.[41] A trial which compared early CPAP in spontaneously breathing infants born at 25–28 weeks with intubation[42] showed no difference in mortality between the two groups. Interestingly, at 28 days, the CPAP-group had a significantly lower incidence of death or oxygen treatment, although at 36-weeks gestation, differences disappeared. However, the CPAP-group had significantly fewer days on ventilation. In addition, there were no significant differences in any complications of prematurity except where there was an increased rate of pneumothorax in the CPAP-group. Thus, preterm infants of 25–29 weeks who breathe spontaneously at birth should initially be ventilated with CPAP titrating pressures and FIO_2 to meet HR and oxygen saturation targets. Oxygen saturation targets in the very preterm infants are 70% at 5 min and 85% at 10–15 min after cord clamping as has been shown in recent studies.[44–46] In case of respiratory failure, intubation and positive pressure with PEEP should be administered.

Laryngeal mask

Laryngeal masks (LMA) are rarely used in newborn resuscitation, though they have been successfully employed in even preterm newborns, but not below 1500 g. With increasing use of noninvasive ventilation in the DR and in the NICU, intubation skill might be difficult to maintain. Therefore, LMA insertion should be considered a valid alternative for problematic intubations and should be included in every RCP program.

Oxygen use in resuscitation

Regarding oxygen use in the delivery room, the ILCOR 2005 statement concluded that there was insufficient evidence to specify the FIO_2 for initiation of resuscitation.[6] Recently, a new meta-analysis was published which included ten studies under which six randomized controlled trials in European countries fulfilled strict methodological criteria.[43] A subgroup analysis of these European studies showed a reduction in mortality from 3.9% to 1.1% with a number needed to harm of 36. Taking into consideration the recent published evidence, the ILCOR 2010 guidelines have acknowledged the evidence supporting the use of air instead of 100% oxygen in the delivery room for the resuscitation of asphyxiated term or near term newborn infants.[49] Nevertheless, a subgroup of newborn infants will benefit from the additional supply of oxygen (e.g. persistent pulmonary hypertension). At present, no scientific guidelines are available for the use of oxygen in newborns not responding to the initial steps of newborn resuscitation. Therefore, it seems reasonable to start supplying additional oxygen whenever a newborn is not responding despite adequate ventilation with room air. It is important that lung inflation/ventilation should be the priority. Once adequate ventilation is established, if HR remains low, there is no evidence to support or refute a change in the oxygen concentration initiated. Monitoring of SpO_2 by pulse oximetry makes it possible to adjust FIO_2 to achieve more or less physiologic levels of oxygen saturation. Recently, a series of studies reported that very preterm infants especially <27 weeks gestation will need additional oxygen in most cases.[44-46] Therefore, for preterm infants, a higher initial FIO_2 may be needed, although evidence is currently not sufficient to recommend an optimal initial oxygen fraction.

Recommendations for therapeutic use of oxygen during and after resuscitation:

1. Positive-pressure ventilation should be initiated with 21% oxygen.
2. Supplemental oxygen should be used if the baby remains cyanotic or the heart rate <100 bpm at 90 seconds of age.
3. Blended gases should be available in the DR and during transport to the NICU.
4. To avoid hyperoxemia, pulse oximetry should be available in DR where babies <32 weeks are delivered. It seems reasonable to avoid saturations >95% when supplemental oxygen is used.

Circulation

In the newborn infant, cardiac output correlates with HR and rates of <100 bpm will not support tissue oxygenation. If HR is absent or intense bradycardia (<60 bpm) is nonresponsive to adequate ventilation, chest compressions (CC) should be provided. The main goal of CC is to achieve or sustain sufficient diastolic blood pressure to assure coronary perfusion and restore effective myocardial function. The two-thumb method, which is generally considered more effective than the two-finger method, is performed by placing both thumbs on the lower third of the sternum, gripping the chest with the hands and supporting the back with the fingers (Fig. 8). General consensus (although not evidence-based) is that CC should be coordinated with ventilation at a ratio of 3:1 and a rate of 120 "events" per minute to achieve approximately 90 compressions and 30 breaths per minute. However, CC are only effective if the lungs have first been successfully aerated, making the quality of the breaths and compressions more important than the rate.

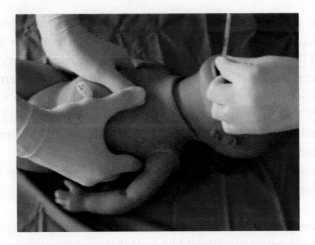

Figure 8. Two-thumb technique seems to be the most efficacious means to administer chest compression in the neonate, especially preterm ones.

Medication and Fluids

Epinephrine

Medications and fluids are rarely indicated for resuscitation of newborn infants. Bradycardia is usually caused by hypoxia and inadequate ventilation, and apnea is due to insufficient oxygenation of the brainstem. Hence, if bradycardia (<60 bpm) persists despite adequate ventilation and chest compressions, drugs may be needed to improve cardiac contractility. Epinephrine is a sympathetic monoamine produced by the adrenal gland. It exerts its effects through the α_1-adrenoreceptors, causing peripheral vasoconstriction and the β_1-adrenoreceptors to increase HR, cardiac output and cerebral brain blood flow. Cardiac effects are obtained by epinephrine's direct action on the myocardial fibers; therefore it is essential to administer it as close to the heart as possible.

The umbilical vein seems to be the most accessible and recommended site for administering drugs and fluids. The umbilical artery is disregarded because of serious concerns of side effects due to vasoactive or hypertonic solutions administered into an artery. The access to peripheral veins in a shocked newborn is extremely difficult, and only very expert caregivers can approach this route rapidly enough. The intraosseous lines are not commonly used in neonates because of the fragility of small bones and the small intraosseous space, particularly in the preterm infant. The intratracheal route should be used only for epinephrine.[47]

Epinephrine is recommended via the intravenous route (preferably via the umbilical venous catheter) and the dosage should be 0.01–0.03 mg/kg. The dosage can be repeated every one to three minutes. Intratracheal route may be used at higher dose (100 mcg/kg).[47] Canadian guidelines[23] recommend the use of the intratracheal route first flushed with 5 mL of saline while preparing for insertion of the umbilical catheter. The other doses if necessary should be administered by the umbilical vein.

A flow diagram of newborn resuscitation is represented in Fig. 9.

Volume expanding fluids

Intravascular fluids should be considered when there is suspected blood loss and/or the infant appears to be in shock (pale, poor perfusion, weak pulse) and has not responded adequately to other resuscitative measures. To compound the problem in a hypovolemic neonate, shock may not be evident at first in the asphyxial process. Early on, there may be peripheral vasoconstriction which helps maintain an adequate perfusion of the vital organs (myocardium and brain). If resuscitation renders this effective, then perhaps clinical signs of shock will become evident and the clinician will be able to indicate fluid expanders with greater acuity.

In the absence of suitable blood for neonatal transfusion (preferably O-negative blood cross-matched against the mother's blood), isotonic crystalloid (normal saline) should be used. The initial dose is 10 mL/kg given by quick IV push. This dose may be repeated after observation of the response.

General Supportive Management

Glucose

Prompt glucose administration to maintain euglycemia is essential for an adequate brain and cardiac metabolism. Low blood glucose on admission to the NICU after resuscitation is associated with poorer neurological outcome. A glucose rate of 8 mg kg min will assure brain metabolic needs

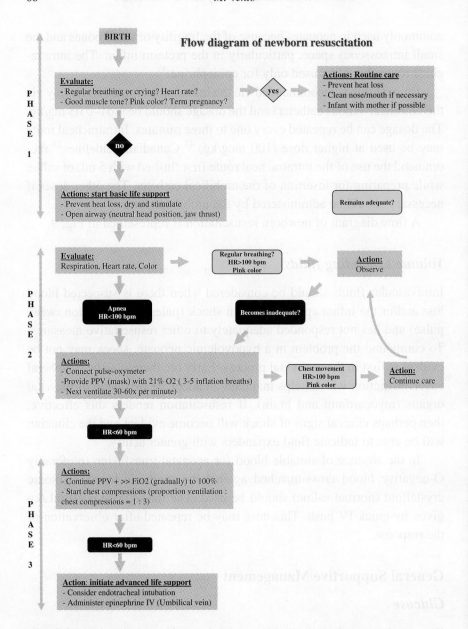

Figure 9. Flow diagram of the resuscitation of the newborn infant in the delivery room (modified from Ref. 21).

and restoration of myocardial glycogen content. Administration of intravenous glucose should be started in the DR when an adequate oxygenation has been achieved because anaerobic metabolism of carbohydrates leads to the formation of additional lactic acid, worsening the acidosis.[9]

Fluids

The urine output of any baby who has gone through an asphyxiated episode should be closely monitored since a certain degree of renal insufficiency may be present in moderate to severe asphyxia.

Feeding

Human studies have reported intestinal injury occurring in 6% to 29% of severely asphyxiated neonates, and newborn animal models of intestinal hypoxia-reoxygenation and ischemia-reperfusion have clearly demonstrated characteristic histopathologic lesions similar to those seen in necrotizing enterocolitis. Therefore, feeding should be cautiously initiated, preferably with human milk after a period of clinical observation.[9]

Ethical Issues

Initiating resuscitation

Mortality and morbidity in the neonatal period is different according to the region and availability of resources. Caregivers should be aware of it before initiating or withholding resuscitation of a newborn with a specific gestational age or clinical condition. Increasingly, parents especially in developed countries want to take part in the decision of starting and continue life support in severely compromised newborns. Religious beliefs and cultural traditions are also factors that should be taken into account.

Resuscitation does not mandate continued support. Therefore, not starting resuscitation and discontinuing of life-sustaining treatment during or after resuscitation are ethically equivalent. Clinicians should not be hesitant to withdraw support when functional survival is highly unlikely. If there is doubt whether to initiate or withhold resuscitation, it is best to start and later withdraw treatment when the situation has been clarified and discussed with the family and other experts. As a general rule, the following guidelines should be interpreted according to local vital statistics and societal principles or beliefs:

> When gestation, birth weight, or congenital anomalies are associated with almost certain early death and an unacceptably high morbidity is likely among the rare survivors, resuscitation is not indicated. Examples from the published literature from developed countries include:
>
> • Extreme prematurity (gestation of <23 weeks or birth weight <400 g).
> • Anomalies such as anencephaly and confirmed trisomy 13 or 18.
> • In conditions associated with a high rate of survival and acceptable morbidity, resuscitation is nearly always indicated.
> • In conditions associated with uncertain prognosis, when there is borderline survival and a relatively high rate of morbidity, and where the burden to the child is high, the parents' views on starting resuscitation should be supported.

Discontinuing resuscitation

It is reasonable to consider discontinuing resuscitation if an infant has not responded with any measurable HR after 10 minutes of maximal resuscitation. In a systematic review, it was shown that 94% of newborns without any sign of life during the first 10 minutes after birth died or had severe neurological handicaps, and only 2% had moderate or minor handicaps.[48] Data for infants of very low birth weight also suggest that survival is negligible if there is no heart beat after 10 minutes of appropriate cardiopulmonary resuscitation.[21] Before resuscitation is stopped, a second opinion should be sought if immediately available and wherever possible by agreement with parent(s). Local discussions are recommended to formulate guidelines consistent with local resources and outcome data.

References

1. Shah PM. (1990) Birth asphyxia: A crucial issue in the prevention of developmental disabilities. *Midwifery* **6**: 99–107.

2. *The World Health Report 1995.* (1997) Geneva, World Health Organization p. 21.
3. Costello AM, Manandhar DS. (1994) Perinatal asphyxia in less developed countries. *Arch Dis Child* **71**: F1–F3.
4. Kumar R. (1995) A community-based study on birth asphyxia risk factors. *IJPSM* **26**: 53–59.
5. Iriondo M, Thio M, Buron E *et al.* (2009) A survey of neonatal resuscitation in Spain: Gaps between guidelines and practice. *Acta Paediatr* **98**: 786–791.
6. 2005 International consensus on cardiopulmonary resuscitation and emergency cardiovascular care science with treatment recommendations. (2005) Part 7: Neonatal resuscitation. *Resuscitation* **67**: 293–303.
7. Maltepe E, Saugstad OD. (2009) Oxygen in health and disease: Regulation of oxygen homeostasis — clinical implications. *Pediatr Res* **65**: 261–268.
8. Fisher DE, Paton JB. (1993) Resuscitation of the newborn infant. In. Klaus MH & Fanaroff AA eds. Care of the high-risk neonate. Philadelphia; WB Saunders Co; 4th ed. pp. 38–61.
9. Bloom RS. Delivery room resuscitation of the newborn. Overview and initial management. In Fanaroff AA, Martin RJ, Walsh MC (eds.), *Neonatal Perinatal Medicine*. Philadelphia; Mosby Elsevier; 8th ed. pp. 483–490.
10. Karlberg P. (1960) The adaptive changes in the immediate postnatal period, with particular reference to respiration. *J Pediatr* **56**: 585–604.
11. Vyas H, Milner AD, Hopkin IE *et al.* (1981) Physiologic responses to prolonged and slow-rise inflation in the resuscitation of the asphyxiated newborn infant. *J Pediatr* **99**: 635–639.
12. Vyas H, Field D, Milner AD, Hopkin IE. (1986) Determinants of the first inspiratory volume and functional residual capacity at birth. *Pediatr Pulmonol* **2**: 189–193.
13. Jobe AH. (2006) The respiratory system. In Fanaroff AA, Martin RJ, Walsh MC (eds) *Neonatal Perinatal Medicine*. Philadelphia; Mosby Elsevier; 8th ed.
14. Jobe AH, Hillman N, Polglase G *et al.* (2008) Injury and inflammation from resuscitation of the preterm infant. *Neonatology* **94**: 190–196.
15. Wiswell TE. (2008) Delivery room management of the meconium-stained newborn. *J Perinatol* **28** Suppl 3: S19–S26.
16. Dawes GS, Jacobson HN, Mott JC *et al.* (1963) The treatment of asphyxiated, mature foetal lambs and rhesus monkeys with intravenous glucose and sodium carbonate. *J Physiol* **169**: 167–184.

17. Saugstad OD. (2004) Physiology of resuscitation. In Polin RA, Fox WW, Abman SH (eds), *Fetal and Neonatal Physiology*. Philadelphia; Saunders; 3rd ed; pp. 765–771.

18. Vento M, Saugstad OD. (2006) Oxygen therapy. In. Fanaroff AA, Martin RJ, Walsh MC (eds.), *Neonatal Perinatal Medicine*. Philadelphia; Mosby Elsevier; 8th ed. pp. 498–500.

19. Sociedad Española de Neonatologia (eds.) (2007) *Manual de Reanimación Neonatal*. Madrid; Ergón Editores; 2nd ed.

20. Australian Resuscitation Council. (2007) Australian Guidelines for Newborn Resuscitation.

21. van den Dungen FAM, van Veenendaal MB, Mulder ALM. (2010) Clinical practice: Neonatal resuscitation. A Dutch consensus. *Eur J Pediatr* **169**(5): 521–527.

22. Berger TM, Pilgrim S. (2009) Reanimation des Neugeborenen. Anaesthesist **58**: 39–50.

23. Recommendations for specific treatment modifications in the Canadian context. Addendum to the 2006 NRP Provider Textbook. Revised March 2007. http://www.cps.ca/ENGLISH/ProEdu/NRP/NRPCommittee.htm Accessed on January 8th 2010.

24. Biarent D, Bingham R, Richmond S *et al.* (2005) European Resuscitation Council Guidelines for Resuscitation 2005. Section 6. Paediatric life support (2005). *Resuscitation* **67**S1: S97–S133.

25. Vento M, Aguar M, Leone TA *et al.* (2008) Using intensive care technology in the delivery room: A new concept for the resuscitation of extremely preterm neonates. *Pediatrics* **122**: 1113–1116.

26. Watkinson M. (2006) Temperature control of premature infants in the delivery room. *Clin Perinatol* **33**: 43–53.

27. Vento M, Cheung PY, Aguar M. (2009) The first golden minutes of the extremely-low-gestational-age neonate: A gentle approach. *Neonatology* **95**: 286–298.

28. Shah PS, Ohlsson A, Perlman M. (2007) Hypothermia to treat neonatal hypoxic ischemic encephalopathy: Systematic review. *Arch Pediatr Adolesc Med* **161**: 951–958.

29. Shankaran S, Pappas A, Laptook AR *et al.* (2008) Outcomes of safety and effectiveness in a multicenter randomized, controlled trial of whole-body hypothermia for neonatal hypoxic-ischemic encephalopathy. *Pediatrics* **122**: e791–e798.

30. Azzopardi DV, Strohm B, Edwards AD *et al.* (2009) Moderate hypothermia to treat perinatal asphyxial encephalopathy. *New Engl J Med* **361**: 1349–1358.

31. Laptook AR, Watkinson M. (2008) Temperature management in the delivery room. *Semin Fetal Neonatal Med* **13**: 383–391.

32. Apgar V. (1953) A proposal for a new method of evaluation of the newborn infant. *Curr Res Anesth Analg* **32**: 260–267.

33. O'Donnell CP, Kamlin CO, Davis PG *et al.* (2006) Interobserver variability of the 5-minute Apgar score. *J Pediatr* **71**: 319–321.

34. Saugstad OD *et al.* (2005) Response to resuscitation of the newborn: Early prognostic variables. *Acta Paediatr* **94**: 890–895.

35. Kamlin CO, O'Donnell CP, Everest NJ *et al.* (2006) Accuracy of clinical assessment of heart rate in the delivery room. *Resuscitation* **71**: 319–321.

36. O'Donnell CP, Kamlin CO, Davis PG *et al.* (2007) Clinical assessment of infant colour at delivery. *Arch Dis Child Fetal Neonatal Ed* **92**: F465–F467.

37. Vain NE, Szyld EG, Prudent LM *et al.* (2004) Oropharyngeal and nasopharyngeal suctioning of meconium-stained neonates before delivery of their shoulders: Multicentre, randomised controlled trial. *Lancet* **364**: 597–602.

38. Boyle DW, Szyld EG, Field D. (2008) Ventilation strategies in the depressed term infant. *Semin Fetal Neonatal Med* **13**: 392–400.

39. Wood FE, Morley CJ, Dawson JA *et al.* (2008) Improved techniques reduce face mask leak during simulated neonatal resuscitation: Study 2. *Arch Dis Child Fetal Neonatal Ed* **93**: F230–F234.

40. Leone TA, Finer NN. (2005) Neonatal resuscitation: Beyond the basics. *Neoreviews* **6**: 177–183.

41. Vanpée M, Walfridsson-Schultz U, Katz-Salamon M *et al.* (2007) Resuscitation and ventilation strategies for extremely preterm infants: A comparison study between two neonatal centers in Boston and Stockholm. *Acta Paediatr* **96**: 10–16.

42. Morley CJ, Davis PG, Doyle LW *et al.* (2008) CPAP or intubation at birth of very preterm infants. *N Engl J Med* **358**: 700–708.

43. Saugstad OD, Ramji S, Soll RF *et al.* (2008) Resuscitation of newborn infants with 21% or 100% oxygen: An updated systematic review and meta-analysis. *Neonatology* **94**: 176–182.

44. Escrig R, Arruza L, Izquierdo I *et al.* (2008) Achievement of targeted saturation values in extremely low gestational age neonates resuscitated with low

or high oxygen concentrations: A prospective, randomized trial. *Pediatrics* **121**: 875–881.

45. Wang CL, Anderson C, Leone TA *et al.* (2008) Resuscitation of preterm neonates by using room air or 100% oxygen. *Pediatrics* **121**: 1083–1089.

46. Vento M, Moro M, Escrig R *et al.* (2009) Preterm resuscitation with low oxygen causes less oxidative stress, inflammation and chronic lung disease. *Pediatrics* DOI: 10.1542/peds.2009-0434.

47. Barber CA, Wyckoff MH. (2006) Use and efficacy of endotracheal versus intravenous epinephrine during neonatal cardiopulmonary resuscitation in the delivery room. *Pediatrics* **118**: 1028–1034.

48. Harrington DJ, Redman CW, Moulden M, Greenwood CE. (2007) The long-term outcome in surviving infants with Apgar zero at 10 minutes: A systematic review of the literature and hospital-based cohort. *Am J Obstet Gynecol* **196**: 463.

49. Perlman JM, Wyllie J, Kattwinkel J *et al.* (2010) Part 11: Neonatal resuscitation: 2010 international consensus on cardiopulmonary resuscitation and emergency cardiovascular care science with treatment recommendations. *Circulation* **122**: S516–S538.

Chapter 4

Transitional Care of the Newborn

Mara G. Coyle

Introduction

The successful transition from the intrauterine to the extrauterine environment, which occurs during the first 12 hours of life, involves significant physiologic changes, the results of which lead to the normal adaptation of the healthy fetus to newborn infant. In the majority of instances, these events occur without the need for significant intervention. However, approximately ten percent of newborns will need some degree of assistance in making this transition, while one percent will need extensive support.[1]

While it is not always clear who will require resuscitation, concerted effort has been made to establish guidelines for those infants who require additional care. The Neonatal Resuscitation Program (NRP), first published in 1987, was a joint effort of the American Academy of Pediatrics and the American Heart Association to address the needs of the neonate in the first minutes of life. With successive additions, NRP recommendations have become increasingly evidenced-based, rather than simply reflecting common practice. As such, the text is re-evaluated on an ongoing basis to incorporate new recommendations as supported through research.

The STABLE Program (**S**ugar and **S**afe Care, **T**emperature, **A**irway, **B**lood Pressure, **L**ab Work, **E**motional support), first introduced by

Dr. Karlsen in 1996, was designed to meet the educational needs of the health care providers responsible for the group of neonates who continue to have difficulty with the transitional period beyond the first few minutes of life.[2] The goal of both NRP and STABLE is to ensure that adequate support is provided to the neonate during this very crucial time period. This chapter will focus on the transitional changes required for normal adaptation, and the evidenced-based recommendations for therapies aimed at ameliorating difficulties experienced by those minority of infants who require additional support.

Adaptation to Extrauterine Life

Thermoregulation

Thermoregulation is the ability to balance heat production with heat loss in order to maintain a stable internal temperature. The fetus does not need to maintain thermoregulation, as heat is transferred via the placenta and the uterus. Fetal temperature is 0.3 to 0.5°C higher than the mother's temperature.[3] Several factors place the infant at risk for temperature imbalance after birth. (Table 1) After delivery, there is a drop in the newborn temperature as the baby is exposed to the cooler environment. In order to maintain normothermia, the infant accelerates heat production through nonshivering thermogenesis and lipolysis of brown fat. Brown fat is deposited around the scapulae, kidneys, adrenals, neck and axilla after 28 weeks gestation. Placental adenosine and prostaglandin E_2 inhibit thermogenesis *in utero*. When the fetus separates from the umbilical cord, these inhibitors are no longer present, allowing for thermogenesis to

Table 1. Factors affecting newborn temperature.

- Fat Stores
  - Small for Gestational Age
  - Prematurity
- Sepsis
- Hypoxia/Asphyxia
- Maternal Fever
- Environmental Temperature

occur.[3] As these processes require oxygen, a distressed hypoxic newborn will be unable to generate sufficient heat and is prone to hypothermia. Infants with minimal fat, be they preterm or growth restricted, are similarly at risk.

A mainstay of newborn resuscitation is to dry the infant immediately after birth in order to minimize evaporative heat loss. The delivery room should be kept sufficiently warm in order to prevent convective heat loss. Conductive heat loss can be avoided if the warmer and other equipment are pre-warmed. The normal axillary temperature should be 36.5–37.5°C (97.7–99.5°F). In an otherwise healthy infant, temperature can be best regulated by skin-to-skin contact with the mother. By placing the naked baby against the mother's skin and covering them with a prewarmed blanket, heat can be directly provided to the newborn through conduction. The effects of skin-to-skin care have been studied in randomized controlled trials, and when compared with routine care, the study infants have been found to have improved temperature,[4] improved sleep and quiet time[5] longer duration of breastfeeding[6] and improved maternal satisfaction.[4] This simple procedure should be encouraged after the delivery of a healthy infant.

Hypothermia

Hypothermia in the newborn increases metabolic stress and can lead to hypoxia, acidosis, respiratory distress, apnea, and hypoglycemia. Efforts to avoid hypothermia in the preterm infant, a group particularly vulnerable, include heating pads, heat shields, special humidified incubators, and covering the infant in plastic wrap/bag. In the EPICure study, 40% of infants born before 26 weeks gestational age were hypothermic on admission.[7] Polyethylene plastic wrap allows for the transmission of radiant heat, but minimizes evaporative losses. By covering very low birth weight infants with polyethylene plastic wrap, Baumgart demonstrated a reduction in oxygen consumption, insensible water loss and the need for exposure to high levels of radiant heat.[8] Wrapping the infant with a plastic wrap or placing the infant in a bag soon after delivery has resulted in improved admission temperature,[9–11] reduced mortality,[9] lessened oxygen requirement in the first 12 hours of life,[10] and improved glucose values[11] when compared to infants managed in the traditional fashion of drying with warm blankets. These findings are most effective for infants born <28 weeks gestation, although plastic wrap has been shown to improve admission temperature in newborns <33 weeks as well.[11]

Induced hypothermia (34–35°C) is a treatment modality for full term infants who have suffered a significant hypoxic ischemic event. This therapy is currently not considered standard of care for all infants at all centers, as ongoing research protocols continue to further optimize the target audience and better define outcome.

Hyperthermia

As previously noted, fetal temperature is dependent on the mother, and at birth, the newborn temperature is on average 0.3–0.5°C warmer. If fetal temperature exceeds maternal temperature, heat produced by the fetus is transferred to the mother. If this process is disrupted for any reason, such as in cord occlusion, fetal temperature will increase. Asakura demonstrated a higher skin temperature in newborns after birth if the umbilical cord was coiled.[12]

Intrapartum maternal fever, whether due to infection or the use of epidural anesthesia[13] may have significant implications for the newborn. In a prospective study of 1218 nulliparous women whose infants were not infected, 123 (10.1%) had a fever >100.4°F, and their infants were more likely to have a one minute APGAR score <7, and be hypotonic after delivery compared to the afebrile newborns. Those infants born to mothers with a temperature >101°F were more likely to require bag mask resuscitation and continued oxygen therapy in the nursery. Furthermore, neonatal seizures were more common in the febrile group.[14] Epidural anesthesia was administered to 98.4% of mothers who developed a temperature of >101°F. No follow-up was performed in this population. In a separate prospective cohort study, infants born with a fever were more likely to require resuscitation, and be admitted to a NICU.[15] Many of the neonatal morbidities described were transient. To better understand the association between neonatal fever and permanent neonatal disability and whether reduction of maternal temperature can prevent these outcomes requires further study.

Glucose regulation

Metabolic changes at birth result in glucose as the main energy source for the brain and vital organs. After the umbilical cord is cut and maternal glucose is no longer available, there is a surge in catecholamines, glucagon and cortisol, and a drop in insulin. Hepatic glycogenolysis and gluconeogenesis are the two means of providing glucose until enteral feedings are established. Gluconeogenesis begins 2 hours after birth and is at its peak by 12 hours. Alanine, from protein breakdown, and glycerol, from triglyceride breakdown, are the two major gluconeogenic substrates.[16] Glucose oxidation can only support 70% of the brain energy needs. Alternative fuels include ketone bodies and lactate, the former of which is felt to provide an alternative fuel for brain metabolism.[16]

A precise definition of hypoglycemia is problematic. A recent workshop conducted by the National Institute of Child Health and Human Development concluded that there are significant gaps of knowledge that preclude a definitive lower blood glucose cut off for the diagnosis of hypoglycemia.[17] Clinicians generally use 30 mg/dL or 20 mg/dL as the cut off for the diagnosis of hypoglycemia based on data published in the older literature.[18,19]

Neonatal hypoglycemia poses a significant risk to the newborn and at its extreme, can lead to seizures and brain injury. In a cohort of 35 term infants with early MRI after symptomatic hypoglycemia, 94% demonstrated white matter abnormalities and 65% demonstrated neurodevelopmental impairment at 18 months, which was related to the severity of white matter injury and involvement of the posterior limb and internal capsule. As such, the authors conclude that early imaging is more instructive than severity or duration of hypoglycemia for predicting neurodevelopmental outcomes.[20]

Healthy asymptomatic newborn infants are at low risk of developing hypoglycemia and therefore do not warrant routine evaluation. Those infants predisposed to hypoglycemia (Table 2) should be evaluated in a timely fashion and treated accordingly.

During early postnatal life, premature infants are at high risk of altered glucose homeostasis.[16] There are limited glycogen stores in infants less than 28 weeks gestation, as glycogen accumulates predominantly in the third trimester. As such, gluconeogeneis is the major source of glucose

Table 2. Risk factors for neonatal hypoglycemia.

- Prematurity
- Large and small for gestational age
- Hyperinsulinism

  — Infant of diabetic mother
  — Pancreatic Nesidioblastosis
  — Beckwith-Wiedemann syndrome

- Infants exposed to Beta adrenergic or oral hypoglycemic agents
- Medically compromised infants

  — Sepsis
  — Asphyxia
  — Hypothermia

- Metabolic

  — Type 1 Glycogen Storage disease
  — Galactosemia
  — Hereditary fructose Intolerance

---

production in the preterm infant. A constant infusion of glucose is required to maintain normoglycemia in the early hours of life given limited glycogen stores and the time required to induce enzymes for gluconeogenesis. Due to limited fat stores in the preterm infant, ketogenesis is less available as an alternative.[16,21]

As a constant glucose infusion is often required before enteral feedings are fully tolerated, the neonate weighing less than 1000 grams at birth is 18 times more likely to become hyperglycemic when compared to infants weighing greater than 2000 grams.[22] There is evidence that the preterm infant is partially resistant to insulin.[23] Should the blood glucose level exceed 200 mg/dl, exogenous insulin should be administered. Treating hyperglycemia by reducing the glucose infusion below basal requirements (4–7 mg/kg/min) is not advised as this significantly reduces caloric intake, which may have long-term effects on growth.

Feeding

Otherwise healthy newborn infants should be fed early and frequently in order to avoid hypoglycemia. Breastfeeding is the recommended nutrition of choice given its benefits for both the infant and the mother. *Healthy*

People 2010 recommends a goal of increasing the proportion of breast-feeding mothers in the early postpartum period from 64% seen in 1998 to 75% by 2010.[24] Well infants should be fed in the delivery room, and every 2–3 hours thereafter. Successful breastfeeding is associated with rooming in,[25] skin-to-skin contact,[26] demand feeding and lactation support. Formula-fed infants may eat less frequently, but no longer than at four-hour intervals for the first few days of life.

During the transition period, the preterm infant is often not in a position to begin enteral feedings, and glucose values are maintained by providing a dextrose solution and ultimately, parenteral nutrition. Early trophic feeding, or feeding small volumes of milk daily for the first days of life, is a strategy used by some to enhance feeding tolerance, minimize the need for intravenous nutrition and ultimately improve outcome. In a randomized controlled trial of 100 preterm infants weighing less than 1750 grams, when compared to infants receiving parenteral nutrition alone, those infants offered trophic feedings from day three had significantly greater energy intake, weight gain, and head circumference gain. In addition, they had fewer episodes of culture positive sepsis, less parenteral nutrition, reached full feedings earlier, and a shorter duration of hospitalization. There was no difference in complications between the groups.[27] However, in a Cochrane review of ten trials comparing trophic feedings to parenteral intake, the relative risk for necrotizing enterocolitis in the fed cohort was 1.16 (CI 0.75–1.79), a finding consistent with a 16% increase in this disease and a number needed to harm of 50.[28] A large, well-designed multi-center trial would be beneficial to compare early trophic feedings to current management with peripheral nutrition, not only to observe short-term effects, but to assess neurodevelopmental sequelae and survival rate without significant gastrointestinal morbidities.

Factors Affecting Normal Transition

Gestational age

The normal physiologic events noted to occur as an infant transitions from the fetal to neonatal state are less tolerated or incomplete as gestational age decreases. The normal cardiopulmonary changes that need to occur in order for the fetus, once dependent on the placenta for gas exchange, to now utilize the lungs for oxygenation and ventilation and the heart to supply adequate pulmonary and system flow, cannot easily occur. Lack of surfactant predisposes the very preterm infant to respiratory distress and failure to close cardiac shunts, particularly the ductus, can exacerbate pulmonary insufficiency. Limited fat stores and substrate predispose the preterm infant to hypothermia and hypoglycemia.

An emerging issue in neonatology is the care of late preterm infants. There is evidence that this population is not as benign as previously thought.[29] They have increased mortality when compared to term infants[30] and are at increased risk for complications, including transient tachypnea of the newborn, respiratory distress syndrome, persistent pulmonary hypertension, respiratory failure, temperature instability, jaundice, feeding difficulties and a prolonged neonatal intensive care unit stay. It is increasingly evident that the care of this group of infants consumes significant health care resources.

Maternal health

Maternal health plays a significant role in neonatal outcome. In 2006, the teen pregnancy rate (15–19 years) rose 3%, the first increase since 1991. In addition, the birth rate for women aged 40–44 also increased by 3%, the highest rate since 1968.[31] Delivering infants at these two age extremes poses a risk to the newborn. In a retrospective cohort study of 3,886,364 nulliparous pregnant women <25 years of age, the rates of preterm delivery, very low birth weight, small for gestational age, very low APGAR scores and neonatal mortality were all higher in teen pregnancies. These findings were consistently increased with decreasing maternal age, with the highest morbidities among infants born to mothers aged 15 or less.[32] Similarly, infants born to mothers older than 35 years had lower one and five minute APGAR scores,[33] were more preterm, had low birth weight and were small for gestational age[34] when compared to infants born to younger mothers. In addition, the mothers developed more pre-eclampsia, antenatal bleeding, premature rupture of membranes, malpresentation and required more Cesarean births, when compared to younger mothers.[33,34]

Many maternal diseases or conditions affect the outcome of a growing fetus and newborn infant. In a retrospective cohort study comparing infants born by Cesarean section between 24 and 33 weeks gestational age because of maternal or fetal indications to infants born at the same gestational age whose mothers developed spontaneous labor, the former group had more complications. Specifically, those infants born because of maternal or fetal complications had a higher mortality, more significant respiratory distress syndrome, and more developed chronic lung disease at one year of age when compared to those infants born after spontaneous labor.[35]

Since 1980, obesity rates have doubled for adults. Obesity in pregnancy poses serious risks to the mother (gestational diabetes, pre-eclampsia, emergency cesarean section, postpartum hemorrhage, urinary tract infection, wound infection) and the infant (large for gestational-age infants and intrauterine death).[36] Optimizing maternal health before pregnancy and maintaining close observation during pregnancy can help minimize the untoward outcomes seen in the newborn.

Maternal analgesia

Most anesthetics and analgesic medications used for pain management during labor cross the placenta, but in an otherwise healthy fetus, are well tolerated. The choice of anesthetics used in order to alleviate the pain of delivery should be based on the individual clinical patient. The advantage of regional anesthesia for operative births is that it allows the mother to be awake and participate in the delivery. There has been a considerable amount of research published looking at the effect of various pain relief strategies that demonstrate conflicting short-term outcomes in the neonate. Specifically, in one large retrospective review comparing the effects of general and regional anesthesia for elective and non-elective Cesarean sections, general anesthesia was associated with a lower 1-minute and 5-minute APGAR score, and greater requirement for intubation and artificial ventilation. There were no differences in mortality.[37] However, in a prospective randomized trial comparing general to spinal anesthesia for Cesarean sections, there was no difference in short-term outcomes, specifically APGAR scores, cord gas, hospital stay, neonatal depression or perinatal asphyxia.[38] In another study, fetal oxygenation and 5-minute APGAR score were not affected by the analgesic method in comparing epidural anesthesia to parenteral opioid analgesia, although infants exposed to maternal opioids required more naloxone and had a lower one minute APGAR score.[39]

Questions have been raised about the negative impact of maternal anesthesia on breastfeeding success. In a review of two prospective cohort studies including 2,364 patients, no correlation was found between parenteral opioid or epidural/spinal anesthesia and breastfeeding success.[40]

Little evidence is available to support long-term morbidities associated with maternal pain relief during labor. However, many women wish to avoid any potential morbidities associated with pharmacologic management. Alternatives to traditional pain management strategies have been reviewed, and acupuncture and hypnosis may be of benefit in managing pain.[41] Future work focusing on long-term neonatal outcomes such as neurobehavior, breastfeeding duration and maternal satisfaction when considering analgesia for delivery would be beneficial when making treatment decisions. Please refer to Chapter 3 for a more in-depth discussion regarding the effects of anesthesia on the fetus and the newborn.

Placental health

During fetal life, the placenta serves as the organ of gas exchange, nutritional delivery and excretion. Although the size of the placenta does not specifically equate with function as there are no adequate measures to assess function, correlations are made between size of the placenta and fetal growth derangements. Abnormalities in the health of this vital organ can have a significant impact on the ability of the fetus to properly develop and normally transition to the newborn state. Specific abnormalities in placental location (placenta previa), placental formation (placenta accreta, vasa previa), or placental separation (placental abruption) can have profound effects on both the mother and infant, particularly if significant bleeding is noted.

The ability of placental volume to predict newborn size is a useful tool in order to identify the at-risk fetus in the perinatal period. In a prospective study of 561 women from the West Indies, placental volume assessed in the early part of the second trimester was positively associated with birth weight, head circumference and length. The authors concluded that low birth weight was often preceded by small placental volume early in the second trimester, which is valuable information when considering management needs during the transition period.[42]

Maternal disease states or maternal habits can also affect placental and ultimately, fetal growth. Maternal hypertensive disease, advanced vascular disease due to diabetes, autoimmune disorders, cigarette smoking, alcohol, and cocaine all can play a role in placental well-being.

Delivery Room Management

Mode of delivery

Approximately ten percent of neonates require resuscitation at birth. While there are conditions known to place the fetus at increased risk of transitional difficulties, this is not always apparent when a mother presents in labor. In general, a vaginal delivery presents less risk to the mother and her infant. However, the US Cesarean delivery rate in 2006 was 31.1%, making operative births the most common surgical procedure performed on American women.[31] Much of this increase is due to a rise in the rate of primary Cesarean deliveries and to the reduction in vaginal births after Cesarean deliveries (VBAC).

In a retrospective cohort study of 672 women with one prior Cesarean section, those neonates born after elective repeat Cesarean delivery had a significantly higher rate of respiratory morbidity, NICU-admission and a longer length of hospital stay, when compared to neonates born after successful VBAC.[43] Of the infants with these morbidities, the 37-week group had the highest rates of oxygen use and admission to the NICU despite also being the group with the greatest number of amniocentesis for fetal lung maturity. These findings are consistent with previous studies demonstrating that, when compared to newborns delivered vaginally or by emergency cesarean section, those infants born by elective Cesarean delivery had an increased risk of respiratory difficulties. This risk increased with decreasing gestational age.[44,45] This data supports the recommendation by the American College of Obstetrics and Gynecology that neonates younger than 39 weeks not be delivered by elective repeat Cesarean delivery.[46]

Despite the data that demonstrates increased morbidities to infants born by elective repeat Cesarean sections, many hospitals no longer offer VBAC as part of a birthing plan, due to the risk of uterine rupture. The odds of uterine rupture depend on the type of uterine incision (low transverse vs low vertical vs classical incision), the number of suturing layers, the time interval between pregnancies and the use of labor inducing drugs.[47] In order to fully evaluate the incidence and consequence of uterine rupture in women with a previous Cesarean delivery, a systematic review of 568 full text articles was conducted to identify 71 eligible studies. Compared to elective Cesarean delivery, trial of labor increased the risk of uterine rupture by 2.7 per 1,000 cases. For those mothers attempting vaginal delivery, the additional risk of perinatal death from rupture of the scar was 1.4 per 10,000 and the additional risk of hysterectomy was 3.4 per 10,000. There were no maternal deaths. The authors conclude that 370 elective Cesarean deliveries would need to occur to prevent one symptomatic uterine rupture. Of note, elective cesarean delivery is not a guarantee that uterine rupture will be prevented.[48]

Instrumented deliveries

The use of forceps or vacuum extraction are generally reserved for complicated vaginal deliveries including, for example, a non-reassuring fetal heart rate, prolonged second stage of labor, or maternal exhaustion. The vacuum is the preferred operative device of choice in the United States, and in 1998, the FDA released a warning that vacuum assisted deliveries may result in fatal complications.[49] In an effort to compare the risk of neonatal morbidities between the use of the forceps and vacuum extraction, Demissie et al. conducted a population-based study involving 10 million singleton live births to examine the association between infant mortality and morbidity and mode of delivery. The risk of birth injuries, neonatal seizures, and third and forth degree perineal tears were lower for vacuum deliveries, while the risk of developing shoulder dystocia and postpartum hemorrhage were lower for the forcep deliveries.[50] Those deliveries in which vacuum was followed by forceps or either procedure was followed by a cesarean delivery had the worse outcomes. Whether the outcome is more a result of a difficult labor versus the use of instrumentation is not clear. Regardless, a pediatric provider should be present at all instrumented deliveries given the increased risks to the infant.

Oxygen vs. room air

One hundred percent oxygen is the commonly used gas for neonatal resuscitation. Understanding the potential dangers associated with the use of 100% oxygen has lead to numerous studies comparing the short and long-term outcomes for infants exposed to 100% oxygen versus room air for resuscitation. In the Resair 2 Study, involving 609 term infants from eleven centers comparing room air to 100% oxygen, resuscitation with room air was as efficient as pure oxygen, but not superior.[51] In a Cochrane review of five studies including 1,302 infants, there was a significant reduction in the death rate for those infants resuscitated in room air. However, the use of back up 100% oxygen was utilized in more than 25% of infants randomized to room air.[52]

Less information regarding oxygen for resuscitation is available in the preterm infant. Untoward effects of hyperoxia, including alterations in cerebral blood flow and reperfusion injury, may be less tolerated in this vulnerable population. However, in a prospective randomized trial of preterm infants ranging from 24 to 31 weeks, all infants assigned to room air received an increase in oxygen to achieve a targeted oxygen saturation. (<70% at three minutes). While the authors conclude that room air should not be used as an initial resuscitating gas for the preterm infant, they recommend starting at 30–40% oxygen instead of 100%.[53]

The American Academy of Pediatrics/American Heart Association in their Neonatal Resuscitation Manual (5th edition)[1] acknowledge that room air may be as effective as 100% oxygen for term infants, but do not recommend this as standard of care. No specific amount of oxygen is recommended for the preterm infant. For those facilities that electively deliver infants <32 weeks, both an oxygen blender and pulse oximetry monitoring are recommended in the delivery room, in order to administer less than pure oxygen. For those centers providing room air resuscitation in the delivery room, a source of 100% oxygen should be available.

Meconium stained amnionic fluid

Meconium staining of the amnionic fluid occurs in 7 to 22% of term infants and meconium aspiration syndrome (MAS) can complicate anywhere from 1.7% to 35% of these deliveries.[54] Several strategies have been used to minimize the chance of developing meconium aspiration at the time of delivery. In a 2001 Cochrane review of amnioinfusion therapy to relieve cord compression or to dilute the meconium, improvements were noted in perinatal outcome variables such as a reduction in meconium aspiration syndrome, neonatal hypoxic-ischemic encephalopathy and ventilation requirement.[55] However, in a more recent large multicenter randomized controlled trial,[56] the use of amnioinfusion did not reduce the risk of moderate or severe meconium aspiration, perinatal death or major maternal or neonatal disorders. As such, amnioinfusion is not routinely performed for all labors involving meconium stained amnionic fluid.

The use of intrapartum suctioning of the mouth and oropharynx before delivery of the shoulders, previously performed routinely by obstetricians, is not universally employed given recent data that has demonstrated no difference in the incidence of meconium aspiration between those children who were and were not suctioned on the perineum.[57] While obstetrical management of the neonatal airway is not specifically addressed in the Academy of Pediatrics Neonatal Resuscitation Textbook (5th Ed.),[1] suctioning of the mouth and nose by the pediatrician to clear the airway once the infant has delivered remains a recommendation for all deliveries.

Guidelines for the management of the vigorous meconium-stained newborn have been revised based on the study by Wiswell that failed to demonstrate a reduction in MAS for those infants intubated after delivery. Furthermore, there were 51 complications of the actual intubation, although they were all mild in nature.[58] Current recommendations for the meconium-stained infant include intubation only if the newborn is not vigorous (depressed muscle tone, depressed respirations, heart rate

<100 beats per minute). There are currently no clinical studies that warrant basing suctioning guidelines on meconium consistency.

Cord clamping

Traditional management after delivery of the newborn includes immediate clamping of the umbilical cord. In a Cochrane review of 11 studies involving 2,989 mothers and their full term infants, delayed cord clamping for two to three minutes resulted in significant increases in hemoglobin at birth (mean difference 2.17 g/dl; 95% CI 0.28 to 4.06; three trials of 671 infants) and elevated ferritin levels at six months. However, the same group was noted to have an increased need for phototherapy for jaundice (RR 0.59, 95% CI 0.38 to 0.92; five trials in 1,762 infants).[59] In a meta-analysis involving 1,912 infants enrolled in 15 controlled trials to determine the benefits and risks associated with delayed cord clamping, the authors concluded that delaying cord clamping for at least two minutes resulted in improved hematocrit, ferritin concentration and stored iron for the first six months, and a clinically important reduction in the risk of anemia. Insignificant differences were noted in the incidence of transient tachypnea, jaundice and polycythemia.[60]

A similar review of delayed cord clamping for 120 seconds in the preterm population (<37 weeks gestation) noted the need for fewer transfusions for anemia and hypotension and less intraventricular hemorrhage in those infants afforded the intervention. No differences in long-term outcome were observed.[61] In order to fully endorse the practice of delayed cord clamping for all deliveries, a multi-centered randomized controlled trial sufficiently powered to detect both short and long-term beneficial and potential adverse effects is necessary.[62] In addition, techniques for care and early stabilization of the newborn with the cord intact should be developed and evaluated.[63]

References

1. Kattwinkel J, ed. (2006) Neonatal Resuscitation, 5th edition. *Am Acad Pediatr and Am Heart Assoc.*

2. Karlsen K, ed. (2006) The Stable Program. *Guidelines for Neonatal Healthcare Providers*, 5th edition.

3. Asakura H. (2004) Fetal and neonatal thermoregulation. *J of Nippon Med School*. Dec; **71**(6): 360–370.

4. Carfoot S, Williamson P, Dickson R. (2005) A randomized controlled trial in the north of England examining the effects of skin-to-skin care on breast feeding. *Midwifery* **21**: 71–79.

5. Ferber SG, Makhouol IR. (2004) The effect of skin-to-skin contact (kangaroo care) shortly after birth on the neurobehavioral responses of the term newborn: A randomized, controlled trial. *Pediatr* **113**(4): 858–865.

6. Vaidya K, Sharma A, Dhungel S. (2005) Effect of early mother-baby close contact over the duration of exclusive breastfeeding. *Nepal Med Coll J.* **7**: 138–140.

7. Costeloe K, Hennessy E, Gibson AT *et al.* (2000) The EPICure study: Outcomes to discharge from hospital for infants born at the threshold of viability. *Pediatr* **106**(4): 659–671.

8. Baumgart S. (1984) Reduction of oxygen consumption, insensible water loss, and radiant heat demand with use of a plastic blanket for low-birth-weight infants under radiant warmers. *Pediatr* **74**(6): 1022–1028.

9. Vohra S, Frent G, Campbell V *et al.* (1999) Effect of polyethylene occlusive skin wrapping on heat loss in very low birth weight infants at delivery: A randomized trial. *J Pediatr* **134**: 547–551.

10. Bjorklund LJ, Hellstrom-Westas L. (2000) Reducing heat loss at birth in very preterm infants. *J Pediatr* **137**: 739–780.

11. Lenclen R, Mazraani M, Jugie M *et al.* (2002) Use of a polyethylene bag: A way to improve the thermal environment of the premature newborn at the delivery room. *Arch de Pediatrie* Mar; **9**(3): 238–244.

12. Asakura H. (1996) Thermogenesis in fetus and neonate. *J Nippon Med Sch* **63**: 171–172.

13. Lieberman E, Lang JM, Frigoletto F *et al.* (1997) Epidural analgesia, intrapartum fever, and neonatal sepsis evaluation. *Pediatr* **99**: 415–419.

14. Lieberman E, Lang J, Richardson DK *et al.* (2000) Intrapartum maternal fever and neonatal outcome. *Pediatr* **105**: 8–13.

15. Shalak LF, Perlman JM, Jackson GL *et al.* (2005) Depression at birth in term infants exposed to maternal chorioamnionitis: Does neonatal fever play a role? *J Perinat* **25**: 447–452.

16. Mitanchez D. (2007) Glucose regulation in preterm newborn infants. *Hormone Res* **68**: 265–271.

17. Hay WW Jr., Raju TN, Higgins RD *et al.* (2009) Knowledge gaps and research needs for understanding and treating neonatal hypoglycemia: Workshop report from Eunice Kennedy Shriver National Institute of Child Health and Human Development. *J Pediatr* **155**(5): 612–617.

18. Srinivasan G, Pildes RS, Cattamanchi G *et al.* (1986) Plasma glucose values in normal neonates: A new look. *J Pediatr* **109**: 114–117.

19. Cornblath M, Reisner SH. (1965) Blood glucose in the neonate and its clinical significance. *N Engl J Med* **273**: 378–381.

20. Burns CM, Rutherford MA, Boardman JP *et al.* (2008) Patterns of cerebral injury and neurodevelopmental outcomes after symptomatic neonatal hypoglycemia. *Pediatr* **122**: 65–74.

21. Duvanel CB, Fawer CL, Cotting J *et al.* (1999) Long-term effects of neonatal hypoglycemia on brain growth a development in small-for-gestational-age preterm infants. *J Pediatr* **143**: 389–391.

22. Dweck H, Cassady G. (1974) Glucose intolerance in infants of very low birth weight. Incidence of hyperglycemia on infants of birth weight 1,100 or less. *Pediatr* **53**:189–195.

23. Mitanchez-Mokhtari D, Lahlou N, Kieffer F *et al.* (2004) Both relative insulin resistance and defective islet beta-cell processing of proinsulin are responsible of transient hyperglycemia in extremely preterm infants. *Pediatr* **113**: 537–541.

24. www.healthpeople.gov/document/html/objectives/16-19.htm

25. Procianoy RS, Fernandez-Filho PH, Lazaro L *et al.* (1983) The influence of rooming in on breastfeeding. *J of Tropical Pediatr* Apr **29**(2): 112–114.

26. Moore ER, Anderson GC, Bergman N. (2007) Early skin-to-skin contact for mothers and their healthy newborn infants. *Cochrane Database of Systematic Reviews* **3**; CD003519.

27. McClure RJ, Newell SJ. (2000) Randomized controlled study of clinical outcome following trophic feeding. *Arch Dis Child- Fetal and Neo Ed* Jan **82**: F29–F33.

28. Tyson JE, Kennedy KA. (2005) Trophic feedings for parenterally fed infants. *Cochrane Database for Systematic Reviews*, **3**: CD000504.

29. Ramachandrappa A, Jain L. (2009) Health issues of the late preterm infant. *Pediatr Clin North Am* **56**: 565–577.

30. Pulver LS, Guest-Warnick G, Stoddard GJ. (2009) Weight for gestational age affects the mortality of late preterm infants. *Pediatrics*: 123: 1072–1077.

31. Hamilton BE, Martin JA, Ventura SJ. (Dec 5, 2007) *National Vital Statistics Reports* **56**(7): 1–18.

32. Chen X, Wen SW, Fleming N *et al.* (2007) Teenage pregnancy and adverse birth outcomes: A large population based retrospective cohort study. *Internat. J Epidemiol* **36**(2): 368–373.

33. Ustun Y, Engin-Ustun Y, Meydanli M *et al.* (2005) Maternal and neonatal outcomes in pregnancies at 35 and older age group. *J Turkish Ger Gynecol Assoc* **6**(1): 46–48.

34. Ziadeh SM. (2002) Maternal and perinatal outcomes in nulliparous women aged 35 and older. *Gynecol Obstet Invest* **54**: 6–10.

35. Kurkinen-Raty M, Koivisto M. (2000) Preterm delivery for maternal or fetal indications: Maternal morbidity, neonatal outcome and late sequelae in infants. *British J of Obstet and Gynecol* **107**(5): 648–655.

36. Sebire NJ, Jolly M, Harris JP *et al.* (2001) Maternal obesity and pregnancy: A study of 287,213 pregnancies in London. *Int J Obes Relat Metab Disord* Aug **23**(8): 1175–1182.

37. Ong BY, Cohen MM, Palahniuk RJ. (1989) Anesthesia for cesarean section-effects on neonates. *Anesth Analg* **68**: 270–275.

38. Kavak ZN, Basgul A, Ceyhan N. (2001) Short-term outcome of newborn infants: Spinal versus general anesthesia for elective cesarean section. A prospective randomized study. *Eur J Obstet Gynecol* **100**: 50–54.

39. Leighton BL, Halpern SH. (May 2002) The effects of epidural analgesia on labor, maternal, and neonatal outcomes: A systematic review. *Amer J Obstet & Gynecol* **186**(5) Supplement: S69–S77.

40. Halpern SH, Leighton BL. (2003) Misconceptions about neuraxial analgesia. *Anesthesiol Clin N Amer* **21**: 51–70.

41. Smith CA, Collins CT, Cyna AM *et al.* (2006) Complementary and alternative therapies for pain management in labour. *Cochrane Database for Systematic Reviews*. Issue 4, Art No.CD003521.4

42. Thame M, Osmond C. Wilks R *et al.* (2001) Second-trimester placental volume and infant size at birth. *Obstet & Gynecol* **98**(2): 279–283.

43. Kamath BD, Todd JK, Glazner JE *et al.* (2009) Neonatal outcomes after elective Cesarean delivery. *Obstet & Gynecol* **113**(6): 1231–1238.

44. Dehdashtian M, Riazi E, Aletayeb MH. (July – Sept, 2008) Influence of mode of delivery at term of the neonatal respiratory morbidity. *Pak J of Med Sci* **24**(4): 556–559.

45. Hansen AK, Wisborg K, Uldbjerg N *et al.* (2008) Risk of respiratory morbidity in term infants delivered by elective Caesarean section: Cohort study. *BMJ* **336**: 85–87.

46. American College of Obstetricians and Gynecologists. (2007) ACOG Committee opinion no. 394, Dec. Cesarean delivery on maternal request. **110**(6): 1501.

47. Leiberman E. (2001) Risk factors for uterine rupture during a trial of labor after Cesarean. *Clin Obstet Gynecol* **44**: 609–621.

48. Guise J, McDonagh MS, Osterweil P, *et al.* (2004) Systematic review of the incidence and consequences of uterine rupture in women with previous Caesarean section. *BMJ* **329**: 19(July 3), dol:10.1136/bmj.329.7456.19.

49. FDA Public Health Advisory: Need for CAUTION when using vacuum assisted delivery devices. (May 21, 1998) http://www.fda/gov/MedicalDevices/ safety/AlertsandNotices/PublicHealthNotifications/

50. Demissie K, Rhoads GG, Smulian JC *et al.* (2004) Operative vaginal delivery and neonatal and infant adverse outcomes: Population based retrospective analysis. BMJ 329:24 (3 July), dol:10.1136/bmj.329.7456.24.

51. Saugstad OD, Rootwelt T, Aalen O. (1998) Resuscitation of asphyxiated newborn infants with room air or oxygen: An international controlled trial: The Resair 2 study. *Pediatr* **102**(1): 1–7.

52. Schulze TA, O'Donnell AA, Davis CPF. (2004) Air versus oxygen for resuscitation of infants at birth. *Cochrane Database of Systematic Reviews* Issue 2. Art. No:CD002273.

53. Wang CL, Anderson C, Leone TA *et al.* (2008) Resuscitation of preterm neonates by using room air or 100% oxygen. *Pediatr* **121**(6): 108301089.

54. Wiswell TE, Tuggle JM, Turner BS. (1990) Meconium aspiration syndrome: Have we made a difference? *Pediatr* **85**: 715–721.

55. Hofmeyr GJ. (2002) Amnioinfusion for meconium-stained liquor in labour. *Cochrane Database of Systematic Reviews*. Issue 1, Art No:CD000014.

56. Fraser WD, Hofmeyr J, Lede R *et al.* (2005) Amnioinfusion for the prevention of the meconium aspiration syndrome. *NEJM* **353**: 909–917.

57. Vain NE, Szyld EG, Prudent LM *et al.* (2004) Oropharyngeal and nasopharyngeal suctioning of meconium-stained neonates before delivery of their shoulders: Multicentre, randomised controlled trial. *Lancet* 14 Aug **364**: 597–602.

58. Wiswell TE, Gannon CM, Jacon J *et al.* (2000) Delivery room management of the apparently vigorous meconium-stained neonate: Results of the multicenter international collaborative trial. *Pediatr* **105**(1): 1–7.

59. Middleton M. (2008) Effect of timing of umbilical cord clamping of term infants on maternal and neonatal outcomes. *Cochrane Database of Systematic Reviews*, Issue 2 Art No:CD004074.

60. Hutton EK, Hassan ES. (2007) Late vs early clamping of the umbilical cord in full-term neonates: Systematic review and meta-analysis of controlled trials. *JAMA*. Mar **297**(11): 1257–1258.

61. Rabe H, Reynolds G, Diaz-Rossello J. (2004) Early versus delayed umbilical cord clamping in preterm infants. *Cochrane Database of Systematic Reviews* 4:CD003248.

62. Oh W. (2007) Timing of umbilical cord clamping at birth in full-term infants. *JAMA* **297**: 1257–1258.

63. Duley LMM, Weeks AD, Hey EN *et al.* (May 2009) Scientific Advisory Committee Opinion Paper Clamping of the umbilical cord and placental transfusion. *Royal Coll of Obstet and Gynecol.*

PART

III

Diseases of the Newborn

Chapter 5

Acute Respiratory Disorders in the Neonates

Yuh-Jyh Lin and Tsu-Fuh Yeh

Respiratory problems constitute the major causes of morbidity and mortality in the neonatal period. Of the infants admitted to the special care nursery, 45% of inborn and 80% of transferred babies had respiratory problems. It is estimated that 10 to 15% of infants with respiratory disorders die in the neonatal period. For those who recover, depending on the nature of the disease, complications or sequelae may persist into childhood. Improvement of mortality and morbidity rates depends on a better understanding of the basic physiology, pathology and biochemistry of the respiratory disorders.

Evaluation of the Infant

To understand the respiratory disease process, four different aspects should be considered in the evaluation of the infant:

1. Clinical signs of respiratory distress,
2. Blood chemistry,
3. Chest radiography and
4. Basic pulmonary physiology.

Clinical signs

A respiratory distress score, described by Downes and coworkers, has been used to evaluate the severity of the clinical distress.[1] Respiratory rate, retraction of the chest wall, color, grunting and air entry into the lungs are considered in the evaluation. Tachypnea is a compensatory reaction, but retractions, grunting, and poor airway entry reflect abnormal lung mechanics. Cyanosis is present whenever reduced hemoglobin is greater than 5 gm per cent. Central cyanosis is a consequence of right to left cardiopulmonary shunting. Peripheral cyanosis, denoting poor tissue oxygenation, is usually seen in infants with acidosis, heart failure, shock, or exposure to a cool environment.

Blood chemistry

Upon emerging from the intrauterine environment, the infant has to initiate respiration and modulate the transition of the cardiovascular system. The overall result of this adjustment is to establish good lung volume and pulmonary circulation. The transition normally occurs within 24 hours after birth. Thus the arterial pO_2 obtained from the umbilical artery during the first 24 hours in a normal newborn may vary from 60 to 90 mmHg. It has been estimated that a 20 to 25% shunt may be present in a normal newborn. Nevertheless, because of the high O_2 affinity of fetal hemoglobin and the relatively high hemoglobin level in the neonate, the O_2 content in the newborn is sufficient. Monitoring of pO_2 and pCO_2, and of the pH of arterial or arterialized capillary blood, is an essential part of the management of any infant requiring the administration of oxygen. The arterial pO_2 should be maintained in the range of 50 to 90 mmHg and the pH at more than 7.15. Using pulse oximeter, the O_2 saturation is preferably maintained at 90–95%.

Chest radiography

Chest X-rays are necessary in the diagnosis of respiratory distress. Anteroposterior and lateral views should be obtained. Factors to be considered in evaluating the chest X-ray include age of the infant, film density, phase of respiration, and position of the patient. Although serial films are frequently necessary, radiographs should be taken only when indicated. Correlation of the chest film findings with clinical conditions of the infant is essential for an accurate diagnosis.

Pulmonary physiology

Measurements of pulmonary functions are used more for research than for clinical diagnosis or management. Lung volume, compliance, airway resistance, ventilation/perfusion ratio, and respiration regulation can be measured and evaluated. Measurements of functional residual capacity and crying vital capacity are considered good screening tests for an overall assessment of lung volume and mechanical factors. Stabilization of the chest cavity is also important in order to reserve more lung volume.

Differential Diagnosis

Disturbance in respiration is not always related to primary lesions of the respiratory tract, because the process of breathing is influenced by many other factors, e.g. cardiac, neurological, am metabolic status. Therefore, a thorough evaluation of the infant is necessary for making a correct diagnosis. A list of common causes of acute respiratory distress in neonates is provided (Tables 1–6). For this chapter, the focus is on respiratory distress syndrome (RDS) and meconium aspiration syndrome (MAS).

Respiratory distress syndrome (RDS)

Essentially a disease of preterm infants, RDS is due to a lack of pulmonary surfactant along with functional and structural immaturity of the cardiopulmonary system (Fig. 1). Depending on the size of the baby, the pulmonary insufficiency may occur at or shortly after birth and may increase in severity over the first few days. Clinical features of respiratory distress and a positive chest radiography at or shortly after birth are required for the diagnosis.

Table 1.   Disease of the upper airways.

Congenital anomalies
Choanal atresia
Laryngeal webs or diaphragms
Laryngomalacia
Tracheal aplasia or stenosis
Tracheoesophageal fistula and esophageal atresia
External compression of the upper airways
    Vascular ring or sling
    Tumors and cysts (Table 2)

Trauma
Postextubation laryngeal edema, atelectasis and subglottic stenosis
Vocal cord paralysis
Laryngeal fracture
Tracheal perforation

Table 2.   Tumors and cysts of the upper airway.

Tumors
Teratoma
    tonsilllar
    nasopharyngeal
    cervical
Dermoid
    pharyngeal
Hemangioma
    subglottic
Hemangiopericytoma
    nasopharyngeal
Neuroblastoma
    Cervical
Neurofibroma
    laryngeal
    cervical
Goiter
    hyperthyroidism
    hypothyroidism

(Continued)

Table 2. (*Continued*).

Cysts
Ectopic thyroid tissue
Thyroglossal duct cyst
Lingual cyst
Congenital laryngeal cyst
Lymphangioma and cystic hygroma
Brachial cleft cyst

Table 3. Diseases of the pulmonary parenchyma.

Congenital Anomalies
Lung cysts
Congenital cystic adenomatosis
Lobar emphysema
Hypoplasia and agenesis of the lung
Chylothorax
Congenital pulmonary lymphangiectasis

Acquired Disorders
Transient tachypnea in the newborn
Respiratory distress syndrome (RDS)
Meconium aspiration syndrome (MAS)
Pneumonia
Chronic lung disease (CLD)
Pulmonary hemorrhage

Table 4. Diseases of diaphragm and neuromuscular disorders.

Diaphragmatic hernia and eventration
Phrenic nerve paralysis
Disorders of the central nervous system
Disorders of anterior horn cells
    Werdnig-Hoffman disease
    Poliomyelitis
    Other viral infections

(*Continued*)

Table 4. (*Continued*).

Disorders of peripheral nerves
    Peripheral neuropathy
    Guillain-Barre syndrome
Disorders of neuromuscular junctions
    Myasthenia gravis
Primary myopathies
    Muscular dystrophies
    Congenital non-progressive myopathy
    Inflammatory myopathy
    Myotonic syndrome
    Periodic paralysis
Skeletal and tendinous disorders
Metabolic and infectious disorders

Table 5. Chest wall deformities.

Asphyxiating thoracic dystrophy (Jeune syndrome)
Ellis-van Creveld syndrome
Achondrogenesis
Thanatophoric dwarfism
Homozygous achondroplasia
Osteogenesis imperfecta
Poland's syndrome
Hypophosphatasia
Spondylothoracic dysplasia
Rickets
Congenital hypoparathyroidism

Table 6. Respiratory distress due to congenital heart disease in the newborn.

Hypoxemia due to intracardiac right-to left shunt
Pulmonary edema and/or congestive heart failure
Poor lung mechanics due to massive left-to right shunt
Airway obstruction due to external cardiovascular compression

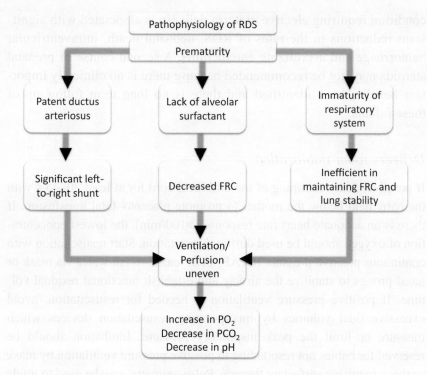

Figure 1. Pathophysiology of respiratory distress syndrome.

Management of respiratory distress syndrome (RDS)

The aim of management of RDS is to provide interventions that will maintain respiratory function and maximize the number of survivors while minimizing potential adverse effects. Some of the following recommendations derived from the recent European Consensus guidelines.[2]

Antenatal corticosteroid

Single course of antenatal betamethasone (two doses of 12 mg given intramuscularly at 24-hour intervals) to women at risk of preterm delivery (before 35 weeks' gestation) including threatened preterm labor, antepartum hemorrhage, preterm rupture of membranes or any condition requiring elective preterm delivery is associated with significant reductions in the rates of RDS, neonatal death, intraventricular hemorrhage and necrotizing enterocolitis. A second course of prenatal steroids may not be recommended because there is no clinically important benefits been identified and there is no long term follow-up of these infants.

Delivery room stabilization

If possible, delay clamping of the umbilical cord for at least 30–45 s with the baby held below the mother to promote placento–fetal transfusion. If there is an adequate heart rate response (>100/min), the lowest concentration of oxygen should be used during resuscitation. Start resuscitation with continuous positive pressure (CPAP) of at least 5–6 cm water via mask or nasal prongs to stabilize the airway and establish functional residual volume. If positive pressure ventilation is needed for resuscitation, avoid excessive tidal volumes by incorporating resuscitation devices which measure or limit the peak inspiratory pressure. Intubation should be reserved for babies not responding to positive pressure ventilation by mask or those requiring surfactant therapy. Pulse oximetry may be used to guide oxygen delivery during resuscitation, aiming to avoid hyperoxic peaks. Prophylatic surfactant may be beneficial when given in the delivery room for those infants under 27 weeks gestation with respiratory distress.

Surfactant therapy

Surfactant treatment reduces mortality and pulmonary air leak for babies with or at high risk of RDS. Prophylactic surfactant is considered in infants under 27 weeks' gestation. Prophylaxis should be considered for babies between 26 and 30 weeks gestation if intubation is required in the delivery room or if the mother has not received prenatal corticosteroids. Early rescue surfactant should be given to untreated babies if there is evidence of RDS. Individual units need to develop protocols for when to intervene as RDS progresses. A second, and sometimes a third dose of surfactant, is often needed if there is ongoing evidence of RDS such as a persistent oxygen requirement and need for mechanical ventilation or if over 50% oxygen is needed on CPAP at 6 cm H_2O. For babies on CPAP, a second dose of surfactant should be given if they are determined to need mechanical ventilation. Natural surfactants should be used in preference to synthetic as they reduce both pulmonary air leaks and mortality. Of the natural surfactants, the bovine products beractant and calfactant seem similar in their efficacy, but poractant alfa in a dose of 200 mg/kg for rescue therapy leads to improved survival compared to beractant. Early surfactant replacement therapy with extubation to NCPAP compared with later selective surfactant replacement and continued mechanical ventilation with extubation from low ventilator support is associated with less need mechanical ventilation, lower incidence of BPD and fewer air leak syndromes. If possible, duration of mechanical ventilation should be shortened by immediate (or early) extubation to CPAP following surfactant administration provided the baby is otherwise stable.

Oxygen supplementation in NICU

Oxygen saturation should be maintained below 95% which may minimize the occurrence of retinopathy of prematurity (ROP) and BPD. After giving surfactant, avoid a hyperoxic peak by appropriately reducing the inspired oxygen concentration. This maneuver will avoid the occurrence of grade I and II intraventricular hemorrhage.

The role of CPAP in the management of RDS

CPAP may be initiated in infants at risk of RDS, because this may stabilize the chest cavity and improve efficiency of ventilation. The use of CPAP with early rescue surfactant should be considered in babies with RDS. Short binasal prongs should be used rather than a single prong and a pressure of at least 6 cmH$_2$O should be applied.

Mechanical ventilation strategies

Mechanical ventilation (MV) should be used to support babies with respiratory failure. All modes of MV can induce lung injury and should be limited to the shortest possible duration. Avoid hypocapnia, wherever possible, as this is associated with increased risks of BPD and periventricular leukomalacia. Following extubation, babies should be put on nasal CPAP as this reduces the need for re-intubation, particularly for extreme low birth weight infants.

High frequency ventilation

High frequency ventilation has been shown to lessen lung injury in experimental studies. A meta-analysis does not show evidence that elective high frequency oscillatory ventilation (HFOV) offers significant advantages over conventional ventilation (CV) when used as the initial ventilation strategy to treat preterm infants with acute pulmonary dysfunction. Subgroups of trials showed a significant reduction in CLD with HFOV when high volume strategy for HFOV was used, when piston oscillators were used for HFOV, when lung protective strategies for CV were not used, when randomisation occurred at two to six hours of age, and when inspiratory:expiratory ratio of 1:2 was used for HFOV. In the meta-analysis of all trials, pulmonary air leaks occurred more frequently in the HFOV group.[3] Currently, HFOV is used for infants who require high setting of IMV or failed to IMV.

For additional information on this issue, please see Chapter 7 of this Handbook.

Inhaled nitric oxide

Randomized controlled trials of inhaled nitric oxide therapy (iNO) in preterm infants can be grouped into three categories depending on the entry criteria; entry in the first three days of life based on oxygenation criteria, routine use in intubated preterm babies and later enrollment based on an increased risk of BPD.[4] Trials of early rescue treatment of infants based on oxygenation criteria demonstrated no significant effect on mortality or BPD. Routine use of iNO in intubated preterm infants demonstrated a marginally significant reduction in the combined outcome of death or BPD. Later treatment with iNO based on the risk of BPD demonstrated no significant benefit for this outcome. Studies of early rescue treatment with iNO demonstrated a trend toward increased risk of severe IVH, whereas the studies with routine use in intubated preterm infants seems to show a reduction in the risk of having either a severe IVH or PVL. Later iNO treatment of infants at risk of BPD is given after the major risk period for IVH and does not appear to lead to progression of old lesions. Two studies presented data on long term neurodevelopmental outcome. The early routine treatment study showed an improved outcome at two years corrected age, while the rescue treatment study showed no effect of iNO.[4] Further studies are needed to confirm these findings, to define groups most likely to benefit, and to describe long term outcomes.

Maintenance of blood pressure

Treatment of hypotension is recommended when it is accompanied by evidence of poor tissue perfusion. Doppler-ultrasound assessment of systemic hemodynamics should be used to guide treatment. In the absence of cardiac ultrasound, volume expansion with 10 mL/kg normal saline should be used as first line treatment to exclude hypovolemia. Dopamine (2–20 mcg/kg/min) should be used if volume expansion fails to satisfactorily improve blood pressure. Dobutamine (5–10 mcg/kg/min) or epinephrine (0.01–1 mg/kg/min) infusions may also be used if the maximum dose dopamine fails to satisfactorily improve blood pressure. Hydrocortisone (1 mg/kg, 8 hourly) should be used in cases of refractory hypotension where conventional therapy has failed.[2]

Management of persistent ductus arteriosus

Indomethacin prophylaxis reduces PDA and severe IVH, but there is no evidence of differences in long-term outcome. Indomethacin or ibuprofen have been shown to be equally efficacious in closing the PDA.

For additional information on this issue, please see Chapter 9 of this Handbook.

Meconium aspiration syndrome (MAS)

Although the incidence of meconium staining of the amniotic fluid varies from 10 to 15% of all deliveries, the overall incidence of meconium aspiration syndrome (MAS) with significant respiratory distress is around one per cent. There is a wide spectrum of severity in this disease, so infants who are admitted to the intensive care unit for MAS represent only a part of those affected by the disease. The clinical manifestations can vary from mild tachypnea to severe respiratory distress starting at birth. Signs of respiratory distress are nonspecific except that the antero-posterior diameter of the chest and pneumothorax tends to increase. The following features are seen: signs of cerebral irritation such as jitteriness, tremors, and seizures and signs, inappropriate ADH secretion such as hyponatremia, weight gain and decreased urinary output. Peeling and parchment-like skin indicate postmaturity. Owing to intrauterine hypoxia, the infant may have a low Apgar score, metabolic acidosis, polycythemia, pulmonary hemorrhage and disseminated coagulopathy. The pathogenesis of MAS is shown in Fig. 2.

In essence, there are four major pulmonary problems:

1. Mechanical obstruction of the airway,
2. Pulmonary hypertension,
3. Bacterial infection of the lungs, and
4. Possible chemical pneumonitis.

Management of MAS

Prevention of meconium aspiration

Antepartum prevention

Most cases of severe MAS are not in fact causally related to the aspiration, but are caused by other pathologic process occurring *in utero*, such as primary chronic asphyxia and infection. Fetal hypoxic stress may stimulate colonic activity, resulting in the passage of meconium and may also stimulate fetal gasping movements that result in meconium aspiration.

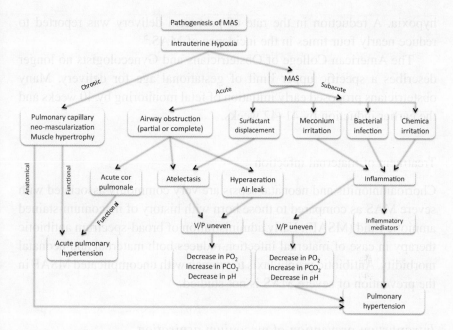

Figure 2. Pathogenesis of meconium aspiration syndrome.

Prevention of intrauterine hypoxia

The incidence of MAS has decreased over the last decade. The improvement has been attributed to the reduction rate of post-term delivery, the aggressive management of fetal distress and the decreased number of infants with low Apgar scores.[5,6] In case the pregnancy is complicated with meconium-stained amniotic fluid, continuous electronic fetal monitoring is indicated.[7] If fetal distress, especially non-assuring fetal tracing, is present, timely intervention should be initiated.

Fetal pulse oximetry is a new modality for antepartum fetal surveillance. The membrane must be ruptured and the cervix dilated to at least 2–3 cm before the probe can be inserted.

Reduction in the rate of post-term delivery

Post-term delivery has been shown to be associated with an increase in the number of infants passing meconium and in the rate of intrauterine hypoxia. A reduction in the rate of post-term delivery was reported to reduce nearly four times in the incidence of MAS.[5]

The American College of Obstetricians and Gynecologists no longer describes a specific upper limit of gestational age for delivery. Many obstetricians proposed early initiation of fetal monitoring by 40 weeks and the earlier induction by 41–42 weeks.

Treatment of maternal infection

Chorioamnionitis and neonatal sepsis are very commonly associated with severe MAS as compared to those born with history of meconium-stained amniotic fluid (MSAF). Early administration of broad-spectrum antibiotic therapy in case of maternal infection reduces both maternal and neonatal morbidity. Antibiotic prophylaxis to woman with uncomplicated MSAF in the prevention of severe MAS is not studied.

Intrapartum prevention of meconium aspiration

The MAS was believed to result from aspiration of meconium during intrauterine gasping or at the first breath. Interventions such as the amnioinfusion, oropharyngeal suction and tracheal aspiration were common practices in the past two decades after reports showed these procedures decreased the incidence and severity of MAS.[8-10] Recently, several well-organized, large-scale randomized trials of these strategies have not shown to reduce the incidence of MAS.[11-13] These interventions are now reserved in infants born with MSAF with other complications.

Amnioinfusion-transcervical infusion of saline

Amnioinfusion is very effective to treat pregnancies complicated with oligohydramnios and variable decelerations. During the procedure, a sterile catheter is introduced transcervically to a depth of 30 cm and a bolus of 800 ml of sterile saline at room temperature is infused under the force of gravity at a rate of 20 ml per minute over a period of 40 minutes. The infusion then is continued at a rate of 2 ml per minute to a maximum of 1500 ml.

Wenstrom *et al.* proposed amnioinfusion as a way of diluting the thickness of the meconium, preventing umbilical cord compression to prevent MAS in 1989.[10]

Review of previous studies shows that this strategy decreases the meconium found below the cords in infants born to mothers with MSAF, but failed to show a reduction in the incidence of MAS.[14,15] Fraser *et al.* conducted an international, multicenter randomized trial involving 2000 women in labor with thick MSAF and concluded that amnioinfusion did not reduce the risk of moderate to severe MAS and perinatal death for women in labor who had thick MSAF.[11]

There is insufficient evidence that amnioinfusion reduces meconium-related neonatal morbidity. Therefore, it is not recommended for women with MSAF alone unless there is evidence of variable fetal heart rate decelerations.

Oropharyngeal and nasopharyngeal suctioning of meconium-stained neonates

Observations in the 1970s and the 1980s showed that pharyngeal and tracheal intubation suctioning decreased the incidence and severity of MAS.[8,9] Until recently, suctioning the pharynx through the mouth and the nose by the obstetricians after the delivery of the head, but before the delivery of the shoulder, was a common practice; routine intubation and tracheal suctioning was recommended in infants with thick meconium or low Apgar scores.[16] However, recent studies do not support universal aggressive suctioning unless infants are depressed. Since 2005, the American Heart Association and the Neonatal Resuscitation Program recommends tracheal suctioning only if infant is not vigorous, has absent or depressed respiration, has decreased muscle tone or has a heart rate less than 100 beats/min.[16]

A 10-Fr to 13-Fr-sized suction catheter or a Delee device is connected to a negative pressure of 150 mmHg. Oropharynx of the neonate is suctioned first, followed by bilateral nasopharyngeal suctioning after the head is delivered, but before the shoulder is delivered and before the infant is able to take a breath. Peng *et al.* showed this intervention resulted in reduction of neonatal intubation for MAS.[17] Vain *et al.* in a multicenter, randomized trial, showed that oropharyngeal and nasopharyngeal suctioning of meconium-stained neonates before delivery of their shoulders did not reduce the incidence of MAS, need for mechanical ventilation, mortality, or duration of ventilation, oxygen treatment or hospital stay.[13] In a multicenter, international collaborative trial, Wisewell *et al.* concluded that intubation and suctioning of the apparently vigorous meconium-stained infants does not result in a decreased incidence of MAS or other respiratory disorders.[12]

As a result of these trials, endotracheal intubation and suctioning of meconium is no longer recommended for vigorous babies born with MSAF. However, meconium-stained, depressed infants should receive suctioning of the mouth, nose and trachea immediately after birth and before stimulation. Figure 3 shows the current management in our delivery room. This has been done since 1991 and is not much different from the current recommendation from AAP.

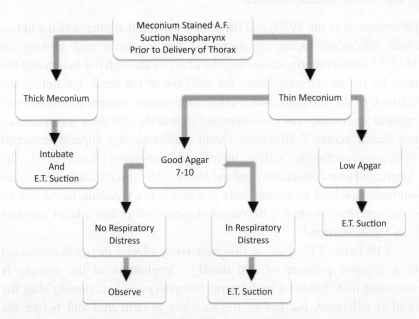

Figure 3. Recommendations for management of meconium aspiration syndrome in the delivery room.

Management of MAS and persistent pulmonary hypertension

Once the infants develop MAS, the management is mainly supportive care. Maintenance of adequate oxygenation, systemic blood pressure and correction of acidosis, hypoglycemia or other metabolic disorders is the mainstay of the treatment. Infants should be cared for in neutral thermal environment and watched closely for the development of persistent pulmonary hypertension. Gentle care is preferred, and excessive handling and agitation should be avoided. Umbilical arterial catheter or radial arterial catheter should be inserted in case of moderate to severe MAS, so blood gases and blood pressure can be monitored accurately and the neonate is not disturbed.

Antibiotics

Bacterial infection might have precipitated the passage and subsequent aspiration of meconium, thus judicious use of antibiotics is indicated. Bacterial pneumonia is indistinguishable radiographically from MAS.

Maintain adequate systemic blood pressure and tissue perfusion

It is important to keep adequate systemic blood pressure in case of moderate to severe MAS. If infants develop PPHN, the systemic blood pressure should be kept higher than pulmonary blood pressure to overcome right to left shunt. In addition to maintaining intravenous fluids, volume expanders such as normal saline and albumin are needed if patients have low blood pressure. Transfusion with packed RBC is indicated to keep hematocrit greater than 40%. Vasopressors are often used. Continuous intravenous drips with dopamine (2–20 mcg/kg/min), dobutamine (2–25 mcg/kg/min) or epinephrine (0.01–0.03 mg/kg/min) are often used separately or in combination to maintain normal systemic arterial blood pressure.

Oxygen therapy and ventilator management

Because hypoxia, acidosis, hypercarbia increase pulmonary vascular resistance, infants should receive oxygen therapy after birth if they show signs and symptoms of oxygen desaturation. Oxygen saturation should be maintained close to 100% or arterial PO_2 be maintained close to 100 mmHg or even higher. In infants with MAS, complication of PPHN is likely to occur during the acute stage. Thus, arterial blood gas should be monitored frequently and weaning of oxygen and ventilator support should be done very cautiously until the acute stage is over and infant's condition is stable. Blood pH should be maintained around 7.35 to 7.45 in order to avoid acidosis and by maintaining PCO_2 at 35 to 45 mmHg in the first 2–3 days. As the ventilatory status is improved, the PCO_2 can be kept between 40–50 mmHg.

Sedation

Term infants may become very agitated with intubation and their breathing may not synchronize with mechanical ventilation. Patients with PPHN are very sensitive to any stimulation. Analgesia and anesthesia agents are indicated. Continuous intravenous infusion with morphine 100 to 150 mcg/kg loading dose over one hour followed by 10 to 20 mcg/kg/hour, or fentanyl at dose 1–5 mcg/kg/hour, or midazolam 10–60 mcg/kg/hour can be initiated. Dosage may be increased after several days of treatment because of development of tolerance. Muscle relaxant with pancuronium 0.1 mg/kg/dose might be needed if patient's breath is not synchronized with mechanical breath.

Veitilator management

Conventional ventilator

Some alveoli in MAS are atelectatic; some are over-distended, resulting in V/Q mismatch. Approximately 30% of infants with MAS require ventilator support.[18] These infants tend to breath on their own to some degree. Compared with non-synchronized ventilation, infants treated with trigger ventilation, either synchronized intermittent mandatory ventilation (SIMV) or assist control ventilation (AC), required less sedation and were associated with shorter duration of mechanical ventilation. There is limited experience with the other two new modes of ventilators — pressure-regulated volume control ventilation (PRVCV) and SIMV plus pressure support (PS).

High frequency ventilation

High frequency ventilation (HFV) uses low tidal volume and high frequency to recruit the collapsed alveoli; HFV also delivers more homogenous pulmonary ventilation and gas exchange. There are two types of high frequency ventilators available now in the United States: the Bunnell Life Pulse high frequency jet ventilator (HFJV) and the SensorMedics high frequency oscillatory ventilator (HFOV). HFV can be used as a primary mode of ventilator therapy or as rescue therapy when patients fail to respond to conventional ventilator. We initially use SIMV; however, if infants require high PIP, high FiO_2, or are at risk of developing air leak, we switch to HFOV. We allow cross-over treatment, since some babies respond differently from time to time. Clark *et al.* showed that among patients with severe respiratory disease, 63% who failed CMV responded to HFOV; and 23%, vice versa.[19]

For more discussion on mechanical ventilation, please see Chapter 7.

Surfactant therapy

Meconium inactivates surfactant. Surfactant deficiency can further complicate MAS. Findlay *et al.* in a randomized, controlled study, concluded that surfactant replacement with three doses of 150 mg/kg (6 ml/kg) beractant within six hours after birth improves oxygenation and reduces the incidence of air leaks, the severity of pulmonary morbidities, the requirement of ECMO treatment and the hospitalization time of term infants with MAS.[20] Another study has showed similar results.[21] The acute side effects include transient oxygen desaturation and endotracheal tube obstruction occurring during bolus administration of the surfactant. Surfactant can be given by bolus or slow infusion, although the dose is not defined. In our practice, we give 100 mg/kg of beractant through intra-tracheal indwelling catheter through the side hole of endotracheal tube to infants with severe MAS.

Inhaled nitric oxide

Nitric oxide (NO) is a potent vasodilator. Inhaled NO (iNO) can be delivered to the alveoli and reach the vascular bed through a ventilator, resulting in selective pulmonary vasodilatation. Once in the blood stream, NO is bound to hemoglobin, thus has limited systemic effects. In general, iNO is initiated when the oxygen index (OI) [The OI is calculated as: OI = mean airway pressure × FiO2 × 100 postductal PO2] exceeds 25 and the starting dose is at 20 ppm. Although brief exposures to higher doses (40 to 80 ppm) appear to be safe, sustained treatment with 80 ppm iNO increases the risk of methemoglobinemia. The lowest effective initial dose for iNO in term newborns who have PPHN has not been determined, but sustained improvement in oxygenation has been demonstrated for doses lower than 10 ppm.[22,23] Methemoglobin and nitrogen dioxide concentration should be monitored from 4–12 hours. Serial echocardiograms are useful in monitoring the pressure gradients and myocardial functions of these infants. Patients usually are maintained on low dose of iNO (5–20 ppm) for 2–6 days and then gradually weaned to avoid rebound hypoxemia.

Initiating iNO treatment early at OI greater than 15 did not change the incidence of ECMO requirement or death, length of hospital stay, duration of mechanical ventilation or incidence of chronic lung disease.[24]

Combination of HFOV and iNO therapy is often more successful than treatment with HFOV or iNO alone in patients with PPHN especially those patients with RDS or MAS as underlying disease.[25]

Steroid

Infants with severe MAS may also suffer from intrauterine hypoxia and have adrenal insufficiency. Physiological replacement with hydrocortisone may be helpful. However, a double-blind trial using hydrocortisone did not show beneficial effect.[26] The anti-inflammatory effect of dexamethasone may decrease the risk of developing PPHN in animal models with MAS.[27]

Phosphodiesterase (PDES) inhibitor: Sildenafil

Sildenafil inhibits cGMP-specific PDES type 5, increases cGMP concentration and may result in pulmonary vasodilatation or enhance the activity of NO. Because PDE-5 is primarily distributed within the arterial wall smooth muscle of the lungs and penis, sildenafil acts selectively in both these areas without inducing vasodilatation in other areas of the body. Sildenafil is only available as enteral form in the market. Revatio, manufactured by Pfizer, was approved by the FDA for the treatment of pulmonary hypertension in adults. Limited data are available in neonates. Baquero *et al.* reported oral sildenafil improved OI in infants with severe PPHN.[28] The dose is 0.3–1 mg/kg/dose via orogastric tube every 6–12 hours. The potential side effects include worsening of oxygenation, systemic hypotension and bleeding tendency.

Extracoporeal membrane oxygenation (ECMO)

The use of adjunctive therapies dramatically decreased the need for ECMO therapy in the last decade,[29] but some infants with MAS and PPHN still developed persistent respiratory failure despite the optimal medical treatments.[19] ECMO provides cardiopulmonary support while allowing the underlying pulmonary or cardiac dysfunction to resolve without the risk of further injury from barotrauma or hyperoxia. This treatment results in 94% survival rate in these high risk infants who had predictive mortality rate of 80% without ECMO therapy.

The selection criteria include:

1. Gestation age of at least 34 weeks.
2. Birth weight of at least 2000 g.
3. Lack of major coagulopathy or active bleeding.
4. No major intracranial bleeding.
5. Mechanical ventilation of less than 10–14 days duration and reversible lung disease.
6. Failure of optimal medical management and who have a high predicted mortality rate.

Oxygen index (OI) and alveolar-arterial difference in oxygen tension (A-aDO$_2$) are commonly used to predict the likelihood of mortality. An OI of 40 or greater and/or an A-aDO$_2$ greater than 600 mmHg are predictive of 80% mortality risk.

Outcome of meconium aspiration syndrome

The case fatality rate of MAS-related illness declined over the decades: from 4.2% during 1973–1987 in the USA to 2.5% during 1995–2002 in Australia and New Zealand.[5,6] The perinatal deaths are related to perinatal depression, airway obstruction and development of PPHN.

Pulmonary sequalae are common in infants with severe MAS. Nearly 50% of the infants had episodes of reactive airway diseases during the first six months of life. Mild airway obstruction or exercise-induced asthma was more common in these children at six to eight years.[30,31]

The long-term neurological outcome of infants with MAS depends upon the underlying disorders. The neurologic outcomes are related to the presence or the absence of intrauterine asphyxia, hypoxic-ischemic encephalopathy and PPHN. Infants who required ECMO treatment had more complications than those who did not.

References

1. Downes JJ, Vidyasagar D, Boggs TR *et al.* (1970) Respiratory distress syndrome of newborn infants. I. New clinical scoring system (RDS score) with acid–base and blood-gas correlations. *Clin Pediatr Phila* 9: 325–331.

2. Sweet D, Bevilacqua G, Carnielli V *et al.* (2007) Working Group on Prematurity of the World Association of Perinatal Medicine, European Association of Perinatal Medicine 2007 European consensus guidelines on the management of neonatal respiratory distress syndrome. *J Perinat Med* 35: 175–186.

3. Cools F, Henderson-Smart DJ, Offringa M *et al.* (2009) Elective high frequency oscillatory ventilation versus conventional ventilation for acute pulmonary dysfunction in preterm infants. *Cochrane Database Syst Rev* CD000104.

4. Barrington KJ, Finer NN. (2007) Inhaled nitric oxide for preterm infants: A systematic review. *Pediatrics* 120: 1088–1099.

5. Dargaville PA, Copnell B. (2006) The epidemiology of meconium aspiration syndrome: Incidence, risk factors, therapies and outcome. *Pediatrics* 117: 1712–1721.

6. Yoder BA, Kirsch EA, Barth WH *et al.* (2002) Changing obstetric practices associated with decreasing incidence of meconium aspiration syndrome. *Obstet Gynecol* **99**: 731–739.

7. Shaw K, Clark SL. (1988) Reliability of intrapartum fetal heart rate monitoring in the postterm fetus with meconium passage. *Obstet Gynecol* **72**: 886–889.

8. Gregory GA, Gooding CA, Phibbs RH *et al.* (1974) Meconium aspiration in infants — A prospective study. *J Pediatr* **85**: 848–852.

9. Carson BS, Losey RW, Bowes WA, Jr., *et al.* (1976) Combined obstetric and pediatric approach to prevent meconium aspiration syndrome. *Am J Obstet Gynecol* **126**: 712–715.

10. Wenstrom KD, Parsons MT. (1989) The prevention of meconium aspiration in labor using amnioinfusion. *Obstet Gynecol* **73**: 647–651.

11. Fraser WD, Hofmeyr J, Lede R *et al.* (2005) Amnioinfusion for the prevention of the meconium aspiration syndrome. *N Engl J Med* **353**: 909–917.

12. Wiswell TE, Gannon CM, Jacob J *et al.* (2000) Delivery room management of the apparently vigorous meconium-stained neonate: Results of the multicenter, international collaborative trial. *Pediatrics* **105**: 1–7.

13. Vain NE, Szyld EG, Prudent LM *et al.* (2004) Oropharyngeal and nasopharyngeal suctioning of meconium-stained neonates before delivery of their shoulders: Multicentre, randomised controlled trial. *Lancet* **364**: 597–602.

14. Eriksen NL, Hostetter M, Parisi VM. (1994) Prophylactic amnioinfusion in pregnancies complicated by thick meconium. *Am J Obstet Gynecol* **171**: 1026–1030.

15. Spong CY, Ogundipe OA, Ross MG. (1994) Prophylactic amnioinfusion for meconium-stained amniotic fluid. *Am J Obstet Gynecol* **171**: 931–935.

16. Kattwinkel J. (2000) Neonatal resuscitation program. *American Academy of Pediatrics*, Elk Grove Village, IL.

17. Peng TC, Gutcher GR, Van Dorsten JP. (1996) A selective aggressive approach to the neonate exposed to meconium-stained amniotic fluid. *Am J Obstet Gynecol* **175**: 296–301.

18. Wiswell TE, Tuggle JM, Turner BS. (1990) Meconium aspiration syndrome: Have we made a difference? *Pediatrics* **85**: 715–721.

19. Clark RH, Yoder BA, Sell MS. (1994) Prospective, randomized comparison of high-frequency oscillation and conventional ventilation in candidates for extracorporeal membrane oxygenation. *J Pediatr* **124**: 447–454.

20. Findlay RD, Taeusch HW, Walther FJ. (1996) Surfactant replacement therapy for meconium aspiration syndrome. *Pediatrics* **97**: 48–52.
21. Lotze A, Mitchell BR, Bulas DI *et al.* (1998) Multicenter study of surfactant (beractant) use in the treatment of term infants with severe respiratory failure. Survanta in Term Infants Study Group. *J Pediatr* **132**: 40–47.
22. Roberts JD, Polaner DM, Lang P *et al.* (1992) Inhaled nitric oxide in persistent pulmonary hypertension of the newborn. *Lancet* **340**: 818–819.
23. Clark RH, Kueser TJ, Walker MW *et al.* (2000) Low-dose nitric oxide therapy for persistent pulmonary hypertension of the newborn. Clinical Inhaled Nitric Oxide Research Group. *N Engl J Med* **342**: 469–474.
24. Konduri GG, Solimano A, Sokol GM *et al.* (2004) A randomized trial of early versus standard inhaled nitric oxide therapy in term and near-term newborn infants with hypoxic respiratory failure. *Pediatrics* **113**: 559–564.
25. Kinsella JP, Truog WE, Walsh WF *et al.* (1997) Randomized, multicenter trial of inhaled nitric oxide and high-frequency oscillatory ventilation in severe, persistent pulmonary hypertension of the newborn. *J Pediatr* **131**: 55–62.
26. Yeh TF, Srinivasan G, Harris V *et al.* (1977) Hydrocortisone therapy in meconium aspiration syndrome: A controlled study. *J Pediatr* **90**: 140–143.
27. Wu JM, Yeh TF, Wang JY *et al.* (1999) The role of pulmonary inflammation in the development of pulmonary hypertension in newborn with meconium aspiration syndrome (MAS). *Pediatr Pulmonol Suppl* **18**: 205–208.
28. Baquero H, Soliz A, Neira F *et al.* (2006) Oral Sildenafil in infants with persistent pulmonary hypertension of the newborn: A Pilot randomized blinded study. *Pediatrics* **117**: 1077–1083.
29. Hintz SR, Suttner DM, Sheehan AM *et al.* (2000) Decreased use of neonatal extracorporeal membrane oxygenation (ECMO): How new treatment modalities have affected ECMO utilization. *Pediatrics* **106**: 1339–1343.
30. Macfarlane PI, Heaf DP. (1988) Pulmonary function in children after neonatal meconium aspiration syndrome. *Arch Dis Child* **63**: 368–372.
31. Swaminathan S, Quinn J, Stabile MW *et al.* (1989) Long-term pulmonary sequelae of meconium aspiration syndrome. *J Pediatr* **114**: 356–361.

Chapter 6

Bronchopulmonary Dysplasia: Present Knowledge and Future Directions

Ilene R. S. Sosenko and Eduardo Bancalari

Introduction

Present day neonatology has witnessed the markedly improved survival of extremely low birth weight infants, including those at the borderline of viability. Despite this apparent success, the risk of these infants developing the chronic lung damage of bronchopulmonary dysplasia (BPD) remains unacceptably high. BPD continues to be one of the most common long-term complications of premature infants requiring prolonged mechanical ventilation, with an incidence ranging between 15 and 50 percent of infants weighing less than 1500 grams at birth.[1] Since the original description of BPD by Northway in 1967,[2] its clinical picture, concepts of pathogenesis and approaches to therapy have changed. Consequently, clinical trials, as well as basic translational research, have increased our understanding of this process and have provided new approaches to treatment as well as promising future possibilities for prevention and therapies for BPD.

Changes in Clinical Presentation

In the original description of what they termed "brochopulmonary dysplasia (BPD)," Northway and colleagues described chronic lung

119

damage in a group of surviving premature infants weighing >1500 g at birth, all of whom had received prolonged mechanical ventilation with high airway pressure and high inspired oxygen concentration. This process was felt to be the result of multiple injuries to the immature lung. Characterized by a progression of its clinical and radiological course through four stages, BPD culminated in severe respiratory failure, with radiographic findings of increased densities due to fibrosis and enlarged, emphysematous alveoli, juxtaposed against areas of collapse.

More than 40 years later, with the widespread application of antenatal steroid therapy, postnatal surfactant administration and a more cautious approach to mechanical ventilation, Northway's severe classic presentation of BPD is infrequently seen. More commonly, smaller and more immature infants (400–1000 g) than those originally described (>1500 g) present with a milder form of lung disease. Despite requiring mechanical ventilation early in life, many of these infants initially start out with only minimal or mild RDS. They may require mechanical ventilation with low inspiratory pressures and low inspired oxygen concentrations for pneumonia, apnea or poor respiratory effort and are also often weaned to room air within the first day or days of life. However, these infants have subsequent progressive deterioration in lung function, with increased ventilator and oxygen requirements, often occurring within a few days or weeks after birth, which may be related to inflammation secondary to bacterial infection or colonization and/or the development of a symptomatic patent ductus arteriosus.[3,4] The chronic lung process that these infants develop has been termed the "new BPD." Infants with "new BPD" may require mechanical ventilation and oxygen for several weeks or months. Nonetheless, the majority of infants with this relatively milder form of chronic lung disease have resolved most symptoms by discharge.[1] A small number of "new BPD" infants demonstrate a more severe lung process, with progressive respiratory failure and even death from severe lung damage, pulmonary hypertension and cor pulmonale, as well as severe airway damage, bronchomalacia and airway obstruction.[5] Infants with this more severe form of BPD are at risk for acute bacterial or viral pulmonary infections, which may increase lung damage and may even lead to death.[6]

Changes in Understanding of BPD Pathogenesis

In his original publication, Northway, implicated four major pathogenetic factors in the development of BPD. These included: 1) immaturity, 2) respiratory failure, 3) oxygen supplementation, and 4) positive pressure mechanical ventilation.[2] These same four pathogenetic factors are still felt to play a major role in the evolution of BPD today. However, increased knowledge of processes involved with inflammation and with lung growth, including lung signaling pathways, transcription factors and growth factors, and a greater understanding of genetics have broadened our concepts related to the influences that play a role in the development of BPD (Fig. 1).

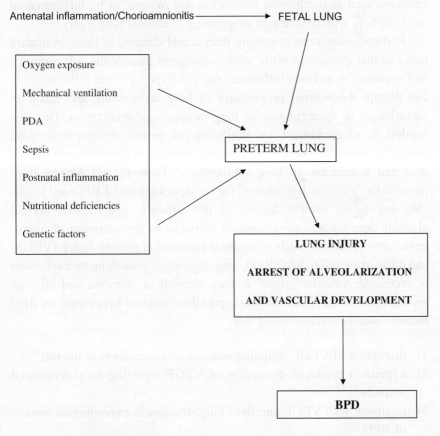

Figure 1. Scheme of factors related to BPD pathogenesis.

Disruption of development of the immature lung: Arrest of alveolar development and the "vascular hypothesis"

The incidence of BPD in premature infants requiring mechanical ventilation is inversely proportional to gestational age and birth weight, making it a disease almost exclusively of the extremely premature infant. In fact, BPD is rarely found in infants beyond 32 weeks of gestation.[1] The immature state of lung development at the time of preterm birth increases its vulnerability to lung damage. At the time of birth, a 24 week gestation premature infant's lung is in the very immature canalicular stage; it is not until 30 weeks that lung development has progressed to the saccular stage. These lungs, at such an immature stage of development, are easily damaged by therapeutic interventions, such as mechanical ventilation and oxygen, or by inflammation and infection, with the damage progressing to chronic lung injury.

Perhaps even more important than actual damage to these immature lungs is that premature birth, with consequent therapeutic interventions and exposure to noxious influences such as hyperoxia and inflammation, can disrupt the normal progression of lung architecture and result in perturbation or dysregulation of lung morphologic maturation. This disruption is characterized by inhibition of acinar development with reduction in numbers of alveoli, resulting in reduced gas exchange surface area and a decrease in lung capillaries.[7,8] Thebaud and Abman have proposed a "vascular hypothesis" for the development of BPD and implicate angiogenic growth factors in this process. Specifically, normal alveolar development progresses in response to the secretion of angiogenic growth factors, such as vascular endothelial growth factor (VEGF) and nitric oxide (NO). With BPD, lung angiogenic growth factor expression is decreased; vascular growth is then arrested or distorted and alveolar growth is impaired.[9] Evidence to support this "vascular hypothesis" of BPD includes studies demonstrating that:

1) disruption of VEGF signaling reduces alveolarization in the rat;[10]
2) hyperoxia produces disruption of VEGF signaling in experimental animals;[11,12]
3) treatment with VEGF improves lung structure in experimental models of BPD.[13]

Furthermore, infants dying of BPD were found to have reduced lung VEGF mRNA and protein expression, reduction of VEGF receptor and decreased expression of other endothelial markers, such as PECAM-1 and tie-2.[14] In addition, endothelial colony-forming cells (EPFC) from preterm infants exposed to hyperoxia showed decreased growth, VEGF receptor and eNOS expression and NO production whereas VEGF treatment and NO treatment restored growth of the cells exposed to hyperoxia.[15] When erythropoietin was administered to experimental animals exposed to hyperoxia, a protective effect on the hyperoxia-induced lung injury was found, characterized by improving alveolar structure, enhancing vascularity and decreasing fibrosis. Here, erythropoietin appears to be functioning as a growth factor to the lung, rather than as an antioxidant.[16]

Role of hyperoxia plus hypoxic spells in BPD pathogenesis

Toxicity from oxygen exposure and trauma due to mechanical ventilation are two other well-accepted pathogenetic mechanisms for BPD, originally proposed by Northway and subsequently supported by studies in experimental animals,[17–19] observational and epidemiologic studies[20–22] and currently the focus of ongoing clinical trials (i.e. SUPPORT trial) (discussed below). In fact, both oxygen exposure and ventilator-induced lung injury are associated with inflammation. However, new evidence suggests that intermittent hypoxic conditions during exposure to hyperoxia may actually play an important role in BPD exacerbation, thought to be related to a worsening of oxidative lung injury. Newborn mice exposed to hyperoxia plus intermittent hypoxia showed increased evidence of alveolar growth arrest and lung oxidative stress compared to those mice exposed to hyperoxia alone,[23] suggesting an additional deleterious effect of hypoxia superimposed on hyperoxia in the development of BPD. In fact, it has been observed that the majority of premature infants requiring oxygen and/or ventilator support manifest intermittent spells of hypoxia during their hospital course, with those infants developing BPD experiencing more frequent episodes of hypoxemia than those who recover without BPD.[24]

Role of inflammation in BPD pathogenesis

Epidemiologic evidence has demonstrated links between infection/inflammation and preterm birth.[25,26] In fact, chorioamnionitis, even in its silent form has been reported in most deliveries prior to 30 weeks of gestation, with the association of chorioamnionitis and preterm delivery increasing with decreasing weeks of gestation.[27] Exposure to antenatal inflammation may paradoxically reduce the incidence of hyaline membrane disease (HMD) in premature infants, but the ultimate effect of inflammation appears to be an increase in the chronic lung damage of BPD.[28] Elevations in amniotic fluid pro-inflammatory mediators such as IL-6, TNF-α, IL-1β and IL-8 within five days of preterm birth were found to correlate with the development of BPD.[29,30] Furthermore, a dose-response effect in relation to chorioamnionitis and BPD has been observed, with a higher risk of developing BPD found in preterms exposed to severe histological chorioamnionitis, compared to those exposed to mild or no chorioamnionitis.[31] However, the association of chorioamnionitis and BPD has not been found consistently, with Van Marter and colleagues demonstrating an actual decrease in BPD risk in a group of preterm infants who had been exposed antenatally to chorioamnionitis, but who did not require mechanical ventilation or develop postnatal infection.[32] Similarly, Soraisham and coworkers used multivariate logistic regression analysis and did not find an increase in BPD incidence associated with clinical chorioamnionitis.[33]

Once exposed to antenatal lung inflammation as a result of chorioamnionitis, the inflammatory stimuli often persist postnatally when the preterm infant continues to be exposed to postnatal inflammation.[34] Infection itself, either antenatal or postnatal, likely plays a major role in the lung inflammation that contributes to the development of BPD. Antenatal colonization with *Ureaplasma urealyticum* may be involved in initiating *in utero* inflammation, since this organism has been isolated from the lungs of infants who develop BPD.[35] Using reverse transcriptase PCR, Kotecha and colleagues explored infants with lung inflammation who subsequently developed BPD and found the majority to have *Ureaplasma urealyticum* in bronchoalveolar lavage fluid at d 10 of age, suggesting that this organism, acquired antenatally, may contribute to early lung inflammation, setting the stage for progression to BPD.[36] Despite these findings, a randomized trial of erythromycin was ineffective at reducing the incidence of BPD, perhaps because *Ureaplasma urealyticum* may not actually have been eradicated from the trachea with this treatment regimen.[37] Other antenatal infections might be related to the inflammation-BPD connection, since increased cord blood IgM levels for viruses such as the adenovirus, were found in infants who later developed BPD.[38] Postnatal infection has also been associated with an increased risk of BPD in preterm infants. For example, Liljedahl and colleagues found that the risk of BPD was significantly higher in premature infants with sepsis due to coagulase negative staphylococcus.[39] This risk is increased even further when the infection occurs concomitantly with the presence of a PDA.[3] Postnatal cytomegalovirus infection has been also associated with an increased risk of BPD,[40] whereas the respiratory syncytial virus infection can produce deleterious effects on the respiratory status of infants with evolving or established BPD.[41]

Inflammation, separate from its relationship to infection, can continue to deleteriously affect the preterm lung. Exposure to oxygen produces not just oxygen free-radicals, but also activates inflammatory cells and synthesis of pro-inflammatory cytokines.[34] Positive pressure ventilation with high tidal volume has also been associated with inflammation.[34] In addition, increased pulmonary blood flow produced by a PDA could initiate the inflammatory cascade by inducing neutrophil margination and activation in the lung, resulting in lung damage.[42] Studies in preterm baboons indicate a deleterious effect of a PDA on alveolar development which was improved with early ibuprofen therapy,[43] possibly related to ibuprofen's effect on ductal closure and/or with other pharmacological functions of ibuprofen, including acting as an anti-inflammatory agent. Interestingly, reversal of alveolarization arrest associated with PDA was not found with PDA ligation.[44]

Role of genetics in BPD pathogenesis

The link of genetic factors to the susceptibility to BPD, using concordance among VLBW twins, was first reported by Parker and coworkers.[45] Delving further, studies by Bhandari and colleagues concluded that genetic factors accounted for 53% of the variance in liability for BPD.[46] As to the specific genes which might be related to the development of BPD, there is evidence that genetic factors related to abnormal airway reactivity may play a role in BPD, since infants with BPD have been found to have a stronger family history of asthma compared to those without BPD.[47] An extensive list of candidate genes that could play a potential role in the pathogenesis of BPD has been proposed and several specific genetic loci have been linked to the development of BPD. These include the SP-B intron 4 deletion (i4del) (which could potentially decrease the ability to produce SP-B, particularly in response to injury),[48] polymorphisms of genes coding for VEGF (-460T allele) (potentially influencing angiogenesis in response to injury),[49] and polymorphisms in the glutathione-S-transferase-P1 gene (which could potentially decrease ability to handle oxidative stress).[50] Future studies linking specific genetic relationships to BPD risk and development will continue to improve our understanding of BPD pathogenesis.

Promising Therapies for Prevention and Treatment

Because the pathogenesis of BPD is complex and multifactorial, it is unlikely that a single modality will successfully treat or completely prevent the lung damage of BPD. The focus of this discussion will be to utilize evidence-based data to identify current approaches to BPD prevention and therapy, emphasizing interventions found to be efficacious vs those found to be ineffective or inconclusive, as well as those showing promise in the experimental setting.

Modalities of ventilator support and BPD prevention and treatment

The majority of premature infants are born with immature lungs and require some form of respiratory support to sustain life. However, the goal is to provide this life-saving respiratory support without further compromising the vulnerable immature lung. The early use of CPAP to avoid mechanical ventilation, examined in a number of clinical trials and by meta-analysis, was not found to reduce the incidence of BPD.[51–53] Data from the recently reported clinical trial examining the effectiveness of early intubation (and surfactant administration) versus early CPAP alone, the SUPPORT (Surfactant Positive Airway Pressure and Pulse Oximetry Trial) trial, failed to demonstrate differences in the primary outcomes of death or BPD between the study groups. However, the CPAP group, as compared with the surfactant group, did require less postnatal corticosteroids and were ventilated for an average of three days less.[54]

A small trial of nasal intermittent positive pressure ventilation (NIPPV) as the primary modality of respiratory support vs CPAP alone in preterm infants did demonstrate a decrease in BPD.[55] Similarly, both a randomized controlled trial of synchronized NIPPV post-surfactant administration vs conventional ventilation in the acute phase of RDS, as well as a retrospective analysis of synchronized NIPPV post-extubation for apnea, were associated with a decrease in BPD compared to those infants managed without NIPPV.[56,57] These studies are suggestive and promising, but hardly definitive in determining protection against BPD with the use of NIPPV.

Another approach to respiratory support for preterm infants at risk for BPD is the use of a low tidal volume strategy to potentially decrease lung injury, with the acceptance of higher values for $PaCO_2$ termed "permissive hypercapnia." Despite theoretical benefits, two randomized controlled trials examining permissive hypercapnia did not show a reduction in incidence of BPD with this ventilatory strategy.[58] High frequency ventilation, another potential ventilatory strategy to limit volutrauma, has not been found to be consistently protective in preventing or decreasing BPD risk.[59,60] Other possible protective modalities of mechanical ventilation which require further investigation include proportional assist ventilation,[61] volume-targeted ventilation,[62] volume guarantee ventilation[63] and the addition of pressure-supported ventilation to SIMV.[64]

Approach to oxygen therapy and BPD prevention and treatment

Despite the known toxicity of oxygen and free-radicals to the lung, evidence that reducing oxygen exposure protects against BPD remains largely circumstantial. Several observational studies found that those

NICUs that attempted to maintain lower levels of oxygen saturation in their treatment of premature infants had less BPD than those with liberal oxygen saturation approaches.[21,65] Two completed prospective trials in premature infants, where randomization of different target oxygen saturation groups occurred, were initiated when infants were already several weeks of age and BPD was already evolving. Neither of these studies was designed with pulmonary endpoints, especially BPD, as the primary outcome. The STOP-ROP trial (Supplemental Therapeutic Oxygen for Prethreshold Retinopathy of Prematurity), randomized infants at ~35 weeks post-menstrual age with prethreshold ROP to a lower oxygen saturation group (target saturations of 89–94%) or a higher oxygen group (target oxygen saturations of 96–99%). Secondary outcome analysis in this study found incidence of pneumonia and/or exacerbations of BPD (manifested as increased need for oxygen, diuretics and hospitalization at three months corrected age) to be greater in infants randomized to the higher oxygen saturations (13.2%) compared to those receiving lower oxygen saturation therapy (8.5%).[66] The BOOST (Benefits of Oxygen Saturation Targeting) trial examined the randomization effect of extremely preterm infants at 32 weeks posmenstrual age with two different oxygen saturation targets (91–94%) and (95–98%), with growth and neurodevelopmental outcome at 12 months corrected age as the primary outcome. Secondary analysis showed those in the higher saturation group to have evidence of adverse pulmonary outcome (increased death and longer requirement for supplemental oxygen, with a 40% increase in infants still requiring oxygen at 36 week postmenstrual age and a 70% increase in infants requiring home oxygen therapy).[67] The definitive question of whether extremely premature infants would have improved pulmonary outcome (decreased incidence or severity of BPD) when randomized to lower oxygen saturations from a very early age (first day or week of life) are currently being addressed by several trials, including the BOOST-II trial, with preliminary data soon to be available. If results from these clinical trials suggest a reduction in BPD with lower saturation limits, tools such as automated regulation of inspired oxygen using a "closed loop" system could potentially improve oxygen stability and perhaps become standard in the clinical care of premature infants.[68]

Potential role for exogenous antioxidants in BPD prevention or therapy

Exogenous antioxidants could have potential benefit in BPD treatment and prevention because of the known toxic effect of oxygen free radicals on the lung and the immaturity of the pulmonary antioxidant enzyme (AOE) system. Although animal studies have shown lung protective effects from exogenously administered AOE, human studies have yielded mostly negative results. A large randomized, placebo-controlled trial of the AOE, recombinant human copper/zinc superoxide dismutase (CuZn SOD) in intubated VLBW infants failed to show a reduction in BPD incidence or death. Surprisingly, when this group of infants returned for follow-up at one year corrected age, those who had received CuZn SOD had a 36% reduction in wheezing episodes requiring bronchodilators, a 55% decrease in emergency room visits and a 44% decrease in subsequent hospitalizations.[69]

Glutathione is a major lung antioxidant known to be deficient in premature infants. The amino acid cysteine serves as a precursor for glutathione, but does not cross cell membranes whereas the formulation of N-acetylcysteine (NAC) is thought to enter cells. In an attempt to explore the potential efficacy of increased intracellular glutathione in preventing BPD, a randomized controlled trial of NAC was conducted in VLBW premature infants. However, no pulmonary improvement was seen in those infants who had received NAC, suggesting either a lack of protection against lung injury or a lack of ability of this compound to increase intracellular glutathione levels.[70] Similarly, a randomized controlled trial of allopurinol, an xanthine oxidase inhibitor which catalyzes reactions generating superoxide radicals, in premature infants between 24 and 32 weeks of gestation, did not produce a decreased incidence of BPD.[71]

Inhaled nitric oxide and prevention of BPD

Although the initial clinical application of inhaled nitric oxide (iNO) to the treatment of critically ill infants was for its vasodilatory role in pulmonary hypertension, NO has been shown to have many positive effects in animal models of lung immaturity and lung injury, including diminution of inflammation, reduction of neutrophil infiltration and enhancement of lung growth and alveolar development.[72-74] Because of these findings in experimental animals, investigators have hypothesized a role for iNO in the amelioration and/or prevention of BPD. Several large randomized controlled trials have explored whether iNO could have a positive effect in terms of BPD prevention. In the study of Schreiber and coworkers, preterm infants <34 weeks who received iNO prior to the 72nd hour of age showed a significant reduction in death or BPD vs placebo (48.6% vs 63.7%).[75] The Ballard study, randomizing infants at a later time point (to those requiring mechanical ventilation at 7–21 days), also showed an increase in survival without BPD in infants receiving iNO.[76] However, neither Kinsella's study nor Van Meurs' groups demonstrated a significant overall decrease in death or BPD in iNO-treated infants. Nonetheless, after *post hoc* analysis, both groups found a reduction in BPD or death in the subgroup of larger infants (>1000 g) that had received iNO.[77,78] The report from the large scale European trial which enrolled 800 VLBW infants and investigated whether iNO prophylaxis could reduce BPD, did not suggest a benefit of iNO in survival without BPD.[79] Though specific subgroups may derive benefit, evidence from these trials and other smaller trials does not support the clinical application of iNO for BPD prevention in VLBW infants at this time.

Nutritional approaches to BPD treatment and prevention

Caloric and protein nutrition

Extremely premature infants often suffer from inadequate nutrition in the days and weeks after birth as a result of their critically-ill state, frequent glucose intolerance, delays in initiating enteral nutrition and attempts at fluid restriction. Findings from experimental animal studies suggest that exposure to general undernutrition, specifically protein malnutrition, impairs tolerance to oxidative lung injury. For example, when rat pups were exposed to conditions of undernutrition and then exposed to seven days of >95% O_2 exposure, these undernourished pups demonstrated 44%

survival rate vs 73% survival for normally nourished pups.[80] Similarly, protein-deficient rats showed earlier deaths in hyperoxia associated with decreased lung glutathione.[81] These data would suggest that early and rigorous provision of adequate caloric and protein intake for premature infants could potentially improve their antioxidant capabilities and decrease their risk for BPD, though definitive clinical trials have not been conducted.

Lipid nutrition

Despite evidence from newborn experimental animals demonstrating protection against hyperoxia with increased lipid intake and increased lung lipid content, specifically lipids high in polyunsaturated fatty acids (PUFA),[82,83] multiple randomized controlled clinical trials in premature infants failed to show BPD protection with early provision of high PUFA intake in the form of intravenous lipid (Intralipid).[84] One possible explanation for failing to show a protective effect against BPD with early Intralipid might be the toxicity of lipid hydroperoxides present in the lipid preparations used at the time these studies were performed, which might have obscured a protective PUFA effect. More recently, Intralipid has been manufactured by a process that virtually eliminates lipid hydroperoxides. Therefore, the question remains unexplored whether early Intralipid, free of lipid hydroperoxides, might have a preventative effect on BPD.

Inositol

A carbocyclic polyol compound, this substance is required for cell growth and survival and is incorporated into cell membranes within the lung and serves as a precursor for synthesis of pulmonary surfactant. Since it has been reported to be deficient in premature infants, Hallman and colleagues addressed the question of whether inositol supplementation could play a potential role in protection against BPD by conducting a double-blind, placebo randomized controlled trial of inositol supplementation in premature infants. They reported improved survival without BPD in inositol-supplemented infants who had not received a surfactant. However, those infants treated with exogenous surfactant derived no benefit from inositol in terms of BPD prevention.[85] Subsequent to that initial report, two additional randomized clinical trials of inositol have been conducted; when the three trials were analyzed together, results continued to demonstrate a significant reduction of death or BPD in infants who had received inositol.[86] Despite these suggestive findings from meta-analysis, inositol supplementation has not become part of the standard care of the VLBW infant.

Vitamin A

Vitamin A is crucial for differentiation and maintenance of airway epithelial cells whereas retinoic acid is important in alveolar development.[87] Because fetal acquisition of vitamin A occurs largely in the third trimester, the very preterm infant is born with lower vitamin A stores than the more mature infant. Early studies have linked low serum levels of vitamin of A with the development of BPD, such as the study of Shenai and coworkers that found infants with lower vitamin A levels in the first weeks of life to be at increased risk of BPD, compared to those with normal vitamin A levels.[88] This hypothesis was strengthened by the findings of similarities between airway epithelial changes seen with both BPD and vitamin A deficiency.[87] These findings provided the basis for several double-blind controlled trials of early vitamin A supplementation in preterm infants at risk for BPD, including the NICHD Neonatal Research Network trial reported by Tyson and coworkers, which revealed a significant reduction (55% vs 62%) in the primary outcome variable, death or BPD in infants supplemented with vitamin A.[89] Meta-analysis of seven trials showed reduction in death or oxygen requirement at one month and at 36-week post-menstrual age with vitamin A supplementation.[90] Despite obstacles such as the necessity to deliver vitamin A by repeated intramuscular injections and the relatively modest reduction in BPD outcome with vitamin A supplementation, its efficacy in decreasing BPD risk is clearly evidence-based.

Trace metals

Deficiencies of trace metals, such as magnesium and selenium, could play a potential role in development of BPD since these trace metals serve as cofactors for antioxidant enzymes, which are crucial in detoxifying oxygen free-radicals that are potentially damaging to the lung. The accretion of trace metals by the developing fetus occurs largely during the third trimester (i.e. ~80% of the accretion of magnesium occurs during the final third of gestation). Thus extremely premature infants, born at the onset of the third trimester, would lack the opportunity to accumulate these crucial trace metals. Caddell and coworkers have suggested a possible role for magnesium deficiency in the pathogenesis of BPD based on data that magnesium deficiency increases the susceptibility of cells to peroxidation and worsens inflammatory reactions.[91] Since the trace metal selenium is an essential cofactor for the antioxidant enzyme glutathione peroxidase, investigators have suggested a role for selenium deficiency in the development of BPD.[92] However, this hypothesis was not substantiated by a recent prospective analysis of selenium levels in preterm infants developing BPD[93] or in a randomized trial of selenium supplementation in VLBW infants.[94]

BPD therapies to reduce lung inflammation

Corticosteroids

The major strategy to reduce the risk of BPD by reducing pulmonary inflammation is with the use of postnatal steroids, which work to inhibit two main products of inflammation, prostaglandins and leukotrienes, as well as inhibiting both cyclooxygenase I and II, decreasing neutrophil recruitment into the lung and decreasing vascular permeability and pulmonary edema.[95] Despite its proven efficacy in reducing extubation failure and oxygen dependence at 28 days and 36 weeks postmenstrual age, as well as death or BPD and discharge home on oxygen, the application of postnatal steroid therapy to clinical practice is fraught with controversy, relating to studies indicating an increase in CP and poorer neurodevelopmental outcome in premature infants exposed to postnatal steroids. For example, in infants receiving early treatment with postnatal steroids (<96 hours of age), the risk of cerebral palsy was approximately double that of infants who did not receive steroids. Grier and Halliday concluded that for every 100 babies receiving early steroids, BPD would be prevented in ten at the expense of an additional six infants with gastrointestinal hemorrhage, twelve infants with cerebral palsy and 14 with an abnormal follow-up neurological exam. However, infants receiving postnatal steroids later in their course failed to show an increased risk of CP.[96] To attempt clarification of which groups of infants would benefit from postnatal steroids without deleterious effects on the brain, Doyle and colleagues reviewed multiple randomized controlled trials of postnatal steroid therapy for treatment or prevention of BPD and conducted meta-regression analysis. They found that both the benefits and deleterious effects of steroid treatment were actually related to an infant's risk for BPD. Specifically, when the risk of BPD was estimated to be less than 35%, postnatal steroid treatment actually increased the risk for CP or death. However, when the risk for BPD was estimated to be greater than 65%, both the risk of death and even CP were found to be reduced.[97] This study suggests that if specific high-risk populations can be identified and targeted for postnatal steroid treatment, benefits could potentially be derived, not just for BPD, but for neurodevelopment as well.

Methylxanthines and BPD prevention

Caffeine

Methylxathines function as phosphodiesterase inhibitors, which play a key role in regulating intracellular levels of second messengers cAMP and cGMP and could purportedly have an anti-inflammatory effect as well. Because of caffeine's use in reducing apnea of prematurity and in facilitating extubation from mechanical ventilation, it was the focus of the recent randomized, placebo-controlled multicenter trial (The CAP trial: **C**affeine for **A**pnea of **P**rematurity) to determine the potential effects of caffeine on long-term developmental outcome at 18–21 months. In this trial, infants were randomized to receive caffeine or placebo if their clinicians determined that they required therapy for apnea or for facilitation of extubation during the first ten days of age. The study's primary outcome was survival without neurodevelopmental disability at 18–21 months corrected age and the results indicated that caffeine did improve disability-free survival. Perhaps surprisingly, *post hoc* analysis revealed that infants who had received caffeine had a significant reduction in BPD (oxygen at 36 week postmenstrual age), with an OR of 0.64 (0.52–0.78). However, because extremely low birth weight infants, already at the highest risk for BPD (i.e. those <27 weeks), tend to remain ventilator-dependent beyond the first ten days of life, they were not candidates for enrollment in this trial.[98–100] Further investigation is required to determine whether early administration of caffeine to these most immature infants would also provide protection against BPD in this highly vulnerable group.

Future directions in BPD prevention

Pentoxifylline

Another member of the methylxanthine group is pentoxifylline, which functions as a phosphodiesterase inhibitor and has been found to inhibit hyperoxic lung injury by stimulating lung antioxidant enzymes and growth factors, as well as reducing inflammation and edema. Studies in newborn rats have demonstrated that pentoxifylline improved survival in hyperoxia, inducing lung antioxidant enzymes, reducing fibrin deposition and reversing downregulation of VEGF.[101,102] There may be a potential role for pentoxifylline in decreasing BPD risk, which will require testing in randomized controlled trials in human premature infants.

Mesenchymal stem cells

Data from experimental animals have shown that bone marrow derived, multipotent mesenchymal sterm cells (MSC) can be efficacious in models of lung injury. These MSCs, administered by either the intravenous or intra-alveolar route in adult animals, reduced lung inflammation and fibrosis and increased survival after endotoxin or bleomycin-induced lung injury.[103] In neonatal animals exposed to hyperoxia, MSC numbers had decreased in lung and blood, leading investigators to suggest that reduced MSC numbers may play a role in BPD pathogenesis.[104] When MSC therapy was tested in a neonatal rat model of BPD, results indicated that MSC were able to decrease lung inflammation and improve lung structure.[104] The finding that apparent lung engraftment of the exogenously delivered MSC was low was of additional interest, suggesting that substances secreted from the MSC, rather than the cells themselves, might explain their protective effect. Similar findings were reported in the neonatal mouse with a protective pulmonary effect of intravenous MSC in hyperoxia-induced lung injury. In fact, a more profound lung protection was demonstrated when the conditioned medium alone (without the presence of MSC) was administered, indicating that the protective function of MSC may be through its "secretome" or paracrine-releasing factors, such as macrophage-stimulating factor-1 and osteopontin.[105] Though these data are both exciting and promising, a more in-depth study of the role of MSC and its "secretome" is required before they are considered for clinical trials investigating a potential role in BPD treatment or prevention.

Conclusion

Over the more than 40 years since BPD was described and the terminology "bronchopulmonary dysplasia" became part of the neonatal lexicon, the clinical process of BPD has evolved and has continued to be a major focus of extensive investigation. From these investigations has emerged increased understanding of the cellular and the molecular processes involved in BPD pathogenesis and the application of present and future therapies that could potentially reduce the risk or severity of BPD, thereby having a major impact on the morbidity, mortality and long-term outcome of premature infants.

References

1. Bancalari E, Claure N, Sosenko IRS. (2003) Bronchopulmonary dysplasia: Changes in pathogenesis, epidemiology and definition. *Seminars in Neonatol* **8**: 63–71.
2. Northway WH Jr., Rosan RC, Porter DY. (1967) Pulmonary disease following respirator therapy of hyaline membrane disease: Bronchopulmonary dysplasia. *N Engl J Med* **276**: 357–368.

3. Gonzalez A, Sosenko IRS, Chandar J *et al.* (1996) Influence of infection on patent ductus arteriosus and chronic lung disease in premature infants weighing 1000 grams or less. *J Pediatr* **128**: 470–478.

4. Hyde I, English ER, Williams JA. (1989) The changing pattern of chronic lung disease of prematurity. *Arch Dis Child* **64**: 448–451.

5. McCubbin M, Frey EE, Wagener JS *et al.* (1989) Large airway collapse in bronchopulmonary dysplasia. *J Pediatr* **114**: 304–307.

6. Groothuis JR, Gutierrez KM, Lauer BA. (1988) Respiratory syncytial virus infection in children with bronchopulmonary dysplasia. *Pediatr* **82**: 199–203.

7. Coalson JJ. (2002) Pathology of chronic lung disease of early infancy. In Bland RJ, Coalson JJ (eds.), *Chronic Lung Disease in Early Infancy*. New York: Marcel Dekker, 85–124.

8. Husain AN, Siddiqui NH, Stocker JT. (1998) Pathology of arrested acinar development in postsurfactant bronchopulmonary dysplasia. *Human Pathol* **29**: 710–717.

9. Thebaud B, Abman SH. (2007) Bronchopulmonary dysplasia: Where have all the vessels gone? Roles of angiogenic growth factors in chronic lung disease. *Am J Respir Crit Care Med* **175**: 978–985.

10. Jakkula M, Le Cras TD, Gebb S *et al.* (2000) Inhibition of angiogenesis decreases alveolarization in the developing rat lung. *Am J Physiol Lung Cell Mol Physiol* **279**: L600–L607.

11. Maniscalco WM, Watkins RH, Chess PR *et al.* (1997) Hyperoxic injury decreases alveolar epithelial expression of VEGF in neonatal rabbit lung. *Am J Res Cell Mol Biol* **16**: 557–567.

12. Klekamp JG, Jarzecka K, Perkett EA. (1999) Exposure to hyperoxia decreases the expression of VEGF and its receptors in adult rat lungs. *Am J Pathol* **154**: 823–831.

13. Thebaud B, Ladha R, Michelakis ED *et al.* (2005) VEGF gene therapy increases survival, promotes lung angiogenesis and prevents alveolar damage in hyperoxia induced lung injury. *Circulation* **112**: 2477–2486.

14. Bhatt AJ, Pryhuber GS, Huyck H *et al.* (2001) Disrupted pulmonary vasculature and decreased VEGF, Flt-1, and TIE-2 in human infants dying with BPD. *Am J Resp Crit Care Med* **164**: 1971–1980.

15. Fujinaga H, Baker CD, Ryan SL *et al.* (2009) Hyperoxia disrupts vascular endothelial growth factor-nitric oxide signaling and decreases growth of

endothelial colony forming cells from preterm infants. *Am J Physiol Lung Cell Mol Physiol* **297**: L1160–L1169.

16. Ozer EA, Kumral A, Ozer E *et al.* (2005) Effects of erythropoietin on hyperoxic lung injury in neonatal rats. *Pediatri Res* **58**: 38–41.

17. Frank L. (1985) Effects of oxygen on the newborn. *Fed Proc* **44**: 2328–2334.

18. Deneke SM, Fanburg BL. (1980) Normobaric oxygen toxicity of the lung. *N Engl J Med* **303**: 76–86.

19. Gerstmann DR, del Lemos RA, Coalson JJ *et al.* (1988) Influence of ventilatory technique on pulmonary baroinjury in baboons with hyaline membrane disease. *Pediatr Pulmonol* **5**: 82–91.

20. Donn SM, Sinha SK. (2006) Minimizing ventilator induced lung injury in preterm infants. *Arch Dis Child Fetal Neonatal Ed* **91**: F226–F230.

21. Tin W, Milligan DW, Pennefather P *et al.* (2001) Pulse oximetry, severe retinopathy, and outcome at one year in babies of less than 28 weeks gestation. *Arch Dis Child Fetal Neonatal Ed* **84**: F106–F110.

22. Finer N, Leone T. (2009) Oxygen saturation monitoring for the preterm infant: The evidence basis for current practice. *Pediatr Res* **65**: 375–380.

23. Ratner V, Slinko S, Utkina-Sosunova *et al.* (2009) Hypoxic stress exacerbates hyperoxia-induced lung injury in a neonatal mouse model of bronchopulmonary dysplasia. *Neonatology* **95**: 299–305.

24. Bolivar JM, Gerhardt T, Gonzalez A *et al.* (1995) Mechanisms for episodes of hypoxemia in preterm infants undergoing mechanical ventilation. *J Pediatr* **127**: 767–773.

25. Wenstrom KD, Andrews WW, Hauth JC *et al.* (1998) Elevated second trimester amniotic fluid interleukin-6 levels predict preterm delivery. *Am J Obstet Gynecol* **178**: 546–550.

26. Watts DH, Krohn MA, Hillier SL. (1992) The association of occult amniotic fluid infection with gestational age and neonatal outcome among women in preterm labor. *Obstet Gynecol* **79**: 351–357.

27. Goldenberg RL, Hauth JC, Andrews WW. (2000) Intrauterine infection and preterm delivery. *N Engl J Med* **342**: 1500–1507.

28. Watterberg KL, Demers SM, Scott SM *et al.* (1996) Chorioamnionitis and early lung inflammation in infants in whom bronchopulmonary dysplasia develops. *Pediatrics* **97**: 210–215.

29. Yoon BH, Romero R, Jun JK *et al.* (1997) Amniotic fluid cytokines (interleukin-6, tumor necrosis factor-a, interleukin-1β, and interleukin-8) and the

risk for the development of bronchopulmonary dysplasia. *Am J Obstet Gynecol* **177**: 825–830.

30. Yoon BH, Romero, Kim CJ *et al*. (1997) High expression of tumor necrosis factor-a and intereukin-6 in periventricular leukomalacia. *Am J Obstet Gynecol* **177**: 406–411.

31. Viscardi RM, Muhumuza CK, Rodriguez A *et al*. (2004) Inflammatory markers in intrauterine and fetal blood and cerebrospinal fluid compartments are association with adverse pulmonary and neurological outcomes in preterm infants. *Pediatr Res* **55**: 1009–1017.

32. Van Marter LJ, Dammann O, Allred EN *et al*. (2002) Chorioamnionitis, mechanical ventilation and postnatal sepsis as modulators of chronic lung disease in preterm infants. *J Pediatr* **140**: 171–176.

33. Soraisham AS, Singhal N, McMillan DD *et al*. (2009) A multicenter study on the clinical outcome of chroioamnionitis in preterm infants. *AJOG* **200**: 372.e1–372.e6.

34. Kallapur SG, Jobe AH. (2006) Contribution of lung inflammation to lung injury and development. *Arch Dis Child Fetal Neonatal Ed* **91**: F132–F135.

35. Van Waarde WM, Brus F, Okken A *et al*. (1997) *Ureaplasma urealyticum* colonization, prematurity and bronchopulmonary dysplasia. *Eur Respir J* **10**: 886–890.

36. Kotecha S, Hodge R, Schraber JA *et al*. (2004) Pulmonary *Ureaplasma urealyticum* is associated with the development of acute lung inflammation and chronic lung disease in preterm infants. *Pediatr Res* **55**: 61–68.

37. Lyon AJ, McColm J, Middlemist L *et al*. (1998) Randomised trial of erythromycin on the development of chronic lung disease in preterm infants. *Arch Dis Child Fetal Neonatal Ed* **78**: F10–F14.

38. Couroucli XI, Welty SE, Ramsay PL *et al*. (2000) Detection of microorganisms in the tracheal aspirates of preterm infants by polymerase chain reaction: Association of adenovirus infection with bronchopulmonary dysplasia. *Pediatr Res* **47**: 225–232.

39. Liljedahl M, Bodin L, Schollin J. (2004) Coagulase negative staphylococcal sepsis as a predictor of bronchopulmonary dysplasia. *Acta Pediatrica* **93**: 211–215.

40. Sawyer MH, Edwards DK, Spector SA. (1987) Cytomegalovirus infection and bronchopulmonary dysplasia in premature infants. *Am J Dis Child* **141**: 303–305.

41. Smith VC, Zupancic JA, McCormick MC *et al.* (2004) Rehospitalization in the first year of life among infants with bronchopulmonary dysplasia. *J Pediatr* **144**: 799–803.

42. Varsila E, Hallman M, Venge P, Andersson S. (1995) Closure of patent ductus arteriosus decreases pulmonary myeloperoxidase in premature infants with respiratory distress syndrome. *Biol Neonate* **67**: 167–171.

43. McCurnin D, Seidner S, Chang LY *et al.* (2008) Ibuprofen-induced patent ductus arteriosus closure: physiologic, histologic, and biochemical effects on the premature lung. *Pediatrics* **121**: 945–956.

44. Chang LY, McCurnin D, Yoder B *et al.* (2008) Ductus arteriosus ligation and alveolar growth in preterm baboons with a patent ductus arteriosus. *Pediatr Res* **63**: 299–302.

45. Parker RA, Lindstrom DP, Cotton RB. (1996) Evidence from twin study implies possible genetic susceptibility to bronchopulmonary dysplasia. *Semin Perinatol* **20**: 206–209.

46. Bhandari V, Bizzarro MJ, Shetty AH *et al.* (2006) Familial and genetic susceptibility to major neonatal morbidities in preterm twins. *Pediatrics* **117**: 1901–1906.

47. Nickerson BG, Taussig LM. (1980) Family history of asthma in infants with bronchopulmonary dysplasia. *Pediatrics* **65**: 1140–1144.

48. Hallman M, Marttila R, Pertille R *et al.* (2007) Genes and environment in common neonatal lung disease. *Neonatology* **91**: 298–302.

49. Przemko K, Miroslaw BM, Zofia M *et al.* (2008) Genetic risk factors of bronchopulmonary dysplasia. *Pediatr Res* **114**: e243–e248.

50. Manar MH, Brown MR, Gauthier TW *et al.* (2004) Association of glutathione-S-transferase-P1 polymorphisms with bronchopulmonary dysplasia. *J Perinatol* **24**: 30–35.

51. Verder H, Robertson B, Greisen G *et al.* (1994) Surfactant therapy and nasal continuous positive airway pressure for newborns with respiratory distress syndrome. *N Engl J Med* **331**: 1051–1055.

52. Ho JJ, Subramaniam P, Henderson-Smart DJ *et al.* (2000) Continuous distending airway pressure for respiratory distress syndrome in preterm infants. *Cochrane Database Syst Rev* (3): CD002271.

53. Morley CJ, Davis PG, Doyle LW *et al.* (2008) Nasal CPAP or intubation at birth for very preterm infants. *N Engl J Med* **358**: 700–708.

54. SUPPORT Study Group of the Eunice Kennedy Shriver NICHD Neonatal Research Network, Finer NN, Carlo WA, Walsh MC *et al.* (2010) Early

CPAP versus surfactant in extremely preterm infants. *N Engl J Med* **362**(21): 1970–1979.

55. Kugelman A, Feferkorn I, Riskin A *et al.* (2007) Nasal intermittent mandatory ventilation versus nasal continuous positive airway pressure for respiratory distress syndrome: A randomized controlled prospective study. *J Pediatr* **150**: 521–526.

56. Bhandari V, Gavino RG, Nedrelow JH *et al.* (2007) A randomized controlled trial of synchronized nasal intermittent positive pressure ventilation in RDS. *J Perinatol* **27**: 697–703.

57. Bhandari V, Finer NN, Ehrenkranz R *et al.* (2009) Synchronized nasal intermittent positive pressure ventilation and neonatal outcomes. *Pediatrics* **124**: 517–526.

58. Woodgate PG, Davies MW. (2001) Permissive hypercapnia for the prevention of morbidity and mortality in mechanically ventilated newborn infants. Cochrane Database Syst Rev (2): CD002061.

59. Courtney SE, Durand DJ, Asselin JM *et al.* (2002) High frequency oscillatory ventilation versus conventional mechanical ventilation for very low birth weight infants. *N Engl J Med* **347**: 643–652.

60. Johnson AH, Peacock JL, Greenough A *et al.* (2002) High frequency oscillatory ventilation for the prevention of chronic lung disease of prematurity. *N Engl J Med* **347**: 633–642.

61. Schulze A, Bancalari E. (2001) Proportional assist ventilation in infants. *Clin Perinatol* **28**: 561–578.

62. Sinha SK, Donn SM, Gavey J *et al.* (1997) Randomised trial of volume controlled versus time cycled, pressure limited ventilation in preterm infants with respiratory distress syndrome. *Arch Dis Child Fetal Neonatal Ed* **77**: F202–F205.

63. Cheema I, Ahluwalia J. (2001) Feasibility of tidal volume-guided ventilation in newborn infants: A randomized crossover trial using the volume guarantee modality. *Pediatrics* **107**: 1323–1328.

64. Reyes ZC, Claure N, Tauscher MK *et al.* (2006) Randomized controlled trial comparing synchronized intermittent mandatory ventilation and synchronized intermittent mandatory ventilation plus pressure support in preterm infants. *Pediatrics* **118**: 1409–1417.

65. Sun RC. (2002) Relation of target SpO2 and clinical outcome in ELBW infants on supplemental oxygen. *Pediatr Res* **51**: A350.

66. STOP-ROP Multicenter Study Group. (2000) Supplemental therapeutic oxygen for prethreshold retinopathy of prematurity (STOP-ROP), A randomized controlled trial. I: Primary outcomes. *Pediatrics* **105**: 295–310.
67. Askie LM, Henderson-Smart DJ, Irwig L *et al.* (2003) Oxygen-saturation targets and outcomes in extremely preterm infants. *N Engl J Med* **349**: 959–967.
68. Claure N, D'Ugard C, Bancalari E. (2009) Automated Adjustment of Inspired Oxygen in Preterm Infants with Frequent Fluctuations in Oxygenation: A Pilot Clinical Trial. *J Pediatr* **155**: 640–645.
69. Davis JM, Parad RB, Michele T *et al.* (2003) Pulmonary outcome at one year corrected age in premature infants treated at birth with recombinant human CuAn superoxide dismutase. *Pediatrics* **111**: 469–476.
70. Sandberg KI, Fellman V, Stigson L *et al.* (2004) N-acetylcysteine administration during the first week of life does not improve lung function in extremely low birth weight infants. *Biol Neonate* **86**: 275–279.
71. Russell GA, Cooke RW. (1995) Randomised controlled trial of allopurinol prophylaxis in very preterm infants. *Arch Dis Child Fetal Neonat Ed* **73**: F27–F31.
72. Kinsella JP, Parker TA, Galan H *et al.* (1997) Effects of inhaled nitric oxide on pulmonary edema and lung neutrophil accumulation in severe experimental hyaline membrane disease. *Pediatr Res* **41**: 457–463.
73. ter Horst SA, Walther FJ, Poorthuis BJ *et al.* (2007) Inhaled nitric oxide attenuates pulmonary inflammation and fibrin deposition and prolongs survival in neonatal hyperoxic lung injury. *Am J Physiol Lung Cell Mol Physiol* **293**: 135–144.
74. Lin YJ, Markham NE, Balasubramaniam V *et al.* (2005) Inhaled nitric oxide enhances distal lung growth after exposure to hyperoxia in neonatal rats. *Pediatr Res* **58**: 22–29.
75. Schreiber MD, Gat-Mestan K, Marks JD *et al.* (2003) Inhaled nitric oxide in premature infants with respiratory distress syndrome. *N Engl J Med* **349**: 2099–2107.
76. Ballard RA, Truog WE, Cnaan A *et al.* (2006) Inhaled nitric oxide in preterm infants undergoing mechanical ventilation. *N Engl J Med* **355**: 343–353.
77. Kinsella JP, Cutter GR, Walsh WF *et al.* (2006) Early inhaled nitric oxide therapy in premature newborns with respiratory failure. *N Engl J Med* **355**: 354–364.

78. Van Meurs KP, Wright LL, Ehrenkranz RA *et al.* (2005) Inhaled nitric oxide for premature infants with severe respiratory failure. *N Engl J Med* **353**: 82–84.

79. Mercier J, Hummler H, Durrmeyer X *et al.* (2010). Inhaled nitric oxide for prevention of BPD in preterm babies (EUNO): A randomized controlled trial. *Lancet* **376**: 346–354.

80. Frank L, Groseclose EE. (1982) Oxygen toxicity in newborns: The adverse effects of undernutrition. *J Appl Physiol* **53**: 1248–1255.

81. Deneke SM, Gershoff SN, Fanberg BL. (1983) Potentiation of oxygen toxicity in rats by dietary protein or amino acid deficiency. *J Appl Physiol* **54**: 147–151.

82. Sosenko IRS, Innis SM, Frank L. (1988) Polyunsaturated fatty acids and protection of newborn rats from oxygen toxicity. *J Pediatr* **112**: 630–637.

83. Sosenko IRS, Innis SM, Frank L. (1991) Intralipid increases lung polyunsaturated fatty acids and protects newborn rats from oxygen toxicity. *Pediatr Res* **30**: 413–417.

84. Sosenko IRS. (1995) Polyunsaturated fatty acids: Do they protect against or promote oxidant lung injury? *J Nutrition* **125**: 1652–1656.

85. Hallman M, Bry K, Hoppu K *et al.* (1992) Inositol supplementation in premature infants with respiratory distress syndrome. *N Engl J Med* **326**: 1233–1239.

86. Howlett A, Ohlsson A. (2003) Inositol for respiratory distress syndrome in preterm infants. *Cochrane Database Syst Rev* (4): CD000366.

87. Takahashi,. Miura,. Takahashi K. (1993) Vitamin A is involved in maintenance of epithelial cells on the bronchioles and cells in the alveoli of rats. *J Nutr* **123**: 634–641.

88. Shenai JP, Chytil F, Stahlman MT. (1985) Vitamin A status of neonates with bronchopulmonary dysplasia. *Pediatr Res* **19**: 185–189.

89. Tyson JE, Wright LL, Oh W *et al.* (1999) Vitamin A supplementation for extremely low birth weight infants. *N Engl J Med* **340**: 1962–1968.

90. Darlow BA, Graham PJ. (2002) Vitamin A supplementation for preventing morbidity and mortality in very low birthweight infants. *Chochrane Database Syst Rev* **4**: CD000501.

91. Caddell JL. (1996) Evidence for magnesium deficiency in the pathogenesis of bronchopulmonary dysplasia. *Magnesium Res* **9**: 205–216.

92. Falciglia HS, Johnson JR, Sullivan J *et al.* (2003) Role of antioxidant nutrients and lipid peroxidation in premature infants with respiratory distress syndrome and bronchopulmonary dysplasia. *Am J Perinatol* **20**: 97–107.

93. Merz U, Peschgens T, Dott W *et al.* (1998) Selenium status and bronchopulmonary dysplasia in premature infants. *Zeit Geburt Neonatol* **202**: 203–206.

94. Darlow BA, Inder TE, Sluis KB *et al.* (1998) Randomised controlled trial of selenium supplementation in New Zealand VLBW infants. *Pediatr Res* **43**: 258A.

95. Rhen T, Cidlowski L. (2005) Anti-inflammatory action of glucocorticoids: New mechanisms for old drugs. *N Engl J Med* **353**: 1711–1723.

96. Grier DG, Halliday HL. (2003) Corticosteroids in the prevention and management of bronchopulmonary dysplasia. *Seminars in Neonatol* **8**: 83–91.

97. Doyle LW, Halliday HL, Ehrenkranz RA. (2005) Impact of postnatal systemic corticosteroids on mortality and cerebral palsy in preterm infants: Effect modification by risk for chronic lung disease. *Pediatrics* **115**: 655–661.

98. Schmidt B, Roberts RS, Davis P *et al.* (2006) Caffeine therapy for apnea of prematurity. *N Engl J Med* **354**: 2112–2121.

99. Bancalari E. (2006) Caffeine for apnea of prematurity. *N Engl J Med* **354**: 2179–2181.

100. Davis PG, Schmidt B, Roberts RS *et al.* (2010) Caffeine for apnea of prematurity: Benefits may vary in subgroups. *J Pediatr* **156**: 382–387.

101. ter Horst SA, Wagenaar GT, de Boer E *et al.* (2004) Pentoxifylline reduces fibrin deposition and prolongs survival in neonatal hyperoxic lung injury. *J Appl Physiol* **97**: 2014–2019.

102. Almario B, Wu S, Peng J *et al.* (2006) Pentoxifylline up-regulates lung vascular endothelial growth factor (VEGF) gene expression and prolongs survival in hyperoxia-exposed newborn rats. *PAS Abstract* **4132**: 8.

103. Abman SH, Matthay MA. (2009) Mesenchymal stem cells for the prevention of BPD: delivering the secretome. *Am J Resp Crit Care Med* **180**: 1039–1041.

104. Van Haaften T, Bryne R, Bonnet S *et al.* (2009) Airway delivery of mesenchymal stem cells prevents arrested alveolar growth in neonatal lung injury in rats. *Am J Resp Crit Care Med* **180**: 1131–1142.

105. Aslam M, Baveja R, Liang OD *et al.* (2009) Bone marrow stromal cells attenuate lung injury in a murine model of neonatal chronic lung disease. *Am J Resp Crit Care Med* **180**: 1122–1130.

Chapter

7

Respiratory Care
of the Newborn

John Kelleher and Waldemar A. Carlo

Pulmonary Mechanics

The mechanical properties of the lungs in part determine the mode and parameters of the ventilator for each infant. In order for effective CO_2 elimination and oxygenation to occur, a pressure gradient between the airway opening and the alveoli must exist. This pressure gradient is determined for the most part by compliance and resistance.

Compliance

This is a measure of the elasticity or distensibility of the lungs plus chest wall. It is determined by the formula:

$$\text{Compliance} = \Delta \text{ volume}/\Delta \text{ pressure.}$$

The total compliance (lungs + chest wall) in newborns with normal lungs ranges from 3 to 5 ml/cm H_2O/kg. Neonates with respiratory distress syndrome (RDS) have "stiffer" or less compliant lungs secondary to surfactant deficiency with total compliance values as low as 0.1 to 1 ml/cm H_2O/kg.

145

Resistance

This describes the inherent ability of the gas conducting system (e.g. airways, endotracheal tube) and tissues to oppose airflow. It is determined by the formula:

$$\text{Resistance} = \Delta \text{ pressure}/\Delta \text{ flow.}$$

Total (airway + tissue) resistance for normal neonatal lungs ranges from 25 to 50 cm $H_2O/L/sec$. In newborns with endotracheal tubes this can range from 50 to 150 cm $H_2O/L/sec$. Airway resistance is determined by the following:

- Length and radii of airways
- Gas flow rate
- Density and viscosity of inhaled gases

Resistance is not typically increased in newborns with RDS, but can be increased if airways are affected by mucosal edema, interstitial edema (decreasing airway lumens), and bronchospasm.

Time constant

The time constant of the respiratory system is the time taken for the alveolar pressure to reach 63% of the change in airway pressure (see Fig. 1). Put simply, it might be considered as the time taken for approximately two-thirds of the gas in the airway to reach the alveoli. The time constant is expressed by the formula:

$$\text{Time constant} = \text{Resistance} \times \text{Compliance.}$$

As depicted by Fig. 1, three to five time constants are required for a relatively complete inspiration or expiration (with associated complete delivery of pressure and volume). For example, if an infant has a total compliance of 2 ml/cm H_2O (0.002 L/cm H_2O) and a resistance of 40 cm $H_2O/L/sec$, the time constant is derived as follows:

$$\text{Time constant} = 0.002 \text{ L/cm } H_2O \times 40 \text{ cm } H_2O/L/sec = 0.08 \text{ seconds.}$$

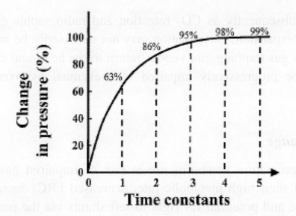

Figure 1. Percentage change in pressure in relation to the time (in time constants) allowed for lung equilibration. The same applies for step-changes in volume. (Modified from Carlo WA, Ambalavanan N. (1999) Conventional mechanical ventilation: Traditional and new strategies. *Pediatrics in Review.* 20:e117–e126, p. e119.)

In calculating the time constant, the compliance is not corrected for unit of weight. If between three and five time constants are required for an infant to achieve complete inspiration or expiration, then in the example given, the time required for either complete inspiration or expiration is 240–400 msec (or 0.24–0.4 seconds). The greater the compliance of the lungs (e.g. term neonates with normal lungs) then the longer the time constant will be. If total resistance is high (e.g. infants with bronchopulmonary dysplasia), then the time constant will be longer. The time constant will be shorter if compliance is decreased (e.g. newborns with RDS).

Understanding of the role of the time constant is fundamental in determining an appropriate ventilatory mode and strategy. An infant with a short time constant will ventilate appropriately with a short inspiratory and expiratory times and a high ventilator rate. On the other hand, an infant with a longer time constant will necessitate longer inspiratory and expiratory times and a lower rate. Too short an inspiratory time can result in both hypercapnia and hypoxemia. If the expiratory time is too short (less than 3–5 time constants), the result will be an increase in functional residual capacity (FRC), inadvertent PEEP and gas trapping. This may manifest subsequently as CO_2 retention and radiographic evidence of lung hyperexpansion. Oxygenation may not necessarily be immediately affected by gas trapping, but venous return to the heart and cardiac output may be progressively impaired with eventual hypoxemia at the tissues.

Gas exchange

Sick and premature newborns are at risk of impaired gas exchange because of their high metabolic rate, decreased FRC, decreased total compliance and potential for right-to-left shunts via the patent ductus arteriosus and foramen ovale. While both hypercapnia and hypoxemia may exist simultaneously, certain disorders may affect one or the other preferentially.

Hypercapnia

The mechanisms responsible for hypercapnia include hypoventilation, increased physiologic dead space, ventilation–perfusion (V/Q) mismatch and shunt. CO_2 elimination during assisted ventilation is determined by the following equation:

Alveolar minute ventilation = Frequency × Alveolar tidal volume.

The alveolar tidal volume is determined by the tidal volume minus the dead space. The tidal volume (V_T) is the volume of gas inhaled (or exhaled) with each breath. Frequency is the number of breaths per minute. The dead space is the volume of the V_T that is not involved in gas exchange (e.g. the volume of gas that fills the conducting airways). As the dead space volume is relatively unchanged during assisted ventilation, changes in either frequency and/or V_T can be used clinically as the determinants of CO_2 elimination.

In a volume-limited (volume-targeted or guaranteed) ventilator, the V_T is a parameter that the clinician can directly program into the ventilator. On a pressure-limited ventilator, the V_T is usually not directly programmed into the machine by the clinician. Rather, the V_T is determined by

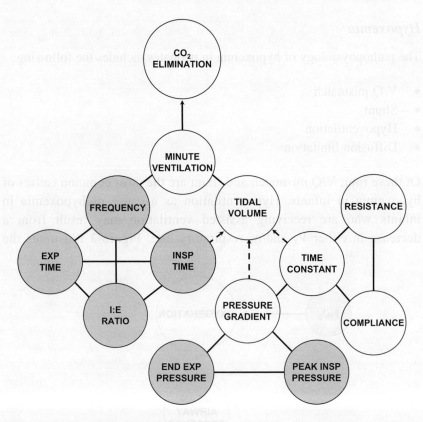

Figure 2. Ventilator-controlled parameters (shaded circles) and pulmonary mechanics (non-shaded circles) that determine alveolar minute ventilation during time-cycled, pressure-limited ventilation. Relationships between circles joined by solid lines are mathematically derived. The dashed lines represent relationships that cannot be precisely calculated without considering other variables such as pulmonary mechanics. (Modified from Carlo WA, Greenough A, Chatburn RL. Advances in mechanical ventilation. In Boynton BR, Carlo WA, Jobe AH (eds) (1994) *New Therapies for Neonatal Respiratory Failure: A Physiologic Approach.* Cambridge (UK): Cambridge University Press; p. 133.)

the pressure gradient between the airway opening and the alveoli. This pressure gradient or amplitude (ΔP) is derived from the peak inspiratory pressure (PIP) minus the positive end-expiratory pressure (PEEP). Figure 2 depicts the interaction between both ventilator-controlled parameters and pulmonary mechanics that determine alveolar minute ventilation during time-cycled, pressure-limited ventilation.

Hypoxemia

The pathophysiology of hypoxemia in neonates includes the following:

- V/Q mismatch
- Shunt
- Hypoventilation
- Diffusion limitation

Of these four, V/Q mismatch and shunt are the most common causes of hypoxemia in infants. Hypoventilation as a cause of hypoxemia in infants who are receiving assisted ventilation may result from a decrease in either V_T and/or respiratory rate. Figure 3 illustrates the

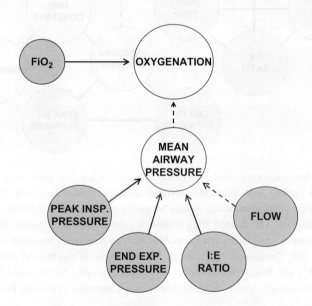

Figure 3. Determinants of oxygenation during pressure-limited, time-cycled ventilation. Shaded circles represent ventilator-controlled variables. Non-shaded circles represent pulmonary mechanics. Solid lines denote the simple mathematical relationships that determine mean airway pressure and oxygenation. Dashed lines represent relationships that cannot be quantified with simple mathematical methods. (Modified from Carlo WA, Greenough A Chatburn RL. Advances in mechanical ventilation. In Boynton BR, Carlo WA, Jobe AH (eds.). (1994) *New Therapies for Neonatal Respiratory Failure: A Physiologic Approach.* Cambridge (UK): Cambridge University Press; p. 134.)

parameters that determine oxygenation during pressure-limited, time-cycled ventilation. V/Q mismatch is an important cause of hypoxemia in infants who have either RDS or other causes of respiratory failure. It is the result of inadequate ventilation of alveoli relative to their degree of perfusion. Supplemental O_2 can often overcome the hypoxemia from V/Q mismatch.

Shunting poorly oxygenated blood away from the alveoli where oxygen is readily available is a common cause of hypoxemia in infants. It can be intracardiac (e.g. persistent pulmonary hypertension of the newborn and cyanotic congenital heart disease), or extracardiac (e.g. lung atelectasis). It can be considered as a V/Q = 0 and supplemental O_2 cannot readily reverse the resultant hypoxemia.[1] The role of inhaled nitric oxide (iNO) will be discussed later in the context of shunting secondary to pulmonary hypertension.

Nasal CPAP

Nasal CPAP improves pulmonary function because it

(1) increases FRC and improves oxygenation.[2]
(2) dilates the larynx, reduces supraglottic airway resistance and the incidence of obstructive apnea.
(3) improves the synchrony of respiratory thoracoabdominal movements.
(4) enhances the Hering–Breuer inflation reflex following airway occlusion.[3]

CPAP for infants with RDS

A Cochrane meta-analysis has shown that the use of nasal CPAP in preterm infants with RDS is associated with less death or use of IPPV (intermittent positive pressure ventilation) (RR 0.65, 95% CI 0.52, 0.81) (NNT 5, 95% CI 4, 10) and less overall mortality (RR 0.52, 95% CI 0.32, 0.81) (NNT 7, 95% CI 4, 25).[4] There is an associated increased risk of pneumothorax (RR 2.64, 95% CI 1.39, 5.04) (NNH 17, 95% CI 17, 25). Most of the trials featured in this meta-analysis were from a time before the frequent use of surfactant and antenatal steroids.

Prophylactic surfactant or early CPAP: The evidence

Two meta-analysis and other trials provide substantial evidence that either early surfactant and brief ventilation (no more than one hour)[5-7] or prophylactic surfactant administration (within the first 15 minutes of life)[8] for preterm infants < 30–32 weeks gestation, when compared to late selective surfactant therapy based upon oxygenation and respiratory clinical criteria, result in a lower incidence of subsequent mechanical ventilation,[5,6,9] fewer pneumothoraces,[8] less pulmonary interstitial emphysema (PIE),[6,8] less BPD at 28 days,[6,8] less mortality and less mortality or BPD at 28 days.[8] There is evidence from a meta-analysis that selective administration of surfactant at higher O_2 treatment criteria versus $\leq 45\%$ was associated with an increased risk of PDA requiring treatment.[6] However, in most of these trials the infants randomized to no surfactant did not consistently receive early CPAP.

Several trials have evaluated the role of early/delivery room nasal CPAP. The trial by Verder *et al.* examined 60 premature infants < 30 weeks' gestation who were all initially managed on nasal CPAP at a median age of 17 minutes in the NICU.[5] This trial was stopped when an interim analysis showed that nasal CPAP with early surfactant administration (median age 5.2 versus 9.9 hours) significantly reduced the need for mechanical ventilation during the first week of life. In a large multicenter trial by Sandri F *et al.* 230 less immature preterm neonates (28–31 weeks' gestation) were randomized to either prophylactic nasal CPAP (within 30 minutes) of age or rescue nasal CPAP.[10] The rescue group received CPAP when the O_2 requirement exceeded 40%. The trial showed a similar requirement for surfactant of 22% in both prophylactic and rescue CPAP groups with no differences between the two groups with regards to pneumothorax, mortality, or need for subsequent mechanical ventilation.

The use of prophylactic nasal CPAP in the delivery room for extremely preterm infants (23 to 27 weeks) was shown to be feasible in a randomized multicenter trial by the NICHD in 104 infants < 28 weeks' gestation.[11] Nasal CPAP was found to be feasible in supporting many of these extremely preterm infants. However, there were no short term benefits of prophylactic CPAP.

A meta-analysis in 2005 addressed the question of prophylactic (early) or nasal CPAP initiated soon after birth in very preterm infants compared to either nasal CPAP or IPPV for a defined respiratory condition.[12] The standard of care was considered as the use of either nasal CPAP or IPPV for a defined respiratory condition. The authors reviewed two trials and found that prophylactic CPAP did not decrease the use of IPPV or the incidence of BPD.

The recent COIN (Cpap Or INtubation) Trial by the Australasian Trial Network addressed the effectiveness of delivery room CPAP versus early surfactant.[13] The trial comprised 610 newborns of gestational age 25 to 28 completed weeks who were breathing spontaneously at five minutes of age. There was a trend for a lower rate of death or BPD at 36 weeks in the infants who received CPAP (34%) versus those who received intubation (39%) (OR 0.8, 95% CI 0.58–1.12, $p = 0.19$). However, the CPAP group had a higher incidence of pneumothorax than the intubation group (9% versus 3%, $p < 0.001$).

The recently published SUPPORT (Surfactant, Positive Pressure, and Pulse Oximetry Randomized) Trial by the NICHD compared delivery room initiated nasal CPAP and a subsequent strategy of limited ventilation versus intubation and surfactant administration within 60 minutes of birth.[14] The study comprised 1316 newborns between 24 to 27 weeks 6 days of gestation. There was a statistically non-significant yet clinically important reduction in the primary outcome of death or BPD (defined as the need for supplemental oxygen at 36 weeks) at 48.7% in the CPAP group compared to 54% in the surfactant group (RR 0.91, 95% CI 0.83–1.01, $p = 0.07$). Furthermore, the trial showed a significantly lower mortality during hospitalization for the CPAP infants in the 24 to 25 week stratum (23.9%) compared to the surfactant group (32.1%) (RR 0.74, 95% CI 0.57–0.98, $p = 0.03$). The trial demonstrated that nasal CPAP is an effective and evidence-based delivery room ventilatory strategy for premature newborns. The recent DRM (Delivery Room Management) trial by the Vermont Oxford Network (VON) reported on 648 newborns between 26 to 29 weeks 6 days of gestation.[15] The study was stopped prior to the target sample size of 895 neonates. In contrast to the SUPPORT study, not only was the study population inclusive of less immature premature neonates but three different ventilatory strategies were studied. The trial found no statistically significant differences between newborns managed by either nasal CPAP in the delivery room or prophylactic surfactant followed by extubation to nasal CPAP compared to those who are managed by prophylactic surfactant followed by assisted mechanical ventilation. The addition of results from the COIN,[13] SUPPORT[14] and DRM[15] trials will add substantially to the meta-analysis[12] and provide further evidence for early nasal CPAP with/without prophylactic surfactant as management strategies for premature newborns at high risk.

Delivery of nasal CPAP

There are two types of devices that are generally used to deliver nasal CPAP to infants. These are variable flow and continuous flow CPAP devices. This distinction is based upon their gas flow characteristics. Both mechanical ventilators and bubble CPAP (Fisher and Paykel HealthCare, Auckland, New Zealand) are continuous flow devices. The Infant Flow Driver (IFD) CPAP (Electro Medical Equipment, Sussex, UK) is a variable flow device. The IFD CPAP uses a dedicated flow driver with a unique fluidic flip mechanism to adjust gas flow throughout the respiratory cycle. Studies to date have compared CPAP delivered by mechanical ventilators versus the IFD.[3] These studies have failed to show any significant differences in reintubation rates between IFD and mechanical ventilator provided nasal CPAP. A study by Gupta *et al.* compared bubble CPAP to the IFD in preterm infants who were intubated and ventilated for RDS.[16] The study outcome was successful maintenance of extubation for at least 72 hours following the initial period of intubation and mechanical ventilation. The study found no difference between the two modes of nasal CPAP with regards to successful extubation rates post initial mechanical ventilation for RDS.

Noninvasive Ventilation

Noninvasive ventilation is a mode of assisted ventilation that provides either synchronized or non-synchronized phasic increases in positive airway distending pressure throughout breathing without intubation.[17]

Dempsey *et al.* have described the numerous confusing acronyms within this modality including the following:

- NIV (noninvasive ventilation) or NPPV (noninvasive positive pressure ventilation)
- NIMV (nasal intermittent mandatory ventilation) or NIPPV (nasal intermittent positive pressure ventilation)
- SNIMV (synchronized nasal intermittent mandatory ventilation) or SNIPPV (synchronized nasal intermittent positive pressure ventilation)

NIV works by providing CPAP with the benefit of additional breaths. While providing CPAP it delivers tidal volumes by augmenting inspiratory transpulmonary pressures. A patent airway is essential for NIV to be effective. The indications for the use of NIV include:

- Post-extubation and apnea of prematurity
- Primary mode of ventilation in RDS

The actual and theoretical benefits of NIV include avoidance of intubation, a reduction of re-intubation rates post extubation and a decrease in apnea events post extubation. Potential adverse effects include skin and/or nasal tissue damage, tube displacement and/or blockage with secretions and subsequent impairment of ventilation and abdominal distention if an orogastric tube is not simultaneously utilized. A single case control study of NIMV as a primary ventilation mode for RDS in 15 patients showed an increase in gastric perforations.[18] This has not been shown in subsequent randomized trials.[12]

NIV and apnea: The evidence

A Cochrane systematic review was performed and last updated in 2007.[19] This review examined the trials to date comparing NIPPV (delivered by either short nasal prongs or nasopharyngeal tube) versus nasal CPAP for apnea of prematurity in premature infants who had not been intubated and ventilated. A total of 54 infants from two eligible trials in 1989 and 1998 were reviewed. The meta-analysis of both trials showed that only one infant

experienced failure of therapy (either CPAP or NIPPV) and required intubation. Unfortunately the two trials reported only examined the outcome of
failed treatment for 4–6 hours post randomization. Gastric perforations were
not reported. NIPPV reduced apnea events (weighted mean difference –1.19,
95% CI, –2.31, –0.07) (p = 0.038). A recent small, randomized controlled
trial has shown that either NIPPV or nasal CPAP delivered by a variable flow
device decreased bradycardias and desaturation events than NIPPV delivered via a constant flow device (a conventional ventilator).[20] The role of NIV
in the management of post extubation apnea was shown by Barrington *et al.*
in a randomized trial that more premature infants who were weaned from
mechanical ventilation to nSIMV were successfully extubated compared to
those weaned to nasal CPAP (15 of 27 infants vs 4 of 27, p < 0.05).[21]

NIV and RDS/BPD: The evidence

Randomized trials of infants with RDS managed with early NIPPV or
NIMV versus nasal CPAP have shown that failure rates of extubation and
the subsequent need for reintubation are lower with either NIPPV[22,23] or
NIMV[24] and the number of apnea events fewer with NIPPV versus nasal
CPAP.[18] However, these trials were small and had other limitations so further research is needed in this area. A single center randomized controlled
trial[25] and an NICHD Neonatal Network retrospective observational study[26]
demonstrated that newborns who receive surfactant with early extubation
to NIV have lower mortality or BPD than those maintained on either nasal
CPAP post-extubation[26] or continued for longer on conventional ventilation.[25] A trial is ongoing in Canada comparing NIPPV versus nasal CPAP
in VLBW infants with respect to the combined outcome of survival
without moderate/severe BPD at 36 weeks PMA.[27]

Conventional Ventilation

Mechanical ventilation for newborns with respiratory failure due to pulmonary disease was first introduced in the 1960s. A Cochrane meta-analysis
updated in 2005 examined 5 trials that compared mechanical ventilation
(MV) versus no mechanical ventilation.[28] All of these trials published
between 1967 and 1970. The review concluded that in newborns with birth

weights above 2 kg there was a significant reduction in mortality with MV compared to no MV (RR 0.67, 95% CI 0.52, 0.87) (NNT 4, 95% 2, 10).

Methods to achieve ventilator synchrony: HFPPV and PTV

High Frequency Positive Pressure Ventilation (HFPPV)

The use of conventional mechanical ventilation with ventilation rate greater than 60 breaths per min with associated low tidal volumes is known as HFPPV. This form of ventilation utilizes low tidal volumes and therefore low peak inspiratory pressure (PIP).

Table 1 illustrates some of the theoretical advantages and disadvantages of such a ventilator strategy.

HFPPV is likely to be associated with synchronous ventilation in the preterm infant. Synchrony of ventilation means that the mechanical ventilator delivered positive pressure ventilation coincides with the infant's spontaneous inspiration. A Cochrane systematic review updated in 2008[29] revealed that a strategy of HFPPV resulted in less air leaks than compared to CMV (28% versus 19%; RR 0.69; 95% CI 0.51, 0.93) (NNT 11) and a trend towards increased survival.

While HFPPV may be an effective strategy to facilitate a preterm infant in achieving synchronous ventilation, an alternative strategy or mode of ventilation that may theoretically achieve synchrony is *triggering*. This is a ventilator feature whereby the patient uses some variable to initiate the phase of inspiration. The ventilation mode that incorporates this variable is commonly referred to as *patient-triggered ventilation* (PTV).[30] The

Table 1.   High rate, Low tidal volume (Low PIP)

PROS	CONS
• Decreased air leaks	• Gas trapping/inadvertent PEEP
• Decreased volutrauma	• Generalized atelectasis
• Decreased cardiovascular side effects	• Maldistribution of gas
• Decreased risk of pulmonary edema	• Increased resistance

Reproduced from Carlo WA, Ambalavanan N. (1999) Conventional mechanical ventilation: Traditional and new strategies. *Pediatric Rev.* **20**:e117–e126.

variables that are most commonly utilized to trigger infant inspiration on a ventilator include pressure, volume, flow or time. Flow triggering perhaps requires less effort on behalf of the infant and is widely used in the ventilation of infants.[31] Under the umbrella heading of PTV there exists many different ventilation modes including[29]:

- Synchronized intermittent mandatory ventilation (SIMV) where mandatory ventilator inspirations are synchronized to the onset of spontaneous breath from an infant, should the infant meet a trigger threshold and initiate a breath. In the case of infant apnea, a defined number of mandatory breaths will be delivered by the ventilator.
- Assist-control ventilation (ACV) also known as synchronous intermittent positive pressure ventilation (SIPPV) where a patient can either trigger spontaneous inspirations from the ventilator or receive mandatory ventilator-initiated breaths if the patient experiences apnea.
- SIMV with *pressure support ventilation* (PSV) is a mode of ventilation where every spontaneous breath triggered by the patient is reinforced with additional inspiratory pressure. PSV can exist with or without the backup mandatory ventilation rate provided by SIMV.
- Pressure-regulated volume-control ventilation (PRVC) is a mode of ventilation whereby a predefined volume is delivered to the patient by regulating the pressure necessary to generate a tidal volume either in assist (patient-triggered) or in a control (mandatory) fashion.

In addition to the above modes of PTV, many volume-controlled ventilators utilize either patient-triggered or *mandatory* delivered inspirations should the infant become apneic.[32]

A Cochrane meta-analysis has been performed of trials comparing various modes of PTV to CMV with respect to outcomes including mortality, air leaks, severe IVH (grades 3 and 4), BPD (oxygen dependency beyond 28 days), BPD as defined by oxygen dependency beyond 36 weeks PMA and duration of ventilation and ventilator weaning.[29] The meta-analysis of six trials showed that ACV/SIMV, compared to CMV, was associated with a significantly shorter duration of ventilation (weighted mean difference — 34.8 hours, 95% CI −62.1, −7.4), but no significant differences in major clinical outcomes, such as mortality or

BPD, were found. The same meta-analysis also examined four trials that compared either ACV or PRVC ventilation to SIMV and showed that ACV compared to SIMV was associated with significantly shorter duration of ventilator weaning (weighted mean difference −42.4 hours, 95% CI −94.4, 9.6). In addition, the Cochrane meta-analysis examined trials that compared SIMV plus PS, to SIMV alone. In this comparison, there has been to date only one randomized controlled trial.[33] This study was a single-center, randomized controlled trial of 107 ELBW preterm infants who required mechanical ventilation during the first week of life. The trial compared infants who were ventilated with SIMV plus PS to those who received SIMV alone and found no significant differences in major clinical outcome such as mortality, severe IVH, air leaks or BPD.

Little is known regarding differences in time-cycled versus flow-cycled synchronized ventilation in infants. A recent prospective randomized crossover trial in ten preterm infants by De Luca *et al.* suggested that flow-cycling is perhaps as effective as time cycled SIPPV (or assist/control), but further research is needed in this area.[34]

Volume Limited Ventilation

Volume-limited (or controlled) ventilation is a form of newborn ventilation that is rapidly acquiring increasing popularity as newer ventilator and microprocessor technologies have evolved. There is limited evidence that volume-limited ventilation has a role to play in reducing the incidence of BDP.[35] In a study by Sinha *et al.* in 1997, 50 premature infants with RDS and birth weights ≥ 1200 g were randomized to either volume-controlled ventilation (VCV) or time-cycled, pressure-limited ventilation (TCPLV).[36] The VCV group had a shorter mean duration of ventilation and a trend towards a reduced incidence of IVH and BPD than the TCPLV. A Cochrane review of volume ventilation versus pressure ventilation updated as of 2005, reported a trend for reduction in the incidence of BPD (RR = 0.34, 95% CI 0.11, 1.05) ($p = 0.06$).[37]

A more recent study included 109 infants with RDS and birth weights between 600 and 1500 g.[38] The infants were randomized to receive either VCV or TCPLV. There was no difference in weaning parameters or total duration ventilation. A recent publication of the developmental follow up of these 109 preterm infants revealed a trend towards improved survival and better respiratory outcomes (fewer treatments with inhaled steroids and bronchodilators) in the VCV group at a median postmenstrual age of 22 months.[39]

High-Frequency Ventilation

High-frequency ventilation (HFV) utilizes tidal volumes for ventilation that may be smaller than the anatomic dead space. There are three basic designs of HFV that are widely used in neonatology:

- High-Frequency Oscillatory Ventilation (HFOV): This form of ventilation uses rates of (180–1200 breaths/minute). In HFOV, gas is actively "sucked" from the infant's lungs during expiration.
- High-Frequency Jet Ventilation (HFJV): This utilizes pulses of high velocity air/oxygen at a frequency range of between 240–660 breaths/minute with expiration being passive and relying upon the patient.
- High-Frequency Flow Interrupter

In general, there are two different strategies that have been historically utilized with HFV. First of all, there is a low lung volume strategy that minimizes mean airway pressure and lung inflation but often with a higher inspired O_2 fraction. On the other hand, a high lung volume strategy features a higher mean airway pressure, with associated recruitment of alveoli and minimization of lung atelectasis. This tends to improve oxygenation by increasing lung surface area and decreasing pulmonary shunting.[40]

Indications for HFV: The evidence

In term and near-term infants with respiratory failure, either "rescue" or "elective" HFOV has been found to be no better or worse than CMV.[41] A similar conclusion has been reached for the use of rescue HFJV in preterm infants with respiratory failure.[42]

In 2005, Thome et al. performed a meta-analysis of all available randomized trials of elective HFV versus conventional mechanical ventilation (CMV).[40] The authors examined important outcome such as BPD at

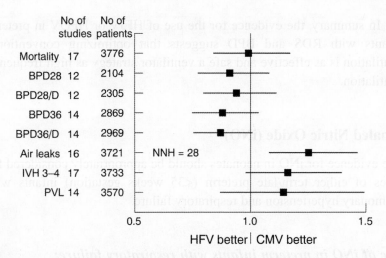

Figure 4. Overall results showing odds ratios and 95% confidence intervals, calculated according to a fixed effect model, for the analyzed outcome parameters. The significant difference in the incidence of air leaks remained significant in a random effects model. Air leaks: pneumothorax, pneumomediastinum, or pulmonary interstitial emphysema; BPD28: bronchopulmonary dysplasia, defined as oxygen or ventilator dependency at 28 days post-natal age; BPD28/D: BPD28 or death; BPD36: bronchopulmonary dysplasia, defined as oxygen or ventilator dependency at 36 weeks postmenstrual age; BPD36/D: BPD36 or death; IVH 3–4: intraventricular hemorrhage grade 3–4 according to Papile *et al.* NNH: number needed to harm; PVL: periventricular leukomalacia. (Modified from Thome UH, *et al.* (2005) Ventilatory strategies and outcome in randomized trials of high frequency ventilation. *Arch Dis Child Fetal Neonatal Ed.* 90:F466–F473. p. F467.)

36 weeks and mortality, but also included an in-depth analysis of outcomes such as IVH and pulmonary air leaks. Figure 4 illustrates some of the important findings. HFV was associated with an increase in pulmonary air leaks, with a number needed to harm of 28 infants treated with HFV.

A Cochrane meta-analysis was last updated in 2007 and included only one trial of rescue HFOV in preterm infants with respiratory failure.[43] This review concluded that rescue HFOV compared to conventional ventilation was associated with a reduction in the rate of new onset pulmonary air leaks (RR 0.73, 95% CI 0.55, 0.96) (number needed to treat: 6, 95% CI 3, 7). The rate of IVH of any grade was increased in HFOV such that for every six infants treated with rescue HFOV, one infant developed an IVH of any grade.

In summary, the evidence for the use of HFJV or HFOV in preterm infants with RDS and BPD suggests that optimizing conventional ventilation is as effective and safe a ventilator strategy as high frequency ventilation.

Inhaled Nitric Oxide (iNO)

The evidence for iNO in neonates should be appropriately considered for cases of either term/late preterm (<35 weeks gestation) infants with pulmonary hypertension and respiratory failure.

Use of iNO in preterm infants with respiratory failure: The evidence

A Cochrane systematic review has analyzed 11 randomized trials of iNO in preterm infants (<35 weeks) with respiratory failure.[44] The trials of iNO in this study population can be broadly grouped into three categories of iNO usage:

- Early rescue treatment during the first three days of life based upon oxygenation criteria
- Routine use at an early stage in intubated preterm neonates
- Use in preterm neonates at increased risk of developing BPD

The reviewers concluded that early iNO rescue treatment offered no significant benefit towards decreased mortality and BPD. In addition there was a trend towards an increase in severe IVH. Similarly, late treatment of neonates who are at increased risk of BPD showed no significant benefits towards reducing BPD. Since the last meta-analysis the recently published EUNO (European Union Nitric Oxide) examined early use of iNO within 24 hours of birth in newborns between 24 and 28 weeks 6 days.[45] The duration of iNO therapy was for a minimum of 7 and a maximum of 21 days in a total of 800 newborns. The study showed no significant difference between placebo and iNO therapy in survival without BPD.

Use of iNO in term infants with respiratory failure: The evidence

A total of 14 trials were analyzed in a Cochrane meta-analysis.[46] The use of iNO in term or near-term infants whether or not they have echocardiographic evidence of pulmonary hypertension, significantly decreases the combined outcome of death or need for ECMO (RR 0.68, 95% CI 0.59, 0.79) ($p < 0.0001$).

Surfactant Therapy

Surfactant therapy reduces mortality most effectively in preterm newborns with RDS at <30 weeks' gestation or with birth weights <1250 g. Surfactant also reduces the incidence of pneumothorax, pulmonary interstitial emphysema (PIE) and the combined outcome of death or BPD.[47] The decrease in the combined outcome of BPD or death is statistically significant from the meta-analysis of animal-derived, but not synthetic surfactant.[48–50] Prophylactic surfactant therapy is typically defined as intubation and surfactant administration most often following initial resuscitation in the delivery room, but within 30 minutes following delivery. Rescue treatment is defined as surfactant administration within the first 12 hours of life after specific criteria such oxygen and ventilatory parameters are reached.[51] Prophylactic surfactant in preterm infants results in lower mortality, pneumothorax, PIE and death or BPD than rescue treatment.[6,8] Surfactant treatment improves oxygenation and reduces the need for extracorporeal membrane oxygenation (ECMO) in neonates with meconium aspiration,[52] sepsis or pneumonia.[53] The possible role of surfactant therapy in the treatment of pulmonary hemorrhage is based upon retrospective observational studies and cannot be strongly recommended at this time.[51] There is no good clinical evidence that surfactant treatment improves respiratory outcomes in congenital diaphragmatic hernia.

Permissive Hypercapnia (PHC)

A strategy of ventilation with higher pCO_2 has been examined by three studies to date.[54–56] The largest of these was the SAVE trial by the NICHD

Neonatal Network.[54] This trial found that at 36 weeks postmenstrual age the use of mechanical ventilation was 1% in the PHC group compared to 16% in the routine ventilation group ($p < 0.01$). PHC may be a potentially better practice to impact upon the prevalence of BPD, but further research is needed.

Respiratory Stimulants — Methylxanthines and Doxapram

Methylxanthines including aminophylline/theophylline and caffeine compared to either no drug or placebo are very effective in treating apnea in premature infants with a decrease in the use of intermittent positive pressure ventilation (IPPV).[57] Methylxanthines result in a reduction in failure of extubation with a number needed to treat (NNT) of four to prevent one case of failed extubation (95% CI, 3, 7).[58] There have been concerns that caffeine could have adverse effect in neurodevelopment, but a large multicenter randomized trial showed that restriction of caffeine compared to routine caffeine dosage increased mortality/ neurodevelopmental delay at 18–21 months corrected age in VLBW infants.[59] Another trial of high versus usual caffeine dose reported short-term improvements and trends for improved neurodevelopmental outcome at one year in the high caffeine dose infants without adverse effects.[60] Methylxanthines are effective in improving short and longer term outcomes in preterm infants.

A randomized trial showed that both doxapram and theophylline resulted in a short term reduction in apnea of prematurity that is not sustained beyond one week.[61] A meta-analysis of two trials of 85 preterm infants randomized to either doxapram or placebo showed no significant effect of doxapram in the reduction of failed extubation.[62] This study showed a trend towards such adverse effects such as hypertension or irritability resulting in termination of doxapram treatment.

References

1. Carlo WA, Ambalavanan N. (1999) Conventional mechanical ventilation: Traditional and new strategies. *Pediatr Rev* **20**: e117–126.

2. Morley CJ. (2006) In: Donn SM, Sinha SK, (eds.) Continuous Positive Airway Pressure. *Manual of Neonatal Respiratory Care.* 2nd ed. Philadelphia: Mosby Elsevier, pp. 183–190.

3. De Paoli AG, Davis PG, Faber B *et al.* (2008) Devices and pressure sources for administration of nasal continuous positive airway pressure (NCPAP) in preterm neonates. *Cochrane Database Syst Rev* CD002977.

4. Ho JJ, Subramaniam P, Henderson-Smart DJ *et al.* (2002) Continuous distending pressure for respiratory distress syndrome in preterm infants. *Cochrane Database Syst Rev* CD002271.

5. Verder H, Albertsen P, Ebbesen F *et al.* (1999) Nasal continuous positive airway pressure and early surfactant therapy for respiratory distress syndrome in newborns of less than 30 weeks' gestation. *Pediatrics* **103**: E24.

6. Stevens TP, Harrington EW, Blennow M *et al.* (2007) Early surfactant administration with brief ventilation vs selective surfactant and continued mechanical ventilation for preterm infants with or at-risk for respiratory distress syndrome. *Cochrane Database Syst Rev* CD003063.

7. Rojas MA, Lozano JM, Rojas MX *et al.* (2009) Very early surfactant without mandatory ventilation in premature infants treated with early continuous positive airway pressure: A randomized, controlled trial. *Pediatrics* **123**: 137–142.

8. Soll RF, Morley CJ. (2001) Prophylactic versus selective use of surfactant in preventing morbidity and mortality in preterm infants. *Cochrane Database Syst Rev* CD000510.

9. Thomson MA. (2002) Continuous positive airway pressure and surfactant: Combined data from animal experiments and clinical trials. *Biol Neonate* **81** Suppl 1: 16–19.

10. Sandri F, Ancora G, Lanzoni A *et al.* (2004) Prophylactic nasal continuous positive airways pressure in newborns of 28–31 weeks gestation: Multicentre randomised controlled clinical trial. *Arch Dis Child Fetal Neonatal Ed* **89**: F394–F398.

11. Finer NN, Carlo WA, Duara S *et al.* (2004) Delivery room continuous positive airway pressure/positive end-expiratory pressure in extremely low birth weight infants: A feasibility trial. *Pediatrics* **114**: 651–657.

12. Subramaniam P, Henderson-Smart DJ, Davis PG. (2005) Prophylactic nasal continuous positive airways pressure for preventing morbidity and mortality in very preterm infants. *Cochrane Database Syst Rev* CD001243.

13. Morley CJ, Davis PG, Doyle LW *et al.* (2008) Nasal CPAP or intubation at birth for very preterm infants. *N Engl J Med* **358**: 700–708.

14. SUPPORT Study Group of the Eunice Kennedy Shriver NICHD Neonatal Research Network, Finer NN, Carlo WA, Walsh MC *et al.* (2010) Early CPAP versus surfactant in extremely preterm infants. *N Engl J Med* **362**(21): 1970–1979.

15. Vermont Oxford Network DRM Study Group, Dunn M, Kaempf J, de Klerk J *et al.* (2010) Delivery room management of preterm infants at risk for respiratory distress syndrome (RDS). *Pediatric Academic Societies'* 2010 Annual Meeting May 1–4. E-PAS2010: 1670.2.

16. Gupta S, Sinha SK, Tin W, Donn SM. (2009) A randomized controlled trial of post-extubation bubble continuous positive airway pressure versus Infant Flow Driver continuous positive airway pressure in preterm infants with respiratory distress syndrome. *J Pediatr* **154**: 645–650.

17. Dempsey EM, Barrington KJ. (2006) Noninvasive Ventilation. In Donn SM, Sinha SK (eds.) *Manual of Neonatal Respiratory Care.* 2nd ed. Mosby Elsevier, Philadelphia, pp. 191–194.

18. Garland JS, Nelson DB, Rice T *et al.* (1985) Increased risk of gastrointestinal perforations in neonates mechanically ventilated with either face mask or nasal prongs. *Pediatrics* **76**: 406–410.

19. Lemyre B, Davis PG, de Paoli AG. (2002) Nasal intermittent positive pressure ventilation (NIPPV) versus nasal continuous positive airway pressure (NCPAP) for apnea of prematurity. *Cochrane Database Syst Rev* CD002272.

20. Pantalitschka T, Sievers J, Urschitz MS *et al.* (2009) Randomised crossover trial of four nasal respiratory support systems for apnoea of prematurity in very low birth weight infants. *Arch Dis Child Fetal Neonatal Ed* **94**: F245–F248.

21. Barrington KJ, Bull D, Finer NN. (2001) Randomized trial of nasal synchronized intermittent mandatory ventilation compared with continuous positive airway pressure after extubation of very low birth weight infants. *Pediatrics* **107**: 638–641.

22. Sai Sunil Kishore M, Dutta S, Kumar P. (2009) Early nasal intermittent positive pressure ventilation versus continuous positive airway pressure for respiratory distress syndrome. *Acta Paediatr* **98**: 1412–1415.

23. Bisceglia M, Belcastro A, Poerio V *et al.* (2007) A comparison of nasal intermittent versus continuous positive pressure delivery for the treatment of

moderate respiratory syndrome in preterm infants. *Minerva Pediatr* **59**: 91–95.

24. Kugelman A, Feferkorn I, Riskin A *et al.* (2007) Nasal intermittent mandatory ventilation versus nasal continuous positive airway pressure for respiratory distress syndrome: A randomized, controlled, prospective study. *J Pediatr* **150**: 521–526.

25. Bhandari V, Gavino RG, Nedrelow JH *et al.* (2007) A randomized controlled trial of synchronized nasal intermittent positive pressure ventilation in RDS. *J Perinatol* **27**: 697–703.

26. Bhandari V, Finer NN, Ehrenkranz RA *et al.* (2009) Synchronized nasal intermittent positive-pressure ventilation and neonatal outcomes. *Pediatrics* **124**: 517–526.

27. ClinicalTrials.gov [Internet]. Ontario: McMaster University; c2007-2009. Efficacy and Safety of NIPPV to increase survival without bronchopulmonary dysplasia in extremely low birth weight infants; 2009 Aug 7. Available from: http://clinicaltrials.gov/ct2/show/NCT00433212.

28. Henderson–Smart DJ, Wilkinson A, Raynes-Greenow CH. (2002) Mechanical ventilation for newborn infants with respiratory failure due to pulmonary disease. *Cochrane Database Syst Rev* CD002770.

29. Greenough A, Dimitriou G, Prendergast M *et al.* (2008) Synchronized mechanical ventilation for respiratory support in newborn infants. *Cochrane Database Syst Rev* CD000456.

30. Donn SM, Sinha SK. (2006) In Donn SM, Sinha SK. (eds.) Synchronized Intermittent Mandatory Ventilation. *Manual of Neonatal Respiratory Care.* 2nd ed. Mosby Elsevier, Philadelphia, pp. 200–202.

31. Carlo WA, Ambalavanam N, Chatburn RL. In: (2006) Donn SM and Sinha SK (eds.), Classification of Mechanical Ventilation Devices. *Manual of Neonatal Respiratory Care.* 2nd ed. Mosby Elsevier, Philadelphia, pp. 74–80.

32. Donn SM, Bandy KP. (2006) In Donn SM, Sinha SK. (eds.) Volume-Controlled Ventilation. *Manual of Neonatal Respiratory Care.* 2nd ed. Mosby Elsevier, Philadelphia, pp. 206–209.

33. Reyes ZC, Claure N, Tauscher MK *et al.* (2006) Randomized, controlled trial comparing synchronized intermittent mandatory ventilation and synchronized intermittent mandatory ventilation plus pressure support in preterm infants. *Pediatrics* **118**: 1409–1417.

34. De Luca D, Conti G, Piastra M *et al.* (2009) Flow-cycled versus time-cycled sIPPV in preterm babies with RDS: A breath-to-breath randomised cross-over trial. *Arch Dis Child Fetal Neonatal Ed* **94**: F397–F401.
35. Sinha SK, Donn SM. (2008) Newer forms of conventional ventilation for preterm newborns. *Acta Paediatr* **97**: 1338–1343.
36. Sinha SK, Donn SM, Gavey J *et al.* (1997) Randomised trial of volume controlled versus time cycled, pressure limited ventilation in preterm infants with respiratory distress syndrome. *Arch Dis Child Fetal Neonatal Ed* **77**: F202–F205.
37. McCallion N, Davis PG, Morley CJ. (2005) Volume-targeted versus pressure-limited ventilation in the neonate. *Cochrane Database Syst Rev* CD003666.
38. Singh J, Sinha SK, Clarke P *et al.* (2006) Mechanical ventilation of very low birth weight infants: Is volume or pressure a better target variable? *J Pediatr* **149**: 308–313.
39. Singh J, Sinha SK, Alsop E *et al.* (2009) Long-term follow-up of very low birthweight infants from a neonatal volume versus pressure mechanical ventilation trial. *Arch Dis Child Fetal Neonatal Ed* **94**: F360–F362.
40. Thome UH, Carlo WA, Pohlandt F. (2005) Ventilation strategies and outcome in randomised trials of high frequency ventilation. *Arch Dis Child Fetal Neonatal Ed* **90**: F466–F473.
41. Henderson–Smart DJ, De Paoli AG, Clark RH *et al.* (2009) High frequency oscillatory ventilation versus conventional ventilation for infants with severe pulmonary dysfunction born at or near term. *Cochrane Database Syst Rev* CD002974.
42. Joshi VH, Bhuta T. (2006) Rescue high frequency jet ventilation versus conventional ventilation for severe pulmonary dysfunction in preterm infants. *Cochrane Database Syst Rev* CD000437.
43. Bhuta T, Henderson–Smart DJ. (2000) Rescue high frequency oscillatory ventilation versus conventional ventilation for pulmonary dysfunction in preterm infants. *Cochrane Database Syst Rev* CD000438.
44. Barrington KJ, Finer NN. (2007) Inhaled nitric oxide for respiratory failure in preterm infants. *Cochrane Database Syst Rev* CD000509.
45. Mercier JC, Hummler H, Durrmeyer X *et al.* (2010) Inhaled nitric oxide for prevention of bronchopulmonary dysplasia in premature babies (EUNO): A randomized controlled trial. *Lancet* **376** (9738): 346–354.

46. Finer NN, Barrington KJ. (2006) Nitric oxide for respiratory failure in infants born at or near term. *Cochrane Database Syst Rev* CD000399.

47. Soll RF. (2000) Prophylactic natural surfactant extract for preventing morbidity and mortality in preterm infants. *Cochrane Database Syst Rev* CD000511.

48. Soll RF, Blanco F. (2001) Natural surfactant extract versus synthetic surfactant for neonatal respiratory distress syndrome. *Cochrane Database Syst Rev* CD000144.

49. Soll RF. (2000) Synthetic surfactant for respiratory distress syndrome in preterm infants. *Cochrane Database Syst Rev* CD001149.

50. Soll R, Ozek E. (2010) Prophylactic protein free synthetic surfactant for preventing morbidity and mortality in preterm infants. *Cochrane Database Syst Rev* CD001079.

51. Engle WA; American Academy of Pediatrics Committee on Fetus and Newborn. (2008) Surfactant-replacement therapy for respiratory distress in the preterm and term neonate. *Pediatrics* **121**: 419–432.

52. El Shahed AI, Dargaville P, Ohlsson A *et al.* (2007) Surfactant for meconium aspiration syndrome in full term/near term infants. *Cochrane Database Syst Rev* CD002054.

53. Finer NN. (2004) Surfactant use for neonatal lung injury: Beyond respiratory distress syndrome. *Paediatr Respir Rev* **5** Suppl A: S289–S297.

54. Carlo WA, Stark AR, Wright LL *et al.* (2002) Minimal ventilation to prevent bronchopulmonary dysplasia in extremely-low-birth-weight infants. *J Pediatr* **141**: 370–374.

55. Mariani G, Cifuentes J, Carlo WA. (1999) Randomized trial of permissive hypercapnia in preterm infants. *Pediatrics* **104**:1082–1088.

56. Thome UH, Carroll W, Wu TJ, *et al.* (2006) Outcome of extremely preterm infants randomized at birth to different PaCO2 targets during the first seven days of life. *Biol Neonate* **90**: 218–225.

57. Henderson–Smart DJ, Steer P. (2001) Methylxanthine treatment for apnea in preterm infants. *Cochrane Database Syst Rev* CD000140.

58. Henderson–Smart DJ, Davis PG. (2003) Prophylactic methylxanthines for extubation in preterm infants. *Cochrane Database Syst Rev* CD000139.

59. Schmidt B, Roberts RS, Davis P *et al.* (2007) Long-term effects of caffeine therapy for apnea of prematurity. *N Engl J Med* **357**:1893–1902.

60. Steer P, Flenady V, Shearman A *et al.* (2004) High dose caffeine citrate for extubation of preterm infants: A randomised controlled trial. *Arch Dis Child Fetal Neonatal Ed* **89**: F499–F503.

61. Peliowski A, Finer NN. (1990) A blinded, randomized, placebo-controlled trial to compare theophylline and doxapram for the treatment of apnea of prematurity. *J Pediatr* **116**: 648–653.

62. Henderson–Smart DJ, Davis PG. (2000) Prophylactic doxapram for the prevention of morbidity and mortality in preterm infants undergoing endotracheal extubation. *Cochrane Database Syst Rev* CD001966.

Chapter 8

Congenital Heart Diseases in the Newborn

Lloyd R. Feit and Sara R. Ford

Acyanotic Congenital Heart Disease

These lesions mainly fall into two categories: shunt lesions, where there is L-R shunt at an anatomical defect, and obstructive lesions.

- **Shunt Lesions** [ventricular septal defect (VSD), atrial septal defect (ASD), Patent ductus arteriosus (PDA), and Endocardial Cushion Defects (ECD)]

  There is increased pulmonary blood flow (left to right shunt). These lesions typically present with a murmur and/or symptoms of congestive heart failure (pulmonary overcirculation).

  Pediatric "congestive heart failure" (CHF) describes a clinical syndrome wherein systemic cardiac output is inadequate to meet the needs of the distal organ beds. In contrast to adult CHF, where symptoms are typically due to pump dysfunction, CHF in infants with L-R shunt lesions is due to diminution of *systemic* cardiac output due to pulmonary overcirculation. The term heart failure is somewhat of a misnomer, as the heart is not failing; in fact, heart function is commonly hyperdynamic. Pediatric CHF primarily manifests as dyspnea and tachypnea at rest or with exertion. Tachypnea can often appear "comfortable," with mild retractions, or with severe respiratory

171

distress. Dyspnea and diaphoresis with feeding and sometimes at rest is also seen, as well as poor feeding or fatigue with feeding. Poor weight gain is a hallmark of symptomatic CHF, due to inadequate caloric intake, and increased metabolic demand/consumption of calories from the increased work of breathing and hyperdynamic myocardial function.

- **Obstructive Lesions** (Pulmonic Stenosis, Aortic Stenosis, Coarctation of the Aorta)

Systemic: diminished cardiac output, poor pulses, despite a hyperdynamic cardiac impulse.

Pulmonary: decreased pulmonary blood flow; most with no symptoms, however, low cardiac output can occur with severe obstruction. Obstructive lesions typically present as a murmur and/or symptoms of systemic or pulmonary obstruction.

Shunt lesions

Ventricular septal defect

Most common congenital heart defect. Incidence as high as 5/1000 in newborn; represents 20–25% of CHD. Septum consists of muscular and membranous portions, defects vary in size and location. The types of VSD include perimembranous, subpulmonary (supracristal), inlet and muscular.

Clinical features

The size and location of the defect will impact its hemodynamic effects and likelihood of spontaneous closure. The majority of small defects will close spontaneously. Downstream resistance to flow, either in the right ventricular outflow tract, or pulmonary vascular bed, also determines the volume of pulmonary blood flow and resultant symptoms.

Symptoms, if present, typically begin at 2–4 weeks of age when pulmonary vascular resistance decreases, and pulmonary overcirculation develops. Symptoms of pulmonary overcirculation include rapid breathing, diaphoresis, poor feeding, and poor weight gain. Symptomatic pulmonary overcirculation is more likely to develop with moderate to large VSDs (Pulmonary blood flow/systemic blood flow ≥2 to 1).

Diagnosis

Physical exam: Grade 2–5/6 holosystolic or nearly holosystolic murmur loudest at left sternal border; location may vary depending on the type of defect and direction of jet.

If the shunt is large, there may be a diastolic flow murmur reflecting increased volume of blood flow across the mitral valve. The pulmonary component of second heart sound may be increased if there is pulmonary hypertension. With significant pulmonary overcirculation, there will be tachypnea, retractions, and diaphoresis.

Electrocardiogram: Normal for small VSDs, Left ventricular hypertrophy due to volume loading or biventricular hypertrophy if VSD is large.

Chest X-ray: Normal or cardiomegaly with increase pulmonary vascular markings if VSD is large.

Echocardiogram: Two dimensional and Doppler echocardiogram is diagnostic: defines the location and size of defect, estimates right ventricular/ pulmonary artery pressure, and the degree of left heart volume loading.

Management

Medical: Symptoms of pulmonary overcirculation can be managed with medications. Diuretics such as furosemide, ± spironolactone are the mainstay of therapy. Occasionally digoxin and afterload reduction with ACE inhibitors are also used.

Surgical: Surgical repair is indicated when symptomatic pulmonary over-circulation ("congestive heart failure") cannot be managed with medications: 1–3 months old for CHF and failure to thrive.

Surgical repair is also indicated if pulmonary hypertension persists at 6–12 months, or for persistent left heart volume loading at 3–5 years old.

Atrial septal defect

Atrial Septal Defect occurs in 1/1500 live births, 6–10% of CHD, and is twice as common in females as in males.

It is the most common defect "escaping" detection in childhood (i.e. initially diagnosed as an adult). The types of ASDs include ostium secundum (most common), ostium primum, superior sinus venosus, and inferior sinus venosus (also called unroofed coronary sinus) depending on the location in the atrial septum.

Clinical features

ASDs, even when large, are usually clinically asymptomatic and detected on evaluation for a murmur, abnormal ECG, or found incidentally on echocardiogram. The majority of small secundum defects will undergo spontaneous closure; ostium primum and sinus venosus defects will not.

Diagnosis

Physical examination: Non-specific systolic ejection murmur is best heard at the upper left sternal border, reflecting increased flow across the pulmonary valve. There is persistently split S2 which does not become single with expiration, also reflecting increased flow across the pulmonary valve which delays pulmonary valve closure (the second component of S2).

Electrocardiogram may be normal if there is only mild right heart volume loading. A rsR' pattern in the anterior precordial leads, right ventricular hypertrophy, and right axis deviation on ECG are typically seen with significant right heart volume loading. Because the ostium primum ASD is a type of endocardial cushion defect, there is a counter clockwise frontal plane vector loop.

Chest X-ray

For small defects the chest X-ray is usually normal. With significant right heart volume loading, there is cardiomegaly and increased pulmonary vascular markings.

Echocardiogram is diagnostic for the location and size of the defect, as well as degree of right heart volume loading. The ostium secundum ASD — center of atrial septum in the region of the fossa ovalis; ostium primum ASD — inferior portion of atrial septum; partial form of A-V canal defect, thus associated with a cleft in anterior leaflet of mitral valve. The superior sinus venosus ASD — near SVC, often overlooked in 4-chamber view, usually PAPVC of right pulmonary veins; inferior sinus venosus ASD seen best in the subcoastal views.

Management

In older patients, closure at diagnosis is recommended, or between two and four years old. Rarely, earlier closure is indicated for respiratory symptoms, failure to thrive, or co-morbidities like chronic lung disease or pulmonary hypertension. Closure options include surgical repair for very large secundum defects, and all primum, superior/inferior sinus venosus defects. Smaller defects are amenable to device closure in a catheter-based approach.

Patent ductus arteriosus (PDA)

The incidence of PDA is inversely proportional to gestational age, occurring in 1–2/5000 live births. With prematurity, the incidence is 8/1000, and increases with decreasing birth weight. The ductus arteriosus connects the pulmonary artery (at the level of the proximal left PA) to the descending aorta, just distal to the origin of the left subclavian artery. This structure shunts a portion of cardiac output away from the lungs during fetal life, and typically closes within several days after birth.

Clinical features

In the term newborn or infant, a characteristic continuous murmur may be detected, and there may be symptoms of pulmonary overcirculation. In the preterm infant, worsening respiratory distress, a murmur, bounding pulses, hypotension, and increasing apnea, may be indicators of a PDA. It is critical to maintain a high index of suspicion for PDA in preemies, as there may be no murmur, and clinical symptoms may be highly variable in the very low birth weight infant.

Diagnosis

Physical examination: Depending on the degree of pulmonary overcirculation, there may be tachypnea, increased precordial impulse, widened pulse pressure (bounding pulses) and a murmur. In the preterm infant there may be no murmur, or the murmur can be systolic and nonspecific. The classic murmur in the term or older infant is a 2–4/6 continuous "machinery-like" murmur at the upper left sternal border or midclavicular region.

Electrocardiogram: Findings are similar to a VSD and reflect degree of left heart volume loading: normal or LVH for smaller shunts, LVH or combined VH for large PDAs. With pulmonary HTN there may be RVH.

Chest X-ray: May be normal with small PDA; with large shunt there will be cardiomegaly and increased pulmonary vascular markings.

Echocardiogram: Two dimensional and Doppler echocardiography is diagnostic and can determine size, degree of left heart volume loading and estimate pulmonary artery pressures.

Management

The management of PDA in the preterm newborn is discussed in detail elsewhere in this Handbook. In general, indomethacin or ibuprofen is used in the preterm newborn. If unsuccessful, surgical ligation may be indicated. In infants and older children, a catheter-based approach using a coil or device, especially if small, is effective. For larger PDAs, ligation is performed via video assisted thoracoscopic surgery (VATS) or surgery using a left lateral thoracotomy approach.

Atrio-ventricular canal defect (AVCD)

Synonyms: Endocardial cushion defect (ECD), atrioventricular septal defect, partial or transitional AV canal defect.

There exist a spectrum of defects resulting from abnormal development of the endocardiocardial cushions *in utero*. The incidence is 0.19/1000, and constitutes 4–5% of CHD. There is a strong association with trisomy 21 (Down syndrome), where it is the most common form of heart disease.

The most common form is complete AVCD, where there is a large primum ASD or common atrium, a single, common atrioventricular valve (with a cleft in the anterior "mitral" leaflet), and inlet VSD of variable size. It should be noted that there is only a single AV valve, comprising of embryologic portions of both the mitral and tricuspid valves. In the partial and transitional forms, there are typically two separate AV valve annuli. In partial AVCD, there is a primum ASD, cleft in the anterior mitral leaflet, with no VSD. Transitional (or incomplete) AVCD includes a primum ASD or common atrium, cleft mitral valve and deficiency in the inlet portion of the ventricular septum with AV valve attachments to the crest of the septum plus/minus a small VSD.

Clinical features

The clinical features are variable and dependent on the type of AVCD. With partial AVCD, the ventricular defect is small or absent, and the atrial component may be large. Thus the clinical features are similar to that of a large ASD and the infant is most often asymptomatic. With complete AVCD, the size of the VSD and degree of pulmonary overcirculation determines the symptomatology, as discussed in the section on VSDs. Patients with complete AVCD and a sizable VSD may have symptomatic pulmonary overcirculation which may be difficult to medically manage. At times, the large VSD contributes to high PA pressures, and there is a delayed fall in pulmonary vascular resistance. This limits symptoms of CHF, and may even obviate an audible murmur. In this setting, pulmonary hypertension is a major complicating issue if not managed, and the absence of a murmur may contribute to missing the diagnosis. The American Academy of Pediatrics currrently recommends an echo evaluation of all newborns with trisomy 21 in the first weeks of life.

Diagnosis

Physical examination: Depending on the type of AVCD, the physical examination may be the same as that of an ASD or VSD. If there is a complete AVCD with a large VSD, there may be no murmur, or a murmur of increased pulmonary blood flow. The degree of pulmonary hypertension (HTN) will also influence the presence and character of the murmur. Oxygen saturation will typically be in the 85–93% range.

Electrocardiogram: All patients with forms of AVCD have a counterclockwise frontal plane vector loop, which can be identified by left axis deviation, Q waves in leads I and aVL, and leads II, III, and aVF will be negative. The presence of right or left ventricular hypertrophy is dependent on the presence of an ASD, VSD, and or pulmonary HTN.

Chest X-ray: May be normal or show cardiomegaly and increased pulmonary vascular markings depending on the degree of pulmonary overcirculation.

Echocardiogram: Two dimensional and Doppler echocardiography is diagnostic and identifies atrial and ventricular components of the defect, presence of a cleft in the anterior mitral leaflet and degree of mitral regurgitation, and characteristics of a common atrioventricular valve. It is also useful in determining the size of the VSD, degree of left heart volume loading and in estimating pulmonary artery pressures.

Management

The management is dependent on the type of AVCD present. For partial AVCD (primum ASD, cleft mitral valve) the management is the same as for other ASDs. Because a primum ASD will not undergo spontaneous closure, elective surgical repair is generally performed after the first year. With complete AVCD, symptomatic pulmonary overcirculation can be managed with medications. Diuretics such as furosemide, ± spironolactone are the mainstay of therapy. Occasionally digoxin and afterload reduction with ACE inhibitors are also used. Failure to thrive associated with CHF can often be managed with fortified calorie feeds. Surgery for complete AVCD is generally performed at greater than three months old but can be performed earlier for CHF that is refractory to medical management.

Obstructive lesions

Pulmonary valve stenosis

Incidence: Pulmonary valve stenosis represents 5–8% of congenital heart disease, with a slight female predominance. The majority of pulmonic stenosis is valvar, but subvalvar (infundibular) or supravalvar can be seen, most often associated with other congenital heart defects or syndromes. Pulmonary valve dyplasia (thickened, stiff leaflets) is seen in Noonan syndrome.

Clinical features

Mild to moderate pulmonary stenosis is almost always asymptomatic and detected only by a murmur or click. Even severe pulmonary stenosis may be asymptomatic or cause exertional dyspnea or rarely, symptomatic right heart failure. The newborn with critical pulmonic stenosis typically presents with cyanosis (atrial right to left "pop-off"), and tachypnea.

Diagnosis

Physical exam: The intensity and duration of the murmur reflects the severity of obstruction. With mild or moderate stenosis, a grade 2–4/6 harsh systolic ejection murmur is heard at the upper left sternal border with radiation to the axillae and posteriorly. Often there is an ejection click at the upper left sternal border. With critical PS, there may be cyanosis and little or no murmur due to minimal antergrade flow across the valve.

ECG: Often normal with mild PS. With moderate PS there may be right axis deviation and RVH, in severe PS a RV strain pattern (upright T waves in the anterior precordial leads) develops.

Chest X-ray: May be normal or show a prominent main pulmonary artery segment due to post-stenotic dilation. Heart size is usually normal and decreased pulmonary vascular markings is seen only in critical pulmonic stenosis.

Echocardiogram: Two dimensional and Doppler echocardiography is diagnostic and identifies the site (valvar, subvalvar, supravalvar) and severity of obstruction. Thickened valve leaflets with systolic doming is often seen. It also demonstrates post-stenotic dilation of the main and branch pulmonary arteries and the degree of right ventricular hypertrophy.

Management

Mild to moderate pulmonary stenosis is asymptomatic and requires no therapy. Cardiac catheterization and balloon valvuloplasty is indicated when the trans-valve peak pressure gradient at catheterization is greater than 40 mmHg, or less if the patient is symptomatic. In newborns with critical pulmonic stenosis, prostaglandin E1 infusion is initiated to provide pulmonary blood flow until catheterization and balloon valvotomy is attempted. Surgery is reserved for patients in whom percutaneous balloon valvotomy is unsuccessful, or when there is significant infundibular or branch pulmonary artery hypoplasia.

Aortic stenosis (AS)

Incidence

Aortic valve stenosis represents about 5% of congenital heart disease and has a male predominance of 4:1. The majority of aortic stenosis is valvar, but subvalvar or supravalvar obstruction can also be seen, most often associated with other congenital heart defects or syndromes.

Clinical features

Mild to moderate aortic stenosis is usually asymptomatic and detected only by a murmur or click. Severe aortic stenosis may be asymptomatic or cause exercise intolerance or syncope. The newborn with critical aortic stenosis typically presents with tachypnea, tachycardia, and cardiogenic shock due to pump dysfunction and inadequate systemic cardiac output when the PDA closes.

Diagnosis

Physical exam: The intensity and duration of the murmur reflects the severity of obstruction. With mild or moderate stenosis, a grade 2–4/6 harsh systolic ejection murmur is heard at the upper right sternal border with radiation to the neck. Often there is an ejection click at the apex or right upper sternal border. With critical aortic stenosis, there may be little or no murmur due to minimal antegrade flow across the valve, and there may be cyanosis if the LV dysfunction is severe.

ECG: Often normal with mild AS. With moderate AS there is left ventricular (LV) hypertrophy, and in severe AS a LV strain pattern (flipped T waves with sagging ST segment in the left precordial leads) develops.

Chest X-ray: May be normal or show dilated ascending aorta. With critical AS there may be cardiomegaly and pulmonary vascular congestion.

Echocardiogram: Two dimensional and Doppler echocardiography is diagnostic and identifies the site (valvar, subvalvar, supravalvar, diffuse "tunnel-like") and severity of obstruction. Typically the valve is thickened with decreased mobility, often with complete or partial fusion of valve leaflets. There may be post-stenotic dilation of the ascending aorta. With severe AS there may be LV hypertrophy and dysfunction as well as endocardial fibroelastosis. In the setting of LV dysfunction and/or mitral regurgitation, Doppler may underestimate the degree of stenosis.

Management

Mild to moderate aortic stenosis is usually asymptomatic and requires no therapy. Cardiac catherization and balloon valvuloplasty is indicated when the mean instantaneous pressure gradient by Doppler echocardiogram is greater than 60 mmHg, or less if the patient is symptomatic. In newborns with critical aortic stenosis, prostaglandin E1 infusion is initiated to provide systemic blood flow until catheterization and balloon valvotomy is attempted. Surgery is reserved for patients in whom percutaneous balloon valvotomy is unsuccessful, or when there is significant associated aortic regurgitation.

Coarctation of aorta

Incidence

Coarctation of the aorta represents about 8% of congenital heart disease with a male predominance of 2:1. The narrowing is most often "juxtaductal" in location; that is just distal to the origin of the left subclavian artery where the ductus arteriosus joins the descending aorta. The narrowing can be discrete (most often related to a "posterior shelf" of tissue) or more diffuse and tubular. Coarctation of the aorta can be seen as an isolated finding, but is often seen in association with bicuspid aortic valve and other more complex left heart obstructive cardiac defects (such as HLHS), or in association with syndromes.

Clinical features

The clinical features are variable and dependent on the age at presentation, severity of obstruction and associated abnormalities. In the newborn, symptoms of poor systemic output (cardiogenic shock) and congestive heart failure are present in the first two weeks of life when the ductus arteriosus closes. As the ductus constricts just opposite the "posterior shelf", obstruction to systemic output becomes severe, causing symptoms of pump dysfunction and CHF. In older infants and children, coarctation of the aorta is usually asymptomatic, presenting as right upper extremity hypertension, a murmur, and/or absent or diminished femoral pulses.

Diagnosis

Physical exam: As described above, the physical exam is variable depending on the age and presentation of the patient. A heart murmur may be present, and an ejection click or systolic ejection murmur suggests associated bicuspid aortic valve and aortic stenosis. In older children, a continuous murmur, heard best posteriorly and medial to the scapulae, reflects increased flow through intercostal collateral vessels. Absent femoral pulses or brachial-femoral pulse delay are typically present.

ECG: Right ventricular hypertrophy or biventricular hypertrophy may be present in infants; in older children ECG is often normal.

Chest X-ray: In infants, cardiomegaly and increased pulmonary vascular markings may be present. In older children heart size is typically normal, and "rib notching" due to dilated intercostal collateral vessels may be seen. Indentation of the aorta at the coarctation site may produce a "3" sign.

Echocardiogram: Two dimensional and Doppler echocardiography is diagnostic and identifies the site, severity, and length of coarctation. In infants, the presence of a discrete "posterior shelf" is typically described. The presence of the ductus arteriosus, arch anatomy, and the presence or absence of associated abnormalities including bicuspid aortic valve, aortic stenosis and a VSD are identified. The characteristic Doppler findings include a "double-envelope" pattern across the coarctation site, as well as continuous diastolic antegrade flow in the distal descending aorta. Rarely, cardiac MRI may be necessary if the coarctation site is difficult to visualize echocardiographically.

Management

In newborn presenting with cardiogenic shock, initial treatment involves prostaglandin infusion to re-open or increase the size of the ductus arteriosus to improve perfusion distal to the coarctation. Correction of acidosis and stabilization of circulation with volume and inotropic support are necessary prior to surgical repair. Surgery involves resection of the coarctation, end-to-end anastomosis of the normal aorta, and occasionally subclavian flap augmentation for long segment coarctation. In symptomatic infants and children, surgery is performed upon diagnosis. Some older children, adolescents, and adults may be candidates for a cardiac catheterization-based approach which typically involves balloon angioplasty and/or stent placement to relieve the obstruction. Restenosis requiring re-intervention may occur in 10–20% of patients, most often in patients repaired in the first month of life. Ballon angioplasty for this restenosis is highly successful. In the long term, patients must be monitored for restenosis, hypertension and aneurysm formation, both in the ascending aorta, and at the coarctation repair site. Older patients treated with patch angioplasty many years ago appear to be at highest risk for aneurysm formation.

Cyanotic Heart Disease in the Newborn

In the newborn, it is critical to make a thoughtful approach to the differential diagnosis of cyanosis, as prompt, appropriate management can be lifesaving. The most important step in making the differential diagnosis lies in determining whether cyanosis is pulmonary or cardiac in origin, although there is a smattering of other, less common diagnostic considerations such as hemoglobinopathies. It is probably most reasonable to begin with a definition of cyanosis. Cyanosis is defined as the appearance of a bluish hue to the patient's skin. Cyanosis is subjective, subject to many other factors including the experience of the observer, skin pigmentation, and fetal hemoglobin concentration. The term cyanosis should be distinguished from hypoxemia or desaturation, which are more quantitative measures of arterial oxygen content.

Distinction must first be made between peripheral and central cyanosis. In *central* cyanosis, this occurs when arterial blood carries 3–5 g/dl of desaturated hemoglobin that does not carry oxygen and is manifest as decreased arterial saturation. *Peripheral* cyanosis occurs when arterial blood carries the normal amount of oxygen, but there is increased oxygen extraction in the tissues, usually from sluggish blood flow in cool extremities or normal newborn vasomotor instability. The skin (often extremities and circumoral area) appears blue due to prominence of venous networks in the skin.

Differential diagnosis and classification: When considering the number of different diagnoses, it is useful to first consider the pathophysiology:

(1) Ventilation/perfusion mismatch:

    a.   Pneumonia, aspiration, hyaline membrane disease, pulmonary hypoplasia, etc.

b. Extrinsic lung compression such as from pneumothorax, diaphragmatic hernia, thoracic cage deformity.

(2) Right-left shunt which can occur at various levels:

a. Intracardiac such as tricuspid atresia or tetralogy of Fallot or congenital anomalies of systemic venous drainage.

b. At the great artery level: through a PDA due to elevated pulmonary vascular resistance (PVR) as in persistent pulmonary hypertension of the newborn.

c. Intrapulmonary R-L shunt such as in pulmonary AV malformations.

(3) Alveolar hypoventilation:

a. CNS hypoventilation with brain injury, asphyxia or sedation.

b. Distal neuromuscular disease such as myasthenia gravis.

c. Airway obstruction or anatomic anomalies of the tracheo-bronchial tree.

(4) Hemoglobinopathies such as methemoglobinemia.

Incidence. Congenital heart disease occurs in approximately 8/1000 live births. The largest percentage of this group are septal defects that are rarely life-threatening, and many are hemodynamically insignificant. Cyanotic heart defects typically make up 20–25% of all types of CHD, but are particularly problematic in the newborn period. Cyanosis usually manifests within the first hours of life, and requires prompt recognition and management.

Assessment. It is important to remember that most forms of cyanotic CHD have diminished pulmonary blood flow due to intracardiac R-L shunt.

Physical examination. Many forms of cyanotic heart disease will have no associated murmur, and generally normal findings on cardiac examination. The absence of a murmur does not rule out CHD!

Chest X-Ray is often helpful in that the prevalent finding (with a few notable exceptions) is a paucity of pulmonary blood flow. Pulmonary vasculature is diminished, with small central pulmonary arteries and little vasculature seen in the periphery. The exceptions are total anomalous pulmonary venous return (TAPVR), especially with obstruction, and the rare patient with transposition of the great arteries or truncus arteriosus.

Hyperoxia test can be useful in discriminating cyanotic CHD from a pulmonary process. Higher FiO2 may be able to override a pulmonary process such as pneumonia, but cannot correct the hypoxemia of cyanotic CHD since intracardiac R-L shunt prevents desaturated systemic venous return from reaching the lungs to pick up oxygen.

Technique: A baseline arterial blood gas is performed from the right arm (pre-ductal), to assess adequacy of oxygenation and ventilation. Elevated pCO2 strongly suggests a pulmonary process. After 10–15 minutes in 100%-oxygen (preferably by ET tube or mask), a repeat ABG is assessed. If the pCO2 is normal, then

• If paO2 is >150, it is likely an intrapulmonary process;
• If paO2 is <120, it is likely cyanotic CHD with intracardiac R-L shunt.

NB: care must be taken to limit the time for hyperoxia test to no more than 10–15 minutes. Oxygen is a potent stimulator of ductal constriction, and may therefore exacerbate limited pulmonary blood flow, with a precipitous fall of oxygen saturation. One should consider having PGE1 infusion on hand to quickly counteract effects of ductal constriction if needed.

ECG: Although it completes the workup, the ECG is highly variable, not clearly diagnostic, though it can be helpful in certain patients. Pulmonary atresia is often associated with right axis deviation; tricuspid atresia is often associated with left axis deviation.

Echocardiography: Cardiac ultrasound is the diagnostic gold standard if cyanotic CHD is suspect. It allows for rapid and real-time assessment of anatomy and physiology. In conjunction with the other tests listed above, it is helpful in determining best options for further management such as need for catheterization or urgent surgery.

List of conditions causing cyanosis

Purely cardiac conditions include the following:

- D-Transposition of the great arteries (D-TGA)
- Tetralogy of Fallot
- Tricuspid atresia and other tricuspid valve abnormalities
- Pulmonary atresia and other forms of right heart hypoplasia
- Hypoplastic left heart syndrome and other left heart obstructions
- Total anomalous pulmonary venous return (TAPVR)
- Truncus arteriosus
- Complex single ventricle variants

Cardiopulmonary conditions include the following:

- Persistent pulmonary hypertension of the newborn (PPHN)

D-Transposition of the great arteries (D-TGA)

This is the most common of all forms of cyanotic CHD. There is a 2:1 male:female predominance and is more common in firstborn child. In this condition the great arteries arise from the contralateral ventricle, so that the RV gives rise to the aorta, and LV gives rise to the pulmonary artery. This results in *parallel circulations*, with little mixing of the two. The only way for oxygen to reach the systemic circulation is via mixing at a patent foramen ovale (PFO), patent ductus arteriosus (PDA) or VSD (when present).

Clinical findings

The characteristic *"big blue boy"* highlights the pathophysiology in that the infant is not premature (with RDS as cause for cyanosis), has little or no symptoms of respiratory compromise, in a male that is quite blue. The cardiac exam is typically normal for age, with a single, sometimes prominent second heart sound. There may be a systolic murmur, especially if a VSD is present.

Laboratory findings

Arterial blood gas will often demonstrate marked hypoxemia in the setting of normal CO_2 representing normal ventilation. Chest X-ray typically demonstrates normal or diminished pulmonary blood flow, but it can show increased flow as well. The classic "egg on a string" is a variable finding representing the common anterior–posterior relationship of the great arteries appearing as a narrowed mediastinum. ECG findings are non-specific. Echocardiography is diagnostic, demonstrating the aorta arising from the anterior RV, parallel to the main pulmonary artery arising from the posterior LV.

Management

Initial management is aimed at improving mixing of the parallel circulations at the PDA and PFO levels to maintain adequate systemic oxygenation. This includes maintenance of ductal patency with PGE1 infusion, which should be done with care, due to rare cases of a restrictive foramen ovale. More definitive stabilization includes balloon atrial septotomy (which can be performed at the bedside with echo guidance or in the catheterization laboratory), which creates a true ASD by disrupting the flap valve of the foramen ovale, thereby promoting more stable mixing. Sometimes fluid bolus with saline, albumin or blood can augment mixing in those that do not respond to septostomy. Definitive surgical management is the arterial switch operation, which typically has excellent short and long term outcomes in the absence of complicating lesions.

Tetralogy of Fallot

Tetralogy of Fallot consists of four findings:

- Malaligned VSD
- Overriding aorta
- Variable RV outflow obstruction (infundibular, valvar and within the pulmonary arterial tree, also known as supravalvar)
- RVH

Most embryologists feel that the latter three findings are secondary to the first abnormality — the malaligned VSD.

Clinical findings

Presentation is dependent on the degree of RV outflow tract obstruction (RVOTO). If mild, blood flow at the VSD level will be L-R, the patient has the murmur of a VSD, and will be fully saturated (also known as "pink tet"). If RV outflow obstruction is significant, flow at the VSD will be R-L, the murmur will be that of RV outflow obstruction — a coarse systolic ejection murmur, and the patient will be cyanotic. The degree of cyanosis and level of desaturation is roughly related to the degree of RVOTO.

Laboratory findings

The typical chest X-ray demonstrates the "boot shaped heart" due to an absent or hypoplastic MPA shadow, in combination with a tipped up apex secondary to RVH. The EKG is usually within normal limits since the normal newborn demonstrates RV dominance, or can demonstrate RVH. Again, the echocardiography is diagnostic, defining the anatomy and any associated abnormalities such as right aortic arch (seen in ~25% of cases), additional VSDs, and coronary anatomy which all have surgical implications.

Management

It is important to determine the degree and location of RVOTO. If severe, the patient will require PGE1 infusion to maintain ductal patency for adequate pulmonary blood flow. Definitive management is surgical, and the larger surgical centers opt for infantile, single-stage complete repair. Some still take a two-stage approach, initially performing a modified BT shunt (Gore-Tex interposition graft) from subclavian artery to pulmonary artery as palliation, with second-stage complete repair at a later date.

Tricuspid atresia and other tricuspid abnormalities

Tricuspid atresia and other tricuspid abnormalities including Ebstein anomaly of the tricuspid valve, are characterized by displacement of one or more tricuspid valve leaflets and "atrialization" of a portion of the RV. The pathophysiology of both lesions is typically that of diminished pulmonary blood flow, with R-L shunting at a PFO. In tricuspid atresia, R-L foramenal flow is obligate and complete. With Ebstein anomaly, there is either functional pulmonary stenosis due to severe TV displacement, or severe tricuspid regurgitation at the dysfunctional valve.

Clinical findings

There is rarely a murmur with tricuspid atresia; there may be a loud holosystolic murmur of tricuspid regurgitation in Ebstein anomaly.

Laboratory findings

For tricuspid atresia, the ECG typically shows left axis deviation, and the chest X-ray demonstrates the non-specific findings of decreased pulmonary blood flow. In Ebstein anomaly, the ECG may demonstrate the classic right atrial enlargement, pre-excitation (WPW) or right bundle branch block. The typical chest X-ray finding of severe Ebstein anomaly is a "wall to wall" heart due to massive right atrial enlargement. Cardiac echo is diagnostic and necessary to define associated lesions and assess hemodynamics.

Management

In tricuspid atresia, initial management depends on the presence of an associated VSD. If a VSD is present, there is usually adequate pulmonary blood flow. If the VSD is small, or absent, then PGE1 infusion is necessary to maintain pulmonary blood flow. Surgical palliation will be the staged modified Fontan procedure, the initial stage being a modified BT shunt. Patients with cyanosis in the setting of Ebstein anomaly can be very problematic to manage. Most improve with the normal transitional fall in pulmonary vascular resistance, though severe cyanosis may necessitate use of PGE1. Surgery is reserved for the most problematic patients, and predicts poor outcome if needed in infancy.

Pulmonary valve atresia with or without hypoplastic right heart

The majority of patients with pulmonary atresia have some degree of associated tricuspid stenosis and right heart hypoplasia. A small subset has a nearly normal sized TV and right ventricle, with plate-like atresia of the pulmonary valve. This latter group may be amenable to biventricular repair.

Clinical findings

Again, these patients rarely present with any findings other than severe cyanosis. There is rarely a murmur.

Laboratory findings

The ECG is often normal, but may demonstrate RVH. The chest X-ray demonstrates non-specific decreased pulmonary blood flow. The echocardiogram is diagnostic and identifies any associated lesions, and the size of the RV.

Management

These patients are clearly dependant on ductal patency for pulmonary blood flow, necessitating early infusion of PGE1. The patients with right heart hypoplasia will require modified BT shunt as part of the staged Fontan. Those with adequate sized right heart structures may be suitable for pulmonary valvuloplasty; the initial procedure often utilizes radiofrequency to create the initial orifice in the atretic pulmonary valve.

Hypoplastic left heart and other left heart obstructions

In contrast to those with diminished blood flow listed above, these patients are ductal dependent for *systemic* blood flow due to variable obstruction in left heart structures. As the PDA closes, systemic flow is reduced, resulting in low cardiac output, metabolic acidosis, pulmonary edema and cyanosis. In hypoplastic left heart syndrome (HLHS), cyanosis is due to a combination of common mixing in the single RV, and low

cardiac output when the ductus closes. In patients with neonatal coarctation, interrupted aortic arch, and Shone's syndrome (multiple left heart
obstructions), cyanosis is solely on the basis of low cardiac output.

The hyperoxia test must be used with care if these lesions are suspect.
The paO2 may improve in patients with a critical coarctation, though
metabolic acidosis may worsen as the ductus constricts in response to
higher arterial oxygen saturation.

Clinical findings

A loud single S2 is common, as manifestation of pulmonary hypertension.
Patients with HLHS usually have no murmur; those with critical aortic
stenosis or coarctation will have the typical murmur of those lesions. A
mottled, grayish skin tone is common in patients with low output and
metabolic acidosis. Blood pressure gradients are hard to measure, especially in the patient with low output. More useful is palpation of femoral
pulses, which are decreased in coarctation. All pulses may be diminished
when cardiac output is critically low.

Laboratory findings

The ECG is often not diagnostic, though may demonstrate RVH. The
chest X-ray will commonly show pulmonary edema, variable pulmonary venous congestion and generalized cardiomegaly. Cardiac
echo is diagnostic, allowing definition of site and severity of left heart
obstruction.

Management

Management is highly variable depending on the lesion. PGE1 infusion is usually needed to maintain systemic flow, often with the
addition of inotropic support with dopamine or dobutamine. Patients
with severe aortic stenosis often respond to balloon valvuloplasty. For
coarctation and interrupted aortic arch, initial surgical repair is definitive, though a percentage requires follow-up angioplasty for recurrent
coarctation. Patients with HLHS will require the stage I Fontan, which

includes aortic arch reconstruction in addition to the modified BT shunt.

Total anomalous pulmonary venous return (TAPVR)

In this lesion, the pulmonary veins drain variably to the systemic venous system. This can be sorted into four main types: supracardiac (most common), retrocardiac, infracardiac, and mixed (least common). Cyanosis occurs due to common mixing of all venous return, with subsequent R-L shunt, though can appear mild if the atrial communication is widely patent.

Clinical findings

Clinical presentation is highly variable and dependant on the presence and degree of obstruction. If TAPVR is unobstructed, symptoms of CHF develop due to the large L-R shunt, but sometimes over days to weeks. These patients have the typical findings of a large ASD, with a systolic ejection murmur at the LUSB, and wide, fixed split S2. The pathophysiology is very different if the TAPVR connection to the systemic veins is obstructed. In this complication, severe pulmonary hypertension develops, with occasional suprasystemic RV pressure and RV failure. The exam is characterized by a prominent RV heave, loud single S2, and possible hepatic congestion as a sign of RV failure.

Laboratory findings

The ECG is non-diagnostic, but can show RVH with strain if there is severe pulmonary hypertension due to obstructed pulmonary veins. The typical "snowman" appearance on chest X-ray is a variable finding, seen when there is a large common vertical vein draining to the innominate vein. If there is obstruction, the heart size is often small, and there are signs of pulmonary venous congestion. Echocardiogram is needed to define the location of pulmonary venous drainage, as well as site and degree of obstruction. On occasion, catheterization is needed to define mixed pulmonary venous return.

Management

A combination of sedation, supplemental O2, and mechanical ventilation is useful as an adjunct to normal transitional fall of PVR. Inotropic support is beneficial for RV failure, but surgical repair is the definitive therapy. Patients with obstructed TAPVR may be particularly tenuous, as a severe low output state may develop despite any form of medical management. These patients require urgent surgical repair or consideration of ECMO if surgery is not available on site.

Truncus arteriosus

In this lesion, there is embryologic failure of septation of the great arteries. A single common arterial trunk arises over a VSD, receiving cardiac output from both ventricles, and the truncal valve is often abnormal, with anywhere from 3–6 cusps. This common truncus gives rise to the normal aortic branches as well as the pulmonary arteries. Presentation for truncus can be variable, depending on the presence and severity of branch pulmonary artery (PA) stenosis. If the branch PAs are of normal caliber and unobstructed, lower pulmonary vascular resistance allows for pulmonary overflow, and the patient presents with signs of CHF and only minimal cyanosis. However, if the pulmonary arteries are hypoplastic or stenotic, then pulmonary blood flow will be diminished, and the presentation will be that of significant cyanosis, with saturation directly proportional to pulmonary blood flow.

Clinical findings

A systolic murmur is invariably present, representing either flow at the VSD, or branch PA stenosis, or both.

Laboratory findings

The chest X-ray will demonstrate the non-specific paucity of vascular markings. Echocardiography is diagnostic, and can be especially helpful in determining the pulmonary artery anatomy.

Management

Surgical repair is indicated within the first week of life, usually with excellent results. Long-term outcomes are largely dependent on function of the truncal (neo-aortic) valve.

Complex single ventricle variants

The highly variable anatomic detail of these defects precludes complete characterization in this text. However, the typical causes of cyanosis in patients with these defects are as follows:

(1) mixing of systemic and pulmonary venous return in a single ventricle, and
(2) reduced pulmonary blood flow secondary to hypoplasia of the branch pulmonary arteries.

Clinical, laboratory findings, and management

Many of these patients will have associated heterotaxy syndromes, and so careful attention should be paid to organ "sidedness" or situs. The typical "babygram" can demonstrate a right sided stomach bubble, left sided liver or reversal of the typical bronchial branching patterns as clues to heterotaxy. The chest X-ray will demonstrate decreased pulmonary vascularity: patients will require advanced imaging (catheterization, and/or cardiac MRI) to define the anatomy and hemodynamic physiology. Surgical management will be some variation of the three-stage modified Fontan procedure.

Persistent pulmonary hypertension of the newborn (PPHN)

This clinical syndrome occurs when there is a clinical scenario that prevents the normal fall in pulmonary vascular resistance (PVR) after birth. Due to a number of diverse causes and variable pathophysiology, PVR remains elevated after birth, resulting in right-to-left flow at either of the fetal shunt pathways (ductus arteriosus and/or foramen ovale). The full discussion of the varied etiologies and specific therapies are covered elsewhere in this Handbook. It should be noted that PPHN with R-L atrial level shunting can easily mimic structural cyanotic congenital heart disease and vice versa. Usually, however, history and clinical presentation can provide clues to the correct diagnosis, since the common precipitating causes are meconium aspiration syndrome, pneumonia, RDS, and congenital diaphragmatic hernia (and other space occupying lesions in the thorax). Still, echocardiography should probably be utilized to rule out structural malformations of the heart. Also, echo has become an important adjunct in managing the patient with PPHN, especially in the setting of congenital diaphragmatic hernia.

References

Acyanotic congenital heart disease

1. Miller RH, Schiebler GL, Grumbar P, Krovetz LJ. (1969) Relation of hemodynamics to height and weight percentiles in children with ventricular septal defects. *Am Heart J* **78**: 523.
2. Alter BP, Czapek EE, Rowe RD. (1968) Sweating in congenital heart disease. *Pediatrics* **41**: 123.
3. Van Praagh R, Geva T, Kreutzer J. (1989) Ventricular septal defects: How shall we describe, name and classify them? *J Am Coll Cardiol* **14**: 1298.
4. Rudolph AM. (2001) Ventricular septal defect. In: *Congenital Diseases of the Heart: Clinical-Physiological Considerations*, Rudolph AM (Ed), Futura Publishing Company, New York, p. 197.
5. Du ZD, Roguin N, Wu XJ. (1998) Spontaneous closure of muscular ventricular septal defect identified by echocardiography in neonates. *Cardiol Young* **8**(4): 500.
6. Perloff JK. (2003) Ventricular septal defect. In: *The Clinical Recognition of Congenital Heart Disease*, 5th edn., W.B. Saunders Company, Philadelphia, p. 311.
7. Gumbiner CH, Takao A. (1998) Ventricular septal defect. In: *The Science and Practice of Pediatric Cardiology*, 2nd edn., Garson A, Bricker JT, Fisher DJ, Neish SR (Eds), Williams & Wilkins, Baltimore, p. 1119.
8. Fyler DC, Rudolph AM, Wittenborg MH, Nadas AS. (1958) Ventricular septal defect in infants and children; a correlation of clinical, physiologic, and autopsy data. *Circulation* **18**: 833.

9. Kidd L, Driscoll DJ, Gersony WM, Hayes CJ, Keane JF, O'Fallon WM, Pieroni DR, Wolfe RR, Weidman WH. (1993) Second natural history study of congenital heart defects. Results of treatment of patients with ventricular septal defects. *Circulation* **87**(2 Suppl): I38–51.

10. Kirklin JW, Dushane JW. (1963) Indications for repair of ventricular septal defects. *Am J Cardiol* **12**: 75.

11. Feldt RH, Avasthey P, Yoshimasu F, *et al.* (1971) Incidence of congenital heart disease in children born to residents of Olmsted County, Minnesota, 1950–1969. *Mayo Clin Proc* **46**: 794.

12. Helgason H, Jonsdottir G. (1999) Spontaneous closure of atrial septal defects. *Pediatr Cardiol* **20**(3): 195.

13. Muta H, Akagi T, Egami K, Furui J, Sugahara Y, Ishii M, Matsuishi T. (2003) Incidence and clinical features of asymptomatic atrial septal defect in school children diagnosed by heart disease screening. *Circ J* **67**(2): 112.

14. Rostad H, Sorland S. (1979) Atrial septal defect of secundum type in patients under 40 years of age. A review of 481 operated cases. Symptoms, signs, treatment and early results. *Scand J Thorac Cardiovasc Surg* **13**(2): 123.

15. Hoffman JI, Kaplan S. (2002) The incidence of congenital heart disease. *J Am Coll Cardiol* **39**(12): 1890.

16. Webb GD, Smallhorn FJ, Terrien J, Redington AN. (2008) Congenital heart disease. In: *Braunwalds' Heart Disease*, 8th edn., Libby P, Bonow RO, Mann DL, Zipes DP (Eds), Philadelphia, p. 1561.

17. Silverman NH. (1993) *Pediatric Echocardiography*. Williams & Wilkins, Baltimore, p. 173.

18. Mendelsohn AM, Crowley DC, Lindauer A, *et al.* (1992) Rapid progression of aortic aneurysms after patch aortoplasty repair of coarctation of the aorta. *J Am Coll Cardiol* **20**: 381.

Cyanotic heart disease

19. Driscoll DJ. (1990) Evaluation of the cyanotic newborn. *Pediatr Clin North Am* **37**(1): 1.

20. Report of the New England Regional Infant Cardiac Program. 1980 *Pediatrics* **65**: 375.

21. Nadas AS. (1992) Hypoxemia. In: *Nadas' Pediatric Cardiology*, Fyler DC (Ed), Hanley & Belfus, Philadelphia, p. 73.

22. Duff DF, McNamara DG. (1998) History and physical examination of the cardiovascular system. In: *The science and practice of pediatric cardiology*, Garson A Jr, Bricker TM, Fisher DJ, Neish SR (Eds), Williams and Wilkins, Baltimore, p. 693.

23. Marino BS, Bird GL, Wernovsky G. (2001) Diagnosis and management of the newborn with suspected congenital heart disease. *Clin Perinatol* **28**(1): 91.

24. Lin AE, Di Sessa TG, Williams RG. (1986) Balloon and blade atrial septostomy facilitated by two-dimensional echocardiography. *Am J Cardiol* **57**(4): 273.

25. Blalock A, Taussig HB. (1945) Surgical treatment of malformations of the heart: In which there is pulmonary stenosis or pulmonary atresia. *Am J Med* **128**: 189.

26. Rashkind WJ, Miller WW. (1966) Creation of an atrial septal defect without thoracotomy. A palliative approach to complete transposition of the great arteries. *JAMA* **196**: 991.

27. Jatene AD, Fontes VF, Souza LC, *et al.* (1982) Anatomic correction of transposition of the great arteries. *J Thorac cardiovasc Surg* **83**: 20.

28. Pigula FA, Khalil PN, Mayer JE, *et al.* (1999) Repair of tetralogy of Fallot in neonates and young infants. *Circulation* **100**(19 Suppl): II157.

29. Tamesberger MI, Lechner E, Mair R, Hofer A, Sames-Dolzer E. (2008) Early primary repair of tetralogy of fallot in neonates and infants less than four months of age. *Tulzer G Ann Thorac Surg*, **86**(6): 1928.

30. Wald RM, Tham EB, McCrindle BW, *et al.* (2007) Outcome after prenatal diagnosis of tricuspid atresia: A multicenter experience. *American Heart Journal*. **153**(5): 772.

31. Keane JF, Fyler DC. (2006) Total anomalous pulmonary venous return. In: *Nadas' Pediatric Cardiology*, 2nd edn., Keane JF, Lock JE, Fyler DC (Eds) Saunders Elsevier, Philadelphia, p. 773.

32. Geva T, Van Praagh S. (2008) Anomalies of the Pulmonary Veins. In: *Moss and Adams' Heart Disease in Infants, Children, and Adolescents: Including the Fetus and Young Adult*, 7th edn., Allen HD, Shaddy RE, Driscoll DJ, Feltes TF (Eds), Wolters Kluwer Health/Lippincott Williams & Wilkins, Philadelphia, p. 761.

33. Noonan JA, Nadas AS. (1959) The hypoplastic left heart syndrome: an analysis of 101 cases. *Pediatr Clin North Am* **5**: 1029.

34. Norwood WI, Lang P, Hansen DD. (1983) Physiologic repair of aortic atresia-hypoplastic left heart syndrome. *N Engl J Med* **308**: 23.

35. Butto F, Lucas RV, Edwards JE. (1986) Persistent truncus arteriosus: Patho-logic anatomy in 54 cases. *Pediatr Cardiol* **7**: 95.
36. Walsh-Sukys MC, Tyson JE, Wright LL, *et al.* (2000) Persistent pulmonary hypertension of the newborn in the era before nitric oxide: Practice variation and outcomes. *Pediatrics* **105**(1 Pt 1): 14.
37. Downard CD, Wilson JM. (2003) Current therapy of infants with congenital diaphragmatic hernia. *Semin Neonatol* **8**(3): 215.

Chapter

9

Patent Ductus Arteriosus in Preterm Infant

Ronald I. Clyman

Introduction

In full-term infants, obliteration of the ductus arteriosus takes place through a process of vasoconstriction and anatomic remodeling. In the preterm infants, the ductus arteriosus frequently fails to close. The clinical consequences of a patent ductus arteriosus (PDA) are related to the degree of left-to-right shunt through the PDA with its associated change in blood flow to the brain, lungs, kidneys and intestine.

Diagnosis

Two-dimensional echocardiography and color Doppler flow mapping are the gold standards for assessing the magnitude and direction of PDA shunting. Ductus diameter ≥1.5 mm, left atrial-to–aortic root (LA/Ao) ratio ≥1.5, reversal of forward blood flow in the descending aorta during diastole and end-diastolic flow velocity in the left pulmonary artery ≥0.20 m/s, are signs consistent with a moderate-to-large PDA left-to-right shunt.

Certain clinical signs such as continuous murmur or hyperactive left ventricular impulse are relatively specific for a PDA but lack sensitivity. Conversely, worsening respiratory status, while a sensitive indicator, is relatively nonspecific for a PDA. Tachycardia is not a useful or reliable indicator of a PDA in preterm infants. In general, the chest X-ray and electrocardiogram are not useful in diagnosing a PDA.

Incidence

Echocardiographic assessments of full term infants indicate that functional closure of the ductus occurs in 90% by 48 hours, and in all by 72 hours. Essentially, all healthy preterm infants (and 90% of those with respiratory distress syndrome) who are ≥30 weeks gestation will close their ductus by the fourth day after birth. Preterm infants of less than 30 weeks gestation, with severe respiratory distress, have a 65% incidence of persistent ductus patency beyond the fourth day of life. Even among these infants, spontaneous closure can occur during the neonatal period. Ninety-four percent of infants weighing between 1000 and 1500 grams at birth will spontaneously close their ductus prior to hospital discharge. On the other hand, spontaneous ductal closure only occurs in 30-to-35% of infants weighing <1000 grams at birth during the neonatal period. Among VLBW infants that are discharged from the hospital with a persistent PDA, 86% will close by one year of age (the rest may require coil occlusion).

Infants who are small for gestational age, develop late-onset septicemia, or receive excessive fluid administration during the first days of life, are also more likely to develop a clinically symptomatic PDA. On the other hand, non-Caucasian infants and infants who receive antenatal glucocorticoids have a reduced risk of PDA. Lowering the "tolerable" range of oxygen saturations in preterm infants has led to an increased incidence of PDA (see below for effects of oxygen on the ductus).

Pathophysiology: Regulation of Ductus Arteriosus Patency and Closure

In the full term infant, closure of the ductus arteriosus occurs in two phases: (1) "functional" closure of the lumen within the first hours after birth by smooth muscle constriction, and (2) "anatomic" occlusion of the lumen over the next several days due to extensive neointimal thickening and loss of smooth muscle cells from the inner muscle media.

Balance between vasoconstriction and vasorelaxation

Ductus arteriosus patency is determined by the balance between dilating and constricting forces. The factors known to play a prominent role in ductus arteriosus regulation involve those that promote constriction (oxygen, endothelin, calcium channels, catecholamines and Rho kinase) and those that oppose it (intraluminal pressure, prostaglandins, nitric oxide, carbon monoxide, potassium channels, cyclic AMP and cyclic GMP). The relative importance of each of these factors depends on the intrauterine and extrauterine environment, the degree of ductus maturation and the genetic background and species being studied.

In utero regulation

The fetal ductus normally has a high level of intrinsic tone. The contractile proteins (smooth muscle myosin, calponin and caldesmon) are more differentiated in the ductus than they are in adjacent fetal arteries. In addition, the fetal ductus arteriosus is more sensitive to the contractile effects of calcium than are the aorta and the pulmonary artery. Endothelin-1 also appears to play a role in producing the elevated basal tone of the fetal ductus arteriosus.

The factors that oppose ductus arteriosus constriction *in utero* are better understood. The elevated vascular pressure within the ductus lumen (due to the constricted pulmonary vascular bed) plays an important role in opposing ductus constriction. The fetal ductus also produces several vasodilators that maintain ductus patency. Vasodilator prostaglandins (PGs) appear to be the dominant vasodilators that oppose ductus constriction in the later part of gestation. Inhibitors of prostaglandin synthesis constrict the fetal ductus both *in vitro* and *in vivo*. Both isoforms of the enzyme responsible for synthesizing prostaglandins (cyclooxygenase (COX)-1 and COX-2) are expressed in the fetal ductus (both nonselective {e.g. indomethacin and ibuprofen} and selective cyclooxygenase inhibitors constrict the ductus). PGE_2 is the most potent prostaglandin produced by the ductus and appears to be the most important prostanoid to regulate ductus patency. The response of the ductus to PGE_2 is unique among blood vessels since it is extraordinarily sensitive to this vasodilating substance. Prostaglandin E2 produces ductus relaxation by interacting with several of the Prostaglandin E receptors (EP2, EP3 and EP4). In contrast with other blood vessels, all of the EP receptors in the ductus can activate adenylate cyclase and relax the vessel. The increased cyclic AMP concentrations inhibit the sensitivity of the contractile proteins to calcium. Inhibitors of phosphodiesterase (the enzyme that degrades cyclic AMP) relax the ductus *in utero*. Low phosphodiesterase levels in the fetal ductus account for its increased sensitivity to PGE2.

In addition to the prostaglandins that are made within the ductus wall, circulating PGE2 concentrations also regulate fetal ductus tone and circulating concentrations of PGE2 appear to be of placental origin. In the late gestation fetal lamb, the circulating concentrations of PGE2 (approximately 1 nM) are close to those that produce maximal relaxation of the ductus. Circulating PGE2 is cleared primarily by the pulmonary endothelium. Decreased pulmonary blood flow in the fetus results in reduced pulmonary clearance and contributes to the elevated fetal plasma PGE2 concentrations.

Nitric oxide (NO), formed mainly by eNOS, is made by the fetal ductus arteriosus. PGE2 and NO appear to be preferentially coupled for reciprocal compensation since cyclooxygenase inhibition upregulates NO.

Carbon monoxide relaxes the ductus arteriosus and both hemoxygenase-1 and -2 (the enzymes that make carbon monoxide) are found within the endothelial and smooth muscle cells of the ductus. Under physiologic conditions, the amount of carbon monoxide made by the ductus does not seem to affect ductus tone; however, in circumstances where its synthesis is upregulated, e.g. endotoxemia, it may exert a relaxing influence on the ductus.

Short-term pharmacologic inhibition of prostaglandin synthesis and signaling *in utero* produces ductus constriction. On the other hand, chronic inhibition of prostaglandin synthesis *in utero* produces the opposite effect, i.e. a persistent PDA that fails to close after birth. The exact mechanisms responsible for the persistent ductus patency that follows chronic inhibition of prostaglandin signaling have yet to be elucidated. Inhibition of prostaglandin signaling may contribute to delayed closure by inhibiting hyaluronic acid production and intimal cushion formation in the ductus. Intimal cushions play an important role in permanent ductus closure after birth (see below). In addition to its function as a vasodilator, PGE2 also plays a significant role in the development of ductus contractility. PGE2 is necessary for the expression of several genes that control postnatal oxygen-induced ductus constriction (see below).

In human pregnancies, inhibition of prostaglandin synthesis induces ductus constriction *in utero* which causes ischemic hypoxia of the ductus wall, increased nitric oxide production and smooth muscle cell death within the ductus wall. These factors prevent the ductus from constricting after birth and make it resistant to the constrictive effects of postnatal indomethacin.

Postnatal regulation

There are several events that promote ductus constriction in the full term newborn following delivery: (1) an increase in arterial PO_2, (2) a decrease in blood pressure within the ductus lumen (due to the postnatal decrease in pulmonary vascular resistance), (3) a decrease in circulating PGE_2 (due to the loss of placental prostaglandin production and the increase in prostaglandin removal by the lung) and (4) a decrease in the number of PGE_2 receptors in the ductus wall. Although the newborn ductus continues to be sensitive to the vasodilating effects of NO, it loses its ability to respond to PGE2. All of these factors promote ductus constriction after birth.

The postnatal increase in arterial PaO2 plays an important role in ductus constriction. The unique oxygen sensor(s) within the ductus wall is still not clearly elucidated and may vary by species. In most species, oxygen appears to constrict the ductus arteriosus through mechanisms that depend on and mechanicms that are independent of smooth muscle depolarization. Oxygen depolarizes the ductus smooth muscle cells by inhibiting K^+ channels. Following the depolarization of the membrane, calcium enters the ductus smooth muscle through L-type and T-type voltage dependent, calcium channels. Several O2 sensitive K^+ channels have been found in the fetal ductus (including Kv1.5 and Kv2.1). These vary with species and gestational age and may account for the differing sensitivity of the ductus to oxygen. Oxygen also appears to have a direct effect on the calcium L-channels themselves and on the store-operated calcium channels. In addition, oxygen may increase smooth muscle sensitivity to calcium by activating Rho kinase-mediated pathways. Elevated oxygen tensions can also increase the formation of the potent vasoconstrictor, endothelin-1. The exact role of endothelin-1 in postnatal ductus closure is still unclear due, in large part, to the marked species variation in its contribution to ductus constriction. The postnatal increase in $PaO2$ also has profound effects on other vasoactive systems. Elevated oxygen tensions can increase the ductus' contractile response to neural mediators and can decrease the formation of vasodilator prostaglandins.

Developmental regulation

In contrast to the full term ductus, the premature ductus is less likely to constrict after birth. This is due to several mechanisms. The intrinsic tone of the extremely immature ductus (<70% of gestation) is decreased compared to the ductus at term. This may be due to the presence of immature smooth muscle myosin isoforms and to decreased Rho kinase expression and activity. Calcium entry through L-type calcium channels appears to be impaired in the immature ductus (especially under hypoxic conditions). Both the type and number of potassium channels that promote ductus relaxation also change during gestation, switching from K_{Ca} channels (which are not regulated by oxygen tension) to K_V channels (which can be inhibited by increased oxygen concentrations).

Premature infants have elevated circulating concentrations of PGE2, which may play a significant role in maintaining ductus patency during the first days after birth. This is due to the decreased ability of the premature lung to clear circulating PGE2. In the preterm newborn, circulating concentrations of PGE2 can reach the pharmacologic range during episodes of bacteremia and necrotizing enterocolitis and are often associated with reopening of a previously constricted ductus arteriosus.

In most mammalian species, the major factor that prevents the preterm ductus from constricting after birth is its increased sensitivity to the vasodilating effects of PGE2 and NO. The preterm ductus' increased sensitivity to PGE2 is due to increased cyclic AMP signaling. There is both increased cyclic AMP production, due to enhanced prostaglandin receptor coupling with adenylyl cyclase and decreased cyclic AMP degradation by phosphodiesterase in the preterm ductus. As a result, inhibitors of prostaglandin production are usually effective agents in promoting ductus closure in the premature infant. Drugs interfering with NO synthesis or function also could become useful adjuncts, especially in situations where indomethacin has proven to be ineffective.

The factors responsible for the changes that occur with advancing gestation are currently unknown. Prenatal administration of vitamin A has been shown to increase both the intracellular calcium response and the contractile response of the preterm ductus to oxygen. However, vitamin A administration does not improve the rate of ductus closure in preterm infants. During normal fetal development, there are increases in the circulating concentrations of cortisol with advancing gestation. Elevated cortisol concentrations in the fetus foster ductus maturation by decreasing the sensitivity of the ductus to the vasodilating effects of PGE_2. Prenatal administration of glucocorticoids significantly reduces the incidence of PDA in premature humans and animals. Postnatal glucocorticoid administration also reduces the incidence of PDA; however, postnatal glucocorticoid treatment also increases the incidence of several other neonatal morbidities.

Genetic regulation

Both species and genetic background play a significant role in determining the relative importance of ductus regulatory pathways. Marked species differences occur in the ductus' dependence on pathways involving endothelin, K_V channels and prostaglandins.

Recently, several genes have been identified (from mouse mutation models and from human genetic syndromes) that are associated with PDA in the full term neonate. These include homeobox genes (Prx1 and Prx2), a region on chromosome 12q24, designated PDA1, the Noonan syndrome gene, PTPN11; genes that regulate myosin heavy chains, filamin 1, prostaglandin signaling (COX2 and EP4), gap junctions (connexin 43) and neural crest transcription factors (TFAP2B and myocardin). Studies that have focused on possible genetic contributions to ductus patency in preterm infants have identified single nucleotide polymorphisms (SNPs) in candidate genes that are associated with PDA in preterm infants: ATR type 1, IFNγ, estrogen receptor-alpha PvuII, TFAP2B, PGI synthase and

TRAF1. The interaction between preterm birth and TFAP2B appears to account for some of the PDAs that occur in preterm infants.

Anatomic closure — histologic changes

In the full term newborn ductus, there is progressive intimal thickening and fragmentation of the internal elastic lamina after delivery. As the intima increases in size, it ultimately forms mounds that occlude the already constricted lumen. The increase in intimal thickening is due (1) to migration of smooth muscle cells from the muscle media into the intima and (2) to proliferation of luminal endothelial cells. The process of intimal cushion formation starts with the accumulation of hyaluron (HA) below the luminal endothelial cells. This is accompanied by the loss of laminin and collagen IV from the basement membrane of the endothelial cells and their subsequent separation from the internal elastic lamina. Laminin and collagen IV ultimately reform under the detached endothelial cells, but HA continues to accumalate in the subendothelial space. The hygroscopic properties of HA cause an influx of water and widening of the subendothelial space; this creates an environment well-suited for cell migration. Hyaluron makes ductus smooth muscle cells migrate faster. Accompanying the increase in HA is an increase in fibronectin (FN) and chondroitin sulfate (CS) in the neointimal space. Fibronectin also plays an important role in facilitating ductus smooth muscle cell migration.

Intimal cushion formation in the ductus is also associated with striking alterations in elastin fiber assembly. The normal elastin fiber assembly in the ductus appears to be disrupted due to a developmental mechanism that reduces insolubilization of elastin and prevents formation of intact elastic laminae. The impaired assembly of thick elastic laminae might facilitate smooth muscle cell migration by removing a physical barrier to which they might attach.

Relationship between vasoconstriction and anatomic closure

In full term animals, loss of responsiveness to PGE_2 shortly after birth prevents the ductus arteriosus from reopening once it has constricted. This is due, in part, to decreased synthesis of PGE2 receptors in the ductus after birth. Both the loss of vasodilator regulation and the anatomic events that lead to permanent closure appear to be controlled by the degree of ductus smooth muscle constriction. Constriction produces ischemic hypoxia of the ductus wall. In the full term newborn ductus, the thickness of the ductus wall requires the presence of intramural vasa vasorum to provide nutrients to the outer half of the vessel wall. These collapsible, intramural vasa vasorum provide the ductus with a unique mechanism for controlling the maximal diffusion distance for oxygen and nutrients across its wall. In the full term newborn, the intramural tissue pressure that develops during ductus constriction obliterates the vasa vasorum flow to the muscle media. The profound ischemic hypoxia that follows the compression of the vasa vasorum inhibits local production of PGE_2 and NO, induces local production of hypoxia inducible factors like HIF1α and vascular endothelial growth factor (VEGF) and produces smooth muscle apoptosis in the ductus wall. VEGF plays a critical role in the migration of the ductus smooth muscle cells into the neointima and in the proliferation of intramural vasa vasorum. Following postnatal ductus constriction, several genes known to be essential for vascular remodeling are increased in the ductus wall. In addition, monocytes/macrophages adhere to the ductus endothelial cells. The inflammatory response that follows postnatal ductus constriction may be necessary for ductus remodeling since the extent of neointimal remodeling is significantly correlated with the degree of mononuclear cell adhesion.

In preterm infants, the ductus frequently remains open for many days after birth, preventing it from developing profound hypoxic ischemia. Although alterations in prostaglandin signaling appear to be responsible for 60–70% of the delayed ductus closures, cyclooxygenase inhibitors become less effective in closing the ductus with increasing postnatal age. A number of factors conspire together to make the preterm ductus increasingly resistant to indomethacin and ibuprofen-induced closure with advancing postnatal age. Following delivery, COX-2 expression and PGE2 production increase in the ductus wall. However, in contrast with the full term ductus (where all of the PGE2 EP receptors are down regulated after birth) the dominant PGE2 receptor, EP4, continues to be synthesized after birth in the preterm ductus, enabling the preterm ductus to relax with prostaglandin stimulation. In addition, there is a progressive decrease in ATP concentrations within the preterm newborn ductus smooth muscle cells that limits its ability to constrict. Mild degrees of hypoxia within the postnatal preterm ductus induce the production of additional vasodilators within its wall (e.g. nitric oxide, TNFα and IL-6) that do not depend on prostaglandin signaling to affect contractility. These "additional" vasodilators produce a change in the balance of vasodilators that maintain ductus patency. These non-prostaglandin-mediated vasodilators explain why the effectiveness of indomethacin wanes with increasing postnatal age. The combined use of a nitric oxide synthase-inhibitor and indomethacin produces a much greater degree of ductus constriction than indomethacin alone.

Even when it does constrict, the premature ductus frequently fails to develop the same degree of profound hypoxia and anatomic remodeling that occurs in the full term newborn ductus. The preterm ductus requires a greater degree of constriction and a more complete degree of luminal closure, than the full term ductus, in order to develop a comparable degree of hypoxia. This is due to the thinness of the preterm ductus wall. In contrast with the full term ductus, the thin-walled preterm ductus does not need intramural vasa vasorum to provide oxygen and nutrients to its wall since it can extract all of the oxygen and nutrients it needs from its luminal blood flow. Prior to 26 weeks gestation, intramural vasa vasorum are absent from the ductus wall. As long as there is any degree of luminal patency and flow, the thin-walled preterm ductus fails to become profoundly hypoxic and fails to undergo anatomic remodeling. The preterm ductus requires that the lumen be completely obliterated before it can develop the same degree of hypoxia found at term. Once the preterm ductus develops profound ischemic hypoxia, it will undergo most of the anatomic changes seen at term. However, if the premature ductus does not develop the degree of ischemic hypoxia needed to induce cell death and anatomic remodeling, it will continue to be responsive to vasodilators and continue to be susceptible to vessel reopening.

Pathophysiology: Hemodynamic and Pulmonary Alterations of a PDA

The pathophysiologic features of a PDA depend both on the magnitude of the left-to-right shunt and on the cardiac and pulmonary responses to the shunt. Preterm newborns are able to increase left ventricular output and maintain their "effective" systemic blood flow, even with left-to-right PDA shunts equal to 50% of left ventricular output. With shunts greater than 50% of left ventricular output, "effective" systemic blood flow falls, despite a continued increase in left ventricular output. The increase in left ventricular output associated with a PDA is accomplished not by an increase in heart rate, but by an increase in stroke volume. Stroke volume increases primarily as a result of the simultaneous decrease in after load resistance on the heart and the increase in left ventricular preload. Despite the ability of the left ventricle to increase its output in the face of a left-to-right ductus shunt, blood flow distribution is significantly rearranged. This redistribution of systemic blood flow occurs even with small shunts. Blood flow to the skin, bone and skeletal muscle is most likely to be affected by the left-to-right ductus shunt. The next most likely organs to be affected are the gastrointestinal tract and kidneys due to a combination of decreased perfusion pressure and localized vasoconstriction. Mesenteric blood flow is decreased in both fasting and fed states in the presence of a PDA. Significant decreases in organ blood flow may occur before there are signs of left ventricular compromise and may contribute to the decreased feeding tolerance and decreased glomerular filtration rate that have been observed with ductus patency.

The decreased ability of the preterm infant to maintain active pulmonary vasoconstriction may be responsible in part for the earlier presentation of a "large" left-to-right PDA shunt. Dopamine increases systemic blood pressure and blood flow in preterm infants with a PDA by increasing pulmonary vascular resistance and decreasing the left-to-right shunt across the ductus. Therapeutic maneuvers like surfactant replacement, or prenatal conditions like intrauterine growth retardation which lead to a rapid drop in pulmonary vascular resistance, can exacerbate the amount of left-to-right shunt and lead to pulmonary hemorrhage.

Depending on the gestational age and the species examined, pulmonary edema and changes in pulmonary mechanics may occur as early as one day after birth or not before several days of exposure to the left-to-right shunt of a PDA. Preterm animals with a PDA have increased fluid and protein clearance into the lung interstitium due to increased pulmonary microvascular filtration pressure. However, a simultaneous increase in lung lymph flow eliminates the excess fluid and protein from the lung. This compensatory increase in lung lymph flow acts as an "edema safety factor," inhibiting fluid accumulation in the lungs. As a result, there is no net increase in water or protein accumulation in the lung and there is no change in pulmonary mechanics. This delicate balance between the PDA-induced fluid filtration and lymphatic reabsorption is consistent with the observation, made in human infants, that closure of the ductus arteriosus, within the first 24 hours after birth, has no effect on the course of the newborn's hyaline membrane disease. However, if lung lymphatic drainage is impaired, as it is in the presence of pulmonary interstitial emphysema or fibrosis, the likelihood of edema increases dramatically. It is not uncommon for infants with a persistent PDA to develop alterations in pulmonary mechanics at 7–10 days after birth. In these infants, improvement in lung compliance occurs following closure of the PDA.

Much of our understanding of the effects of a PDA on pulmonary mechanics comes from studies performed in premature baboons that are delivered at 67% term gestation (equivalent to 26 weeks human gestation) and mechanically ventilated for two weeks. In this animal model, exposure to a persistent PDA for two weeks does not alter surfactant secretion, pulmonary epithelial protein permeability, presence of surfactant inhibitory proteins, or alter the expression of any of the pro-inflammatory or tissue remodeling genes that were examined. The animals with an open ductus had an increased amount and altered distribution of water in their lungs. Closure of the PDA with a cyclooxygenase inhibitor, like indomethacin or ibuprofen, produced an increased expression of alveolar epithelial sodium channels, which facilitated fluid removal from the alveolar compartment. This finding may account for the decreased incidence of significant pulmonary hemorrhage in infants that are treated with prophylactic indomethacin after birth. Pharmacologic closure of the PDA was also associated with improved lung development in the preterm baboons. In contrast to the animals with an open ductus, where an arrest in alveolar development (the hallmark of the new "BPD") was noticeable by two weeks after birth, pharmacological closure of the PDA produced improved alveolarization.

Treatment

Treatment options for closing a PDA

Surgical ligation produces definitive ductus arteriosus closure. However, it is associated with its own set of morbidities: thoracotomy, pneumothorax, chylothorax, scoliosis and infection. The incidence of unilateral vocal cord paralysis (which increases the requirements for tube feedings, respiratory support and hospital stay) has been reported to be as high as 67% in ELBW infants, following PDA ligation. Between 30–50% of infants with birthweights $\leq$1000 gm will require inotropic support for profound hypotension during the postoperative period. Early surgical ligation of the PDA has recently been shown to be an independent risk factor for the development of bronchopulmonary dysplasia.

Inhibition of prostaglandin synthesis with nonselective cyclooxygenase inhibitors appears to be an effective alternative to surgical ligation. However, both indomethacin and ibuprofen have been associated with several potential adverse effects in the newborn. Indomethacin produces significant reductions in renal, mesenteric and cerebral blood flow. Indomethacin also reduces cerebral oxygenation. Alterations in creatinine clearance and oliguria (that are minimally responsive to dopamine or furosemide therapy) are common problems with the initial doses of indomethacin. Renal function returns towards normal after the initial doses of indomethacin or after drug discontinuation.

Although indomethacin produces significant physiologic alterations, none of the randomized controlled trials that have examined the relationship between indomethacin and neonatal morbidity have found an increase in the incidence of necrotizing enterocolitis, gastrointestinal perforation, retinopathy of prematurity, chronic lung disease, or cerebral white matter injury following indomethacin treatment. Although indomethacin, by itself, has not been shown to increase the incidence of gastrointestinal perforations, the combination of indomethacin *and* postnatal steroids, administered simultaneously, has been shown to increase the incidence of gastrointestinal perforations and necrotizing enterocolitis.

Indomethacin's cerebral vasoconstrictive effects are frequently cited as a concern for neonatologists; however, a Cochrane systematic review found that indomethacin prophylaxis is more likely to decrease rather than increase the incidence of periventricular leukomalacia. There is no evidence that prophylactic indomethacin has any adverse effect on neurodevelopmental outcome at 18 months; in fact, there is evidence that it may have long-term benefits at 4.5 and 8 years.

While there may be general consensus on the efficacy of indomethacin for treatment of a PDA, questions about proper dosage, treatment duration, and optimal timing of treatment remain quite controversial. Indomethacin's plasma clearance depends on postnatal age. Therefore, a dosage regime recommended for infants at the end of the first week (when the half life of the drug is 21 hours) may lead to elevated and prolonged plasma concentrations when used in infants on day one (when the half life is 71 hours).

Many variations in dosage regimens have been evaluated. A prolonged low-dose course of indomethacin (0.1 mg/kg every 24 hours for 5–7 days) may increase the rate of permanent closure especially in infants who still have residual ductus flow after completing the standard short course (2–3 doses over 24 hours). This dosage regimen still needs further evaluation since, in some reports, a higher mortality rate was observed in the infants receiving prolonged maintenance indomethacin.

Although some have suggested that the dose of indomethacin be increased when conventional dosing fails to produce ductus closure, a randomized controlled trial examining this issue found that the rate of ductus closure was not substantially improved despite a nearly three-fold increase in serum indomethacin concentrations. In addition, the higher indomethacin concentrations produced significant increases in the incidence of moderate/severe retinopathy of prematurity and late renal dysfunction.

The postnatal age at which indomethacin is administered plays an important role in determining its effectiveness. Even when indomethacin concentrations have been maintained in the "desired" range, the drug's ability to produce ductus closure remains inversely proportional to the postnatal age at the time of treatment. With advancing postnatal age, dilator prostaglandins play less of a role in maintaining ductus patency (see above). As a result, indomethacin becomes less effective in producing PDA closure.

Recurrence of a symptomatic PDA can occur after initial successful treatment. The rate of reopening, which is greatest among the most immature infants, appears to be related to the timing and completeness of ductus closure after the treatment course. Permanent anatomic closure requires tight constriction of the ductus lumen and the development of ductus wall hypoxia (see above). Eighty percent of infants delivered at less than 28 weeks gestation, that constrict their ductus with indomethacin treatment, will reopen their ductus and develop clinical symptoms if there is any evidence of luminal patency on the Doppler examination performed at the end of indomethacin treatment. Unfortunately, there are limitations in the Doppler's ability to detect complete luminal closure. Even when there is no evidence of ductus patency on the Doppler/echocardiogram, a significant number of preterm infants will still have a tiny patent ductus lumen. The more immature the ductus (e.g. the thinner the ductus wall), the greater the likelihood that profound hypoxia and anatomic remodeling will not occur. These vessels will reopen at a later date: 23% of those delivering before 26 weeks reopen in spite of echocardiographic evidence of closure; in contrast, only 9% of those delivering between 26–27 weeks will reopen if the ductus is found to be closed by echocardiography. Early treatment produces a tighter degree of ductus constriction and as a result produces higher rates of ductus wall hypoxia and permanent closure.

Ibuprofen is another nonselective cyclooxygenase inhibitor. It appears to be as effective as indomethacin in producing PDA closure in very low birthweight infants (at least in infants with a mean gestational age of 28 weeks). In contrast with indomethacin, ibuprofen does not appear to affect mesenteric blood flow and has less of an effect on renal perfusion, oliguria and cerebral blood flow. However, aside from its renal-sparing effects, comparison trials have not found ibuprofen to be superior to indomethacin in the prevention of other neonatal morbidities (necrotzing enterocolitis, GI perforation and BPD). In addition, ibuprofen does not appear to have the same intracranial hemorrhage-sparing effects that is seen with indomethacin (see below). The optimal age-appropriate dosing schedule for ibuprofen is still under consideration. Ibuprofen's effects on total and free serum bilirubin concentrations raise concerns about the safety of some of the higher dose options.

Indomethacin and intracranial hemorrhage (ICH)

Previous studies have shown that indomethacin can decrease the incidence of intracranial hemorrhage in preterm infants (this has not been the case with ibuprofen). The effects of indomethacin on ICH do not appear to be due to its effects on ductus patency. Indomethacin decreases cerebral blood flow, decreases reactive post-asphyxial cerebral hyperemia and accelerates maturation of the germinal matrix microvasculature. Since most intracranial hemorrhages occur within the first three days after birth, the beneficial effects only occur when indomethacin is given in a Prophylactic strategy (within the first 18 hours after birth).

Evidence-Based Management: PDA and Neonatal Morbidity — To Treat or Not to Treat

Although a prolonged, persistent left-to-right shunt through a PDA shortens the life span of animals and humans, there has been a growing debate in recent years about whether or not to treat a persistent PDA during the neonatal period. Preterm infants have a high rate of spontaneous PDA closure during the first two years. Therefore, early treatment runs the risk of exposing infants to drugs or procedures they might not need.

Published randomized controlled trials (RCTs) provide only a limited amount of information to help guide current PDA treatment choices. Most RCTs were designed to assess the relationship between "timing," or initiation of indomethacin treatment, and efficiency of PDA closure. They were not designed to address the question of whether or not to treat a symptomatic PDA during the neonatal period.

RCTs have examined the effects of *brief* (*2–6 days*) *exposures* to a PDA in preterm infants that were greater than 2–3 days old. None of these studies observed an increase in serious neonatal morbidities like BPD, NEC or ROP.

Even less information exists about the consequences of a persistent, symptomatic, moderate-large PDA shunt on neonatal morbidity. To date, only two small RCTs, performed almost 30 years ago, have specifically examined the role of a persistent untreated symptomatic PDA on neonatal morbidity. Both studies found that a persistent PDA increased pulmonary morbidity and prolonged the need for respiratory support. Whether these findings are still applicable in the setting of modern neonatal treatment is a matter of controversy among neonatologists.

Although some retrospective, population-based studies have reported an association between PDA and NEC, there is little evidence from RCTs to either support or refute the idea that a PDA plays a role in the development of necrotizing enterocolitis. At this time, there are no RCTs in the medical literature that address this issue. Nor is there information about the advisability of continuing or stopping enteral feeding in the presence of a PDA.

Numerous RCTs have examined the risks and benefits of indomethacin prophylaxis (starting treatment within 12 hours of birth) versus waiting for early PDA symptoms to appear before starting treatment (usually 2–3 days after birth). Indomethacin prophylaxis decreases the incidence of (1) severe early pulmonary hemorrhages, (2) severe grades of IVH, (3) the risk of developing a symptomatic PDA, and (4) the need for surgical PDA ligation. On the other hand, indomethacin prophylaxis results in over-treatment of infants that would normally close their ductus spontaneously.

Although indomethacin has been shown to be effective in producing ductus closure, its long-term benefits have yet to be established. At this time, 95% of US neonatologists believe that a moderate-to-large PDA should be treated if it persists in ELBW infants that still require mechanical ventilation. In contrast, the number of neonatologists that treat a persistent PDA when it occurs in infants that do not require mechanical ventilation varies significantly by geographic region.

Reference

1. Clyman RI. Patent ductus arteriosus in the premature infant. In Gleason CA, Devaskar S (eds), *Avery's Diseases of the Newborn*, 9th ed. W.B. Saunders Co., Philadelphia, PA. (in press).

Chapter

10

Common Gastrointestinal Disorders

Rajan Wadhawan

This chapter provides an overview of the important gastrointestinal (GI) morbidities affecting preterm infants. The focus is on the controversial aspects of these disorders, basing the discussion on available evidence. Surgical disorders affecting the GI tract are presented elsewhere in this Handbook.

Necrotizing Enterocolitis

Necrotizing enterocolitis (NEC) is one of the most severe clinical emergencies affecting primarily premature infants. In term infants, NEC is often associated with predisposing factors such as low Apgar scores, exchange transfusions, congenital heart disease and neural tube defects.[1] In preterm infants, NEC often occurs without an association with these factors. An entity that is often confused with NEC is spontaneous intestinal perforation (SIP). The onset of SIP is typically at an earlier postnatal age than NEC and exposure to glucocorticoids and indomethacin are considered risk factors.[2,3] SIP often occurs prior to the institution of enteral feedings. NEC, on the other hand, occurs commonly after the first week of life and has been associated with aggressive enteral feedings. The differences between NEC and SIP are listed in Table 1.

Table 1. Comparison between NEC and SIP in preterm infants.

	Necrotizing enterocolitis	Spontaneous intestinal perforation
Timing of onset	After first week of life	Often during the first week of life
Localization	Proximal colon and terminal ileum	Terminal ileum-anti-mesenteric position
Histology	Coagulation necrosis	Minimal necrosis
Association with feeds	Yes	No
Other associations	Prolonged rupture of membranes Colonization of the GI tract with pathogenic bacteria, PDA	Use of early dexamethasone in combination with indomethacin, Prolonged rupture of membranes

The incidence of NEC is inversely proportional to the gestational age. Most cases of NEC occur in preterm infants, with a decrease in the incidence of NEC in infants with a birth weight over 1500 g. The incidence of NEC in infants below 1500 g has been reported to be in the range of 4–13%.[4,5] NEC carries a very high mortality rate, often reported to be in the 20–25% range. In addition, it results in considerable morbidity in the form of intestinal dysfunction and short bowel syndrome.

Clinical presentation

The presenting signs and symptoms of NEC include episodes of apnea and bradycardia, abdominal distension and tenderness, bloody stools, pneumatosis intestinalis, portal venous gas, intestinal perforation, sepsis and shock. The clinical presentation of NEC is often categorized based on Bell's classification,[6] with stage 1 being suggestive; stage 2, definitive; and stage 3, severe. Stage 1 is highly nonspecific and may represent other conditions such as sepsis and feeding intolerance. This stage is characterized by nonspecific signs: increased feeding residuals, increased frequency and severity of apneas and bradycardias and mild abdominal distension. These signs may alert the clinician to the possibility of NEC. Stage 2 is definite NEC with pneumatosis intestinalis, a pathognomonic

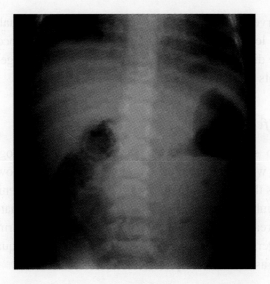

Figure 1. Radiograph of a neonate with NEC showing pneumatosis intestinalis (Arrow).

sign of NEC (Fig.1). Stage 3 is the severe form of NEC, which often needs surgical management. This stage is characterized by signs of intestinal perforation, along with signs of systemic compromise. Intestinal perforation may be evident on abdominal radiographs as pneumoperitoneum. Infants with SIP can however present with signs of stage 3 NEC and it can be confused with NEC. The clinical progression of NEC is variable and often does not follow a step-wise progression from one stage to the next. Some infants may initially present with early signs of NEC and subsequently progress to more severe form of NEC. In other infants, the initial presentation may be that of fulminant NEC, without any early warning signs of NEC.

Radiological findings

The classical radiological hallmark of NEC is pneumatosis intestinalis or gas in the bowel wall. In severe cases of NEC, this may be associated with the extension of air into the portal circulation. Left lateral decubitus films are helpful in evaluating for pneumoperitoneum, thereby indicating intestinal perforation. Pneumoperitoneum is an indication for emergency surgical intervention, whereas pneumatosis alone is usually medically managed, at least initially. Abdominal ultrasound can occasionally be helpful in the diagnosis of NEC, especially in the early stages by showing echogenic dots in the bowel wall.[7]

Laboratory features

There are no specific laboratory findings that are pathognomonic for NEC. Infants with NEC often have an abnormally high or low white blood cell count. As the disease progresses, there may be a worsening neutropenia and thrombocytopenia. In addition, several inflammatory markers, including C-reactive protein has been shown to be abnormal in infants with NEC. Persistently elevated CRP levels despite adequate treatment may indicate associated complications.

Pathogenesis

No ideal animal model is available for NEC in preterm infants. However, epidemiologic studies, individual case evaluations and animal studies suggest that NEC is a result of a close interplay between genetics, intestinal immaturity, microbial environment and feeding. Twin analyses support the fact that NEC is familial in origin.[8] However, the search for genetic markers that predispose to NEC risk has been unsuccessful.[9] Immaturity of the digestive and absorptive capacity and that of the immune function are thought to play an important role in the pathogenesis of NEC. The intestinal innate barrier is important in preventing bacterial translocation and preventing an inflammatory response. Decreased hydrogen ion output and low enterokinase activity in the immature stomach can allow colonization of the intestinal tract with pathogens. In fact, use of H2 blockers has been shown to be associated with an increase in the incidence of NEC.[10] Immature neonates have a higher intestinal permeability as compared to older children and adults, thus perhaps allowing passage of higher molecular weight molecules.[11] The motility of the small intestine in premature infants is less organized than that in term infants, because of the inherent immaturity of the enteric nervous system,[12] which can potentially lead to stasis and bacterial overgrowth. All of these factors can lead to an inflammatory cascade leading to NEC.[13] Several inflammatory mediators are involved in the pathogenesis of NEC, including lipopolysaccharide, platelet-activating factor, several interleukins and tumor necrosis factor.

The majority of preterm newborns in the NICU are treated with broad-spectrum antibiotics soon after birth, which may alter the microbial ecology of the gastrointestinal tract, promoting colonization with resistant microbial species, rather than the usual commensal organisms such as lactobacillus and bifidobacterium.[14] Cohort studies in preterm infants have shown prolonged empiric antibiotics to be related to increased risk of NEC.[15] For similar reasons, probiotics have been explored in the prevention of NEC and the preliminary results have shown efficacy.[16,17] However, routine use of these agents cannot be recommended at the present time, as the safety and efficacy needs to be established in large, well-designed trials.[18]

Management

Treatment strategy for NEC depends on the stage of the disease. In Bell's stage 1, patient should be carefully followed to either confirm or rule out the suspicion of NEC, while instituting bowel rest and the appropriate use of antibiotics. Once NEC is confirmed (Bell's stage 2), the bowel should be decompressed by an indwelling, large-bore orogastric tube. Fluid and electrolyte status needs to be closely monitored. In addition, hematological parameters need to be followed as well. Frequent radiographic evaluations may be necessary during the initial stages of the disease to rule out bowel perforation. If a perforation occurs, surgical intervention is essential. Coordination with pediatric surgeons in monitoring progress for appropriate timing of surgical intervention is essential. In infants without perforation, surgical intervention may be indicated if there is a deterioration of clinical condition with worsening of hematological parameters. Antibiotic coverage for anerobic infection should be considered, especially in the case of bowel perforation.

The choice of surgical intervention remains controversial, with exploratory laparotomy and peritoneal drain placement having been shown to be associated with similar outcomes.[19]

Despite aggressive medical management, outcomes in infants with severe NEC are poor, with a high mortality and morbidity rate. Prevention of NEC has a potential of substantially improving outcomes in preterm infants. Providing human milk to preterm infants has been consistently shown to be associated with a decrease in the incidence of NEC.[20,21] On the other hand, aggressive institution and advancement of enteral feedings has been associated with an increased risk of NEC.[22,23] As stated previously, prevention of NEC with probiotics is promising but requires additional studies and availability of probiotic preparations with the right species and dosages.

Short Bowel Syndrome

Recent improvements in neonatal intensive care have resulted in improved survival of extremely low birth weight infants. This, however, has been accompanied by an increase in infants with short bowel syndrome and intestinal dysfunction as a result of intestinal catastrophies secondary to prematurity, including those who suffer from NEC.

Pathophysiology

Most instances of short bowel syndrome are due to intestinal resection. The important causes of intestinal resection include necrotizing enterocolitits, intestinal atresia, gastroschisis, omphalocele, volvulus, meconium ileus and Hirschsprung's disease. The severity of short bowel syndrome depends on the length of small bowel resected, since the small bowel is responsible for absorption of most of the fluids and nutrients in the gut.[24] Other factors that affect the severity of short bowel are the presence or absence of the ileocecal valve and the adaptive capacity of the remaining small bowel. The remaining length of small bowel that is essential for survival without parenteral nutrition depends on the gestational age of the infant. The preterm infants are more likely to recover with a smaller remaining length of small intestine, presumably a result of increased growth potential of their small bowel.[25] The critical length of remaining small bowel in full term infants has been shown to be 40 cm.[24,26]

Complications

The most important effect of short bowel syndrome is malabsorption. The severity of malabsorption is inversely proportional to the length of small intestine as well as the segment removed. Most of the water absorption takes place in the small intestine. However, in the absence of small intestine, the large intestine can take over the role of substantial absorption of water and electrolytes.[27] Most of the other nutrients are, however, absorbed in the small intestine. There are significant differences in the absorptive capacity of jejunum and ileum. Jejunum has the highest concentration of mucosal disaccharidases and peptidases, in addition to having taller villi, as compared to the ileum. As a result, the resection of jejunum results in a greater loss of absorptive capacity. Ileum, on the other hand, is responsible for absorption of vitamin B12 and bile salts. Ileal resection predisposes to fat malabsorption secondary to bile acid deficiency and need for long term vitamin B12 supplementation.

Most of the complications of short bowel syndrome are secondary to the long-term dependence on parenteral nutrition. These complications are:

1. Infection: Infants with short bowel syndrome need long term central vascular access, predisposing them to increased risk of central line-associated sepsis. The majority of these infections are caused by coagulase negative staphylococci, although other organisms, including candida albicans are also responsible for a substantial number of infections.[28,29]
2. Hypergastrinemia and increased acid production: Small bowel resection is often followed by an increase in gastrin and gastric acid output that may need treatment with acid blocking agents.[30]
3. Noninfectious colitis: This may be manifested by diarrhea with bloody stools. Steroids may be needed for treatment if the colitis is severe.[31]
4. Thrombosis: Since central venous access is essential for a prolonged period of time; venous thrombosis is a major issue. Thrombosis may be spontaneous or related to infections that can lead to superior vena cava syndrome, a serious complication. Extensive thrombosis of

multiple sites can limit the ability to care for these infants and can be a serious challenge over the long term.

5. Cholestasis: This is the most common and serious problem affecting infants with short bowel syndrome. It can occur within 2–4 weeks following initiation of total parenteral nutrition, often manifesting initially as an increase in liver transaminases.[32] The severity of cholestasis is directly related to the degree of prematurity of an infant.[33,34] Septicemia episodes also increase the severity of cholestasis. Several components of parenteral nutrition have been proposed to predispose to cholestasis. This is discussed in greater length further in the chapter. In most infants with short bowel syndrome, choletasis resolves after TPN has been discontinued, but it may take several weeks to resolve. Up to 25% of infants with short bowel syndrome develop cholelithiasis, secondary to a depletion of bile acid pool, especially in infants with loss of terminal ileum.[34]

Management

Management of short bowel syndrome includes dietary management, use of pharmacologic agents and parenteral nutrition. Intestinal transplant is a recent development.

Dietary management

Enteral feedings should be initiated early in order to exert a trophic effect on the remaining bowel. Continuous feeds are generally tolerated better than bolus feeds.[35] There is, however, a higher risk of gallstones with continuous feeds as compared to bolus feeds, presumably because of a lack of contraction of gall bladder.[36] Administration of continuous feeds may also impair the proper development of suck and swallow in preterm newborns. The attempt should be to initiate feeds with continuous feeds and transition over to bolus feeds, as soon as tolerated. Alternatively, a combination of continuous feeds with small intermittent boluses may be explored.

The ideal composition of enteral feeding in infants with short bowel syndrome is also controversial. Breast milk and amino acid based formulas are thought to be beneficial and have been shown to be associated with a shorter duration of TPN.[37] These are also associated with a lower risk of milk protein induced colitis. In addition, glucose needs to be provided as polymers, rather than in the form of lactose, which is poorly tolerated. In addition, fat should be provided as long chain triglycerides, as these are thought to exert a trophic effect on intestinal mucosa. Medium chain triglycerides can be beneficial in conditions with loss of terminal small intestine, as they do not require bile acids for absorption. There are several commercially available formulas, which meet these requirements.

Pharmacological agents

Several pharmacological agents are used in the management of short bowel syndrome. These include bile salt resin binders (cholestyramine), cholerectic agents (ursodeoxycholic acid), antidiarrheal agents (loperamide) and amino acids such as glutamine. Most of these agents are helpful in managing diarrhea secondary to malabsorption, except for ursodeoxycholic acid, which is associated with a decrease in the duration of cholestasis through separate mechanisms.[38]

Parenteral nutrition

Several factors may contribute to the development of TPN induced cholestasis. Abnormalities in enterohepatic circulation by surgery or lack of enteral feedings has been implicated in the development of cholestatic liver disease.[39] The flow of bile, which is secreted by hepatocytes into biliary canaliculi, depends on the volume of fluid in the biliary system. Fluid is drawn into the canaliculi by the osmotic forces of secreted bile salts. Thus, bile flow and bile salt excretion by the liver are interdependent. In addition, all components of TPN have been implicated in the etiology of cholestasis. The risk of hepatic steatosis correlates with dextrose concentration in TPN; increasing periportal fat infiltrate has been shown to be related to increasing glucose concentrations and a high insulin-to-glucagon ratio.[40] Similarly, both protein and lipids have been implicated in the development of cholestasis after prolonged TPN exposure. The standard amino acid preparation currently used for preterm newborns (Trophamine) containing increased cysteine and taurine has decreased the risk of cholestasis as compared to the standard adult preparations, but not eliminated it.[41] Hepatic accumulation of trace elements, including both iron and copper has been seen in these infants.[42,43] It is not clear as to whether the accumulation of these heavy metals contributes to liver injury or occurs secondary to the liver injury. Several approaches have been recommended for infants on long-term parenteral nutrition to decrease the risk and severity of cholestasis. These include limiting the dextrose concentration in TPN, "cycling" TPN and omitting trace elements. None of these however have been shown to have a consistent effect on cholestasis. One novel approach that has been recommended to improve cholestasis has been the use of fish-oil based lipid emulsion containing omega-3 fatty acids, instead of the usual soy-based emulsions, which contain the omega-6 fatty acids. While the initial results are promising, these preparations are currently not widely available in the US and experience is limited so far.[44]

Intestinal transplantation

The results of intestinal transplantation have improved over the past decade, with a one-year patient survival rate currently exceeding 90%.[45] Patients with short bowel syndrome who are TPN dependent, should be considered as a candidate for intestinal transplant if they have recurrent episodes of sepsis, two or more episodes of loss of central venous access, cholestatic liver disease or evidence of portal hypertension. Unfortunately, a substantial percentage of infants listed as transplant candidates often die while awaiting donor organs. Early enlistment in transplant programs could potentially avoid such outcomes.

Gastro-Esophageal Reflux

Diagnosis and management of gastro-esophageal reflux (GER) in preterm newborns is perhaps one of the most controversial aspects of newborn medicine. While there is no doubt that gastro-esophageal reflux occurs frequently in preterm neonates,[46,47] its role in causing neonatal morbidities is less clear.

Pathogenesis

Reflux may occur when the lower esophageal sphincter relaxes. In an upright adult, gas exits the stomach during these transient lower esophageal sphincter relaxations (TLESRs), causing belching. In a subject lying supine, however, the gastroesophageal junction is constantly under water, and liquid instead of gas may enter the esophagus. The quantity of the reflux depends on the fluid volume inside the stomach. The volume of fluid given to an infant (150 mL/kg per day) would correspond to a daily intake of over 10 l/day in an adult. Thus, GER in infants may be a direct reflection of the supine body habitus and relatively high fluid intake. The frequency of TLESR's has been studied using micro-manometric transducer devices and has not shown to be different among infants with and without GER.[48] These authors proposed that there may be some anatomic or sensory variations in some preterm infants that predispose them to a greater degree of acid reflux. The presence of a gastric feeding tube has also been shown to increase the frequency of reflux,[49] presumably secondary to interference with the lower esophageal sphincter function. Delayed gastric emptying is often believed to be contributory to GER, but this claim has been challenged in clinical studies of gastric motility.[48,50]

Diagnosis

The gold standard for diagnosis of GER in older children and adults is pH monitoring. Continuous measurement performed over a period of several hours is essential for the diagnosis of GER. Demonstration of a few reflux episodes on a brief radiologic study should not be taken as evidence of significant reflux, as it only provides a snap-shot in time. The application of pH monitoring in the preterm neonate is complicated by the fact that this technique relies on the presence of gastric pH below four. Some preterm infants may have gastric pH of more than four, more than 90% of the time, thereby making diagnosis difficult based on this technique.[51,52] Another technique, known as multiple intraluminal impedance (MII) has been shown to be a better alternative to pH monitoring in diagnosing GER.[53] This technique relies on intraluminal measurement of electrical impedance, from a number of closely arranged electrodes, during the passage of a food bolus. This technique can identify the retrograde passage of a bolus during GER, without relying on pH measurement. A combination of MII and pH study will likely result in more accurate diagnosis, as compared to either technique alone. Other techniques for diagnosis of GER have been suggested, including a clinical scoring system[54] and testing of pharyngeal secretions for acid.[55] The constant search for the perfect diagnostic tool for GER highlights the controversy surrounding this diagnosis.

Relationship of GER and apnea and airway problems

GER is frequently blamed for apnea of prematurity (AOP) that is refractory to xanthine therapy. The evidence for this relationship between GER and AOP is controversial and largely circumstantial. Both GER and AOP frequently coexist in the same infants and are more likely to occur in the post-prandial phase.[56] There are several anecdotal reports documenting AOP following an episode of GER.[57,58] Several studies have attempted to document an irrefutable temporal relationship between GER and AOP, but have failed to do so.[47,59–62] Similarly, treatment of preterm infants with anti-reflux medications does not consistently improve AOP.[63]

In addition to AOP, there is considerable controversy surrounding the relationship of GER with chronic airway problems. A few studies have proposed an association of GER with stridor and bronchomalacia in older infants, with improvement of these symptoms with anti-reflux treatment.[64,65] The causal relationship between GER and airway problems, however, remains unclear. In addition, it is not clear if the data from term infants can be extrapolated to preterm infants. A study of GER in infants with bronchopulmonary dysplasia (BPD) in preterm infants showed GER to be less frequent in infants with BPD as compared to the ones without BPD.[66] It thus seems unlikely that GER plays a significant role in adverse respiratory outcomes in a majority of preterm infants.

Treatment of gastro-esophageal reflux

Based on current evidence, the common practice of treating preterm infants with recurrent apnea or recurrent regurgitation with anti-reflux therapy seems unwarranted. Reflux may be physiologic in the majority of these infants and apnea may be unrelated to GER. There may be a small proportion of infants with recurrent aspiration or recurrent cyanosis, who may benefit from anti-reflux therapy. A step-wise approach to the management of GER is recommended, starting with left lateral or prone positioning and progressing to thickening of feeds, medications and nasojejunal feeds or surgery for refractory cases.[54] The last option should be reserved for the most severe cases with clear evidence of GER contributing to morbidities. Medications often used in the treatment of GER include prokinetic agents like metoclopramide and erythromycin, histamine-2 blockers like ranitidine and proton pump inhibitors. It is unlikely that erythromycin has any beneficial effects in preterm infants, as the effect of erythromycin on migrating motor complexes is not seen before 32 weeks gestation.[67] In addition, there are concerns about possible side effects of pyloric stenosis and multi-drug resistant sepsis.[68] Similarly, acid-suppressive agents should be used with caution, as they may have a harmful effect on bacterial colonization of the GI tract and thus increase the risk of sepsis.[69] Ranitidine has also been associated with increased risk of NEC in preterm infants.[10]

Cholestasis in Neonates

While unconjugated hyperbilirubinemia is by far the most common type of jaundice in the newborn in the first few days of life, conjugated hyperbilirubinemia does occur. Early diagnosis and treatment of cholestasis, resulting in conjugated hyperbilirubinemia, are important for improved outcomes. A conjugated bilirubin level of greater than 2 mg/dl or greater than 15% of the total serum bilirubin is often used to define conjugated hyperbilirubinemia. The most common cause of conjugated hyperbilirubinemia in infants younger than 60 days of age is biliary atresia, while TPN-induced cholestasis is the most common acquired cause. However, several other less common conditions can be responsible for conjugated hyperbilirubinemia as well and must be considered in the differential diagnosis. A list of causes of cholestasis appears in Table 2. Biliary atresia, an important cause of cholestasis is discussed in detail below. TPN-associated cholestasis is discussed above.

Table 2.   Cholestatic disorders affecting the newborn.

Disorders affecting bile ducts

Biliary atresia
Choledochal cyst and choledochocele
Biliary hypoplasia
Choledocholithiasis
Bile duct perforation
Neonatal sclerosing cholangitis

Disorders affecting intrahepatic bile ducts

Syndromic paucity (Allagille syndrome)
Non-syndromic paucity (Hypothyroidism, Panhypopituitarism)
Bile duct dysgenesis (Congenital hepatic fibrosis, Polycystic kidney disease,
    Caroli's disease, Hepatic cysts)
Cystic fibrosis
Langerhans' cell histiocytosis
Hyper-Ig M syndrome

Disorders affecting Hepatocytes

Sepsis-associated cholestasis
Neonatal hepatitis
Viral infections (Hepatitis B, Cytomegalovirus, Herpes virus, Adenovirus,
    Enterovirus, Parvovirus B19)
Toxoplasmosis
Syphilis
Progressive familial intrahepatic cholestasis syndrome
Bile acid synthetic defects
Urea cycle defects (Ornithine transcarbamylase deficiency, Carbomyl
    phosphate synthetase deficiency)
Tyrosinemia
Fatty acid oxidation disorders
Mitochondrial enzymopathies
Peroxisomal disorders (Zellweger syndrome)
Lipid storage disorders (Niemann-Pick disease, Gaucher's disease,
    Wolman's disease)
Carbohydrate disorders (Galactosemia, Hereditary fructose intolerance,
    Glycogen storge disease)
Alpha-1 antitrypsin deficiency
Neonatal hemochromatosis
Parenteral nutrition (TPN) associated cholestasis

Biliary Atresia

Pathophysiology

Biliary atresia is the end result of an inflammatory and destructive process involving extrahepatic and intrahepatic bile ducts. This leads to obliteration of the biliary tract and eventually cirrhosis. Most of these infants with biliary atresia are normal at birth and develop progressive jaundice in the first weeks of life. Occasionally, a fetal form of biliary atresia may be accompanied by other congenital anomalies.[70,71]

Diagnosis

Conjugated hyperbilirubinemia can be caused by a myriad of conditions and a careful diagnostic workup is indicated to exclude other possible causes. One such algorithm is shown in Fig. 2. Radiological investigations useful in evaluating conjugated hyperbilirubinemia include ultrasonography, radionuclide scintigraphy and MR cholangiography. The pathologic hallmark is the histologic finding of cholestasis, bile duct proliferation and inflammatory infiltrate.[72] In cases where the results are inconclusive with a high index of suspicion, an exploratory laparotomy with intraoperative cholangioraphy may need to be performed.[73]

Management

The natural history of biliary atresia is that of progressive liver failure and death during infancy. Surgical management, in the form of hepatic portoenterostomy (Kasai procedure) during the first 60 days of life provides effective palliation in infants with biliary atresia. The predictors of a good outcome after a Kasai procedure are postnatal age of less than 60 days, extent of liver damage prior to the procedure and degree of surgical expertise.[74] Most of these infants, however, go on to need liver transplant as a long-term solution.[75] Survival following liver transplant in these patients is excellent.[76]

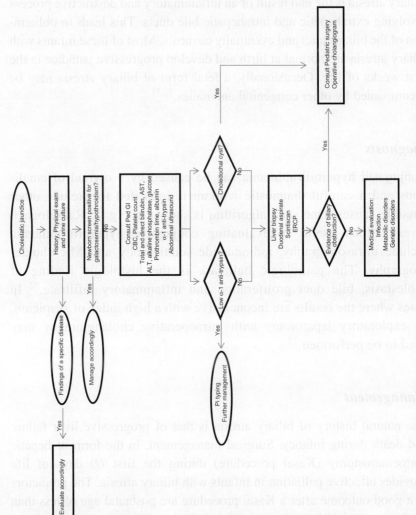

Figure 2. Algorithm for management of direct hyperbilirubinemia.

References

1. Martinez–Tallo E, Claure N, Bancalari E. (1997) Necrotizing enterocolitis in full-term or near-term infants: Risk factors. *Biol Neonate* **71**(5): 292–298.

2. Stark AR, Carlo WA, Tyson JE *et al.* (2001) Adverse effects of early dexamethasone in extremely-low-birth-weight infants. National Institute of Child Health and Human Development Neonatal Research Network. *N Engl J Med* **344**(2): 95–101.

3. Attridge JT, Clark R, Walker MW *et al.* (2006) New insights into spontaneous intestinal perforation using a national data set: (2) Two populations of patients with perforations. *J Perinatol* **26**(3): 185–188.

4. Lemons JA, Bauer CR, Oh W *et al.* (2001) Very low birth weight outcomes of the National Institute of Child health and human development neonatal research network, January 1995 through December 1996. NICHD Neonatal Research Network. *Pediatrics* **107**(1): E1.

5. Kliegman RM, Fanaroff AA. (1984) Necrotizing enterocolitis. *N Engl J Med* **310**(17): 1093–1103.

6. Bell MJ, Ternberg JL, Feigin RD *et al.* (1978) Neonatal necrotizing enterocolitis. Therapeutic decisions based upon clinical staging. *Ann Surg* **187**(1): 1–7.

7. Kim WY, Kim WS, Kim IO *et al.* (2005) Sonographic evaluation of neonates with early-stage necrotizing enterocolitis. Pediatr Radiol **35**(11): 1056–1061.

8. Bhandari V, Bizzarro MJ, Shetty A *et al.* (2006) Familial and genetic susceptibility to major neonatal morbidities in preterm twins. *Pediatrics* **117**(6):1901–1906.

9. Szebeni B, Szekeres R, Rusai K *et al.* (2006) Genetic polymorphisms of CD14, toll-like receptor 4, and caspase-recruitment domain 15 are not associated with necrotizing enterocolitis in very low birth weight infants. *J Pediatr Gastroenterol Nutr* **42**(1): 27–31.

10. Guillet R, Stoll BJ, Cotten CM *et al.* (2006) Association of H2-blocker therapy and higher incidence of necrotizing enterocolitis in very low birth weight infants. *Pediatrics* **117**(2): e137–e142.

11. Beach RC, Menzies IS, Clayden GS *et al.* (1982) Gastrointestinal permeability changes in the preterm neonate. *Arch Dis Child* **57**(2): 141–145.

12. Berseth CL. (1996) Gastrointestinal motility in the neonate. *Clin Perinatol* **23**(2): 179–190.

13. Martin CR, Walker WA. (2006) Intestinal immune defences and the inflammatory response in necrotising enterocolitis. *Semin Fetal Neonatal Med* **11**(5): 369–377.

14. Kosloske AM. (1994) Epidemiology of necrotizing enterocolitis. *Acta Paediatr Suppl* **396**: 2–7.

15. Cotten CM, Taylor S, Stoll B *et al.* (2009) Prolonged duration of initial empirical antibiotic treatment is associated with increased rates of necrotizing enterocolitis and death for extremely low birth weight infants. *Pediatrics* **123**(1): 58–66.

16. Lin HC, Su BH, Chen AC *et al.* (2005) Oral probiotics reduce the incidence and severity of necrotizing enterocolitis in very low birth weight infants. *Pediatrics* **115**(1): 1–4.

17. Deshpande G, Rao S, Patole S *et al.* (2010) Updated meta-analysis of probiotics for preventing necrotizing enterocolitis in preterm neonates. *Pediatrics* **125**(5): 921–930.

18. Soll RF. (2010) Probiotics: Are we ready for routine use? *Pediatrics* **125**(5): 1071–1072.

19. Moss RL, Dimmitt RA, Barnhart DC *et al.* (2006) Laparotomy versus peritoneal drainage for necrotizing enterocolitis and perforation. *N Engl J Med* **354**(21): 2225–2234.

20. Lucas A, Cole TJ. (1990) Breast milk and neonatal necrotising enterocolitis. *Lancet* **336**(8730): 1519–1523.

21. McGuire W, Anthony MY. (2003) Donor human milk versus formula for preventing necrotising enterocolitis in preterm infants: Systematic review. *Arch Dis Child Fetal Neonatal Ed* **88**(1): F11–F14.

22. Anderson DM, Kliegman RM. (1991) The relationship of neonatal alimentation practices to the occurrence of endemic necrotizing enterocolitis. *Am J Perinatol* **8**(1): 62–67.

23. Berseth CL, Bisquera JA, Paje VU. (2003) Prolonging small feeding volumes early in life decreases the incidence of necrotizing enterocolitis in very low birth weight infants. *Pediatrics* **111**(3): 529–534.

24. Wilmore D. (1969) Short bowel syndrome. A comprehensive approach to patient management. I. Pathophysiology following massive intestinal resection. *J Kans Med Soc* **70**(5): 233–237.

25. Weaver LT, Austin S, Cole TJ. (1991) Small intestinal length: A factor essential for gut adaptation. *Gut* **32**(11): 1321–1323.

26. Wilmore D. (1969) Short bowel syndrome. II. Patient management following massive intestinal resection. *J Kans Med Soc* **70**(6): 280–282.

27. Ladefoged K, Olgaard K. (1985) Sodium homeostasis after small-bowel resection. Scand *J Gastroenterol* **20**(3): 361–369.

28. O'Keefe SJ, Burnes JU, Thompson RL. (1994) Recurrent sepsis in home parenteral nutrition patients: An analysis of risk factors. *JPEN J Parenter Enteral Nutr* **18**(3): 256–263.

29. Moukarzel AA, Haddad I, Ament ME *et al.* (1994) Two hundred thirty patient years of experience with home long-term parenteral nutrition in childhood: Natural history and life of central venous catheters. *J Pediatr Surg* **29**(10): 1323–1327.

30. Hyman PE, Everett SL, Harada T. (1986) Gastric acid hypersecretion in short bowel syndrome in infants: association with extent of resection and enteral feeding. *J Pediatr Gastroenterol Nutr* **5**(2): 191–197.

31. Taylor SF, Sondheimer JM, Sokol RJ *et al.* (1991) Noninfectious colitis associated with short gut syndrome in infants. *J Pediatr* **119**(1(Pt 1)): 24–28.

32. Merritt RJ. (1986) Cholestasis associated with total parenteral nutrition. *J Pediatr Gastroenterol Nutr* **5**(1): 9–22.

33. Pereira GR, Sherman MS, DiGiacomo J *et al.* (1981) Hyperalimentation-induced cholestasis: Increased incidence and severity in premature infants. *Am J Dis Child* **135**(9): 842–845.

34. Sondheimer JM, Bryan H, Andrews W *et al.* (1978) Cholestatic tendencies in premature infants on and off parenteral nutrition. *Pediatrics* **62**(6): 984–989.

35. Parker P, Stroop S, Greene H. (1981) A controlled comparison of continuous versus intermittent feeding in the treatment of infants with intestinal disease. *J Pediatr* **99**(3): 360–364.

36. Jawaheer G, Shaw NJ, Pierro A. (2001) Continuous enteral feeding impairs gallbladder emptying in infants. *J Pediatr* **138**(6): 822–825.

37. Andorsky DJ, Lund DP, Lillehei CW *et al.* (2001) Nutritional and other postoperative management of neonates with short bowel syndrome correlates with clinical outcomes. *J Pediatr* **139**(1): 27–33.

38. Chen CY, Tsao PN, Chen HL *et al.* (2004) Ursodeoxycholic acid (UDCA) therapy in very-low-birth-weight infants with parenteral nutrition-associated cholestasis. *J Pediatr* **145**(3): 317–321.

39. Dunn L, Hulman S, Weiner J *et al.* (1988) Beneficial effects of early hypocaloric enteral feeding on neonatal gastrointestinal function: Preliminary report of a randomized trial. *J Pediatr* **112**(4): 622–629.

40. Baserga MC, Sola A. (2004) Intrauterine growth restriction impacts tolerance to total parenteral nutrition in extremely low birth weight infants. *J Perinatol* **24**(8): 476–481.

41. Wright K, Ernst KD, Gaylord MS *et al.* (2003) Increased incidence of parenteral nutrition-associated cholestasis with aminosyn PF compared to trophamine. *J Perinatol* **23**(6): 444–450.

42. Zambrano E, El–Hennawy M, Ehrenkranz RA *et al.* (2004) Total parenteral nutrition induced liver pathology: An autopsy series of 24 newborn cases. *Pediatr Dev Pathol* **7**(5): 425–432.

43. Blaszyk H, Wild PJ, Oliveira A *et al.* (2005) Hepatic copper in patients receiving long-term total parenteral nutrition. *J Clin Gastroenterol* **39**(4): 318–320.

44. Gura KM, Duggan CP, Collier SB *et al.* (2006) Reversal of parenteral nutrition-associated liver disease in two infants with short bowel syndrome using parenteral fish oil: Implications for future management. *Pediatrics* **118**(1): e197–201.

45. Fishbein TM. (2009) Intestinal transplantation. *N Engl J Med* **361**(10): 998–1008.

46. Wenzl TG, Schneider S, Scheele F *et al.* (2003) Effects of thickened feeding on gastroesophageal reflux in infants: A placebo-controlled crossover study using intraluminal impedance. *Pediatrics* **111**(4 Pt 1): e355–9.

47. Peter CS, Sprodowski N, Bohnhorst B *et al.* (2002) Gastroesophageal reflux and apnea of prematurity: No temporal relationship. *Pediatrics* **109**(1): 8–11.

48. Omari TI, Barnett CP, Benninga MA *et al.* (2002) Mechanisms of gastro-oesophageal reflux in preterm and term infants with reflux disease. *Gut* **51**(4): 475–479.

49. Peter CS, Wiechers C, Bohnhorst B *et al.* (2002) Influence of nasogastric tubes on gastroesophageal reflux in preterm infants: A multiple intraluminal impedance study. *J Pediatr* **141**(2): 277–279.

50. Ewer AK, Durbin GM, Morgan ME *et al.* (1996) Gastric emptying and gastro-oesophageal reflux in preterm infants. *Arch Dis Child Fetal Neonatal Ed* **75**(2): F117–F121.

51. Mitchell DJ, McClure BG, Tubman TR. (2001) Simultaneous monitoring of gastric and oesophageal pH reveals limitations of conventional oesophageal pH monitoring in milk fed infants. *Arch Dis Child* **84**(3): 273–276.

52. Grant L, Cochran D. (2001) Can pH monitoring reliably detect gastro-oesophageal reflux in preterm infants? *Arch Dis Child Fetal Neonatal Ed* **85**(3): F155–7; discussion F7–F8.

53. Wenzl TG, Moroder C, Trachterna M *et al.* (2002) Esophageal pH monitoring and impedance measurement: A comparison of two diagnostic tests for gastroesophageal reflux. *J Pediatr Gastroenterol Nutr* **34**(5): 519–523.

54. Birch JL, Newell SJ. (2009) Gastro-esophageal reflux disease in preterm infants: Current management and diagnostic dilemmas. *Arch Dis Child Fetal Neonatal Ed* **94**(5): F379–F383.

55. James ME, Ewer AK. (1999) Acid oro-pharyngeal secretions can predict gastro-oesophageal reflux in preterm infants. *Eur J Pediatr* **158**(5): 371–374.

56. Poets CF, Langner MU, Bohnhorst B. (1997) Effects of bottle feeding and two different methods of gavage feeding on oxygenation and breathing patterns in preterm infants. *Acta Paediatr* **86**(4): 419–423.

57. Herbst JJ, Minton SD, Book LS. (1979) Gastroesophageal reflux causing respiratory distress and apnea in newborn infants. *J Pediatr* **95**(5 Pt 1): 763–768.

58. Leape LL, Holder TM, Franklin JD *et al.* (1977) Respiratory arrest in infants secondary to gastroesophageal reflux. *Pediatrics* **60**(6): 924–928.

59. Walsh JK, Farrell MK, Keenan WJ *et al.* (1981) Gastroesophageal reflux in infants: Relation to apnea. *J Pediatr* **99**(2): 197–201.

60. Newell SJ, Booth IW, Morgan ME *et al.* (1989) Gastro-oesophageal reflux in preterm infants. *Arch Dis Child* **64**(6): 780–786.

61. Kahn A, Rebuffat E, Sottiaux M *et al.* (1990) Sleep apneas and acid esophageal reflux in control infants and in infants with an apparent life-threatening event. *Biol Neonate* **57**(3–4): 144–149.

62. Paton JY, Nanayakkara CS, Simpson H. (1990) Observations on gastro-oesophageal reflux, central apnea and heart rate in infants. *Eur J Pediatr* **149**(9): 608–612.

63. Kimball AL, Carlton DP. (2001) Gastroesophageal reflux medications in the treatment of apnea in premature infants. *J Pediatr* **138**(3): 355–360.

64. Nielson DW, Heldt GP, Tooley WH. (1990) Stridor and gastroesophageal reflux in infants. *Pediatrics* **85**(6): 1034–1039.

65. Bibi H, Khvolis E, Shoseyov D *et al.* (2001) The prevalence of gastro-esophageal reflux in children with tracheomalacia and laryngomalacia. *Chest* **119**(2): 409–413.

66. Sindel BD, Maisels MJ, Ballantine TV. (1989) Gastroesophageal reflux to the proximal esophagus in infants with bronchopulmonary dysplasia. *Am J Dis Child* **143**(9): 1103–1106.

67. Jadcherla SR, Berseth CL. (2002) Effect of erythromycin on gastroduodenal contractile activity in developing neonates. *J Pediatr Gastroenterol Nutr* **34**(1): 16–22.

68. Ng PC, So KW, Fung KS *et al.* (2001) Randomised controlled study of oral erythromycin for treatment of gastrointestinal dysmotility in preterm infants. *Arch Dis Child* Fetal *Neonatal Ed* **84**(3): F177–F182.

69. Beck–Sague CM, Azimi P, Fonseca SN *et al.* (1994) Bloodstream infections in neonatal intensive care unit patients: Results of a multicenter study. *Pediatr Infect Dis J* **13**(12): 1110–1116.

70. Lilly JR, Chandra RS. (1974) Surgical hazards of co-existing anomalies in biliary atresia. *Surg Gynecol Obstet* **139**(1): 49–54.

71. Chandra RS. (1974) Biliary atresia and other structural anomalies in the congenital polysplenia syndrome. *J Pediatr* **85**(5): 649–655.

72. Li MK, Crawford JM. (2004) The pathology of cholestasis. *Semin Liver Dis* **24**(1): 21–42.

73. Senyuz OF, Yesildag E, Emir H *et al.* (2001) Diagnostic laparoscopy in prolonged jaundice. *J Pediatr Surg* **36**(3): 463–465.

74. Kobayashi H, Stringer MD. (2003) Biliary atresia. *Semin Neonatol* **8**(5): 383–391.

75. Lykavieris P, Chardot C, Sokhn M *et al.* (2005) Outcome in adulthood of biliary atresia: A study of 63 patients who survived for over 20 years with their native liver. *Hepatology* **41**(2): 366–371.

76. Chen CL, Concejero A, Wang CC *et al.* (2006) Living donor liver trans-plantation for biliary atresia: A single-center experience with first 100 cases. *Am J Transplant* **6**(11): 2672–2679.

Chapter  11

Blood Disorders of the Newborn

Ted Rosenkrantz

This chapter will primarily focus on the problems of the red blood cell including anemia and polycythemia. Thrombocytopenia will also be covered due to frequency in the newborn, especially those admitted to a NICU.

Erythropoiesis and Changing Hemoglobin Function

The mature red cell is the result of multiple steps that begin with the myeloid stem cell. Under the influence of multiple factors the stem cell evolves into a functional cell in the circulation. The myeloid stem cell becomes the burst-forming unit-erythroid (BFU-E). Under the influence of erythropoietin and insulin-like growth factor 1 (IGF-1), the BFU-E becomes the normoblast, a cell that still contains a nucleus and DNA. Under the influence of Rac GTPase mDia2, the normoblast loses its nucleus and becomes a reticulocyte and, finally, a mature functional RBC.

The mature red cell contains protein, primarily in the form of hemoglobin. Hemoglobin is a tetramer of two pairs of globin chains, which change as the embryo becomes a fetus and newborn. Table 1 summarizes the chain pairs from embryonic to adult life. The alpha and alpha like

Table 1. Globin chains and types of hemoglobin at the various stages of development. Used with permission. *Neonatal Hematology*, de Alarcon P and Werner E (eds), Cambridge University Press, NY, 2005, p. 43.

Stage	Hemoglobin	Composition
Globin-chain development		
Embryo	Gower 1	ε_4 or $\zeta_2 \varepsilon_2$
Embryo	Gower 2	$\alpha_2 \varepsilon_2$
Embryo	Portland	$\zeta_2 \gamma_2$
Embryo	Fetal	$\zeta_2 \gamma_2$
Fetus	Fetal	$\zeta_2 \gamma_2$
Fetus	A	$\alpha_2 \beta_2$
Adult	A	$\alpha_2 \beta_2$
Adult	A2	$\alpha_2 \delta_2$
Adult	F	$\alpha_2 \gamma_2$

chains have their coding on chromosome 16 while the beta and beta-like chains have their coding on chromosome 11. By 12 weeks of age, fetal hemoglobin (HF) predominates and increases. At 34 weeks, there is a decline in HF as the amount of hemoglobin A increases. Concurrent with the changes in hemoglobin composition are changes in the site of formation. In the first few weeks of gestation, cell formation occurs in the yolk sac. By 5–10 weeks of gestation, all red cell formation occurs in the liver. At 15–20 weeks of life, the bone marrow starts to make red cells and is the primary site by 35 weeks gestation and sole site by term.

The primary function of the hemoglobin is to carry oxygen. The oxygen-carrying capacity changes with the type of hemoglobin, from fetal to adult life. Little oxygen is carried in the plasma of the blood. Hemoglobin-carrying capacity is dependent on the type of hemoglobin as well as the interaction with 2–3 DPG and pH. At birth, the maximal oxygen content within the blood is 20 ml/dl due to the predominance of HF. As HF production falls and HA predominates, the carrying capacity of the blood falls to 10 ml/dl. The oxygen-carrying capacity of the blood is also influenced by the amount of hemoglobin or the hematocrit (HCT) of the blood. The hemoglobin and hematocrit increase with gestational age (Table 2).

Table 2. Normal hemoglobin values in the fetus.

Gestation Age (weeks)	Hemoglobin (g/dl)
28–29	14.3
30–31	15.3
32–33	15.7
34–35	16.1
36–37	16.0
38–39	16.4
39–40	16.5

Anemia

Physiologic anemia occurs in all healthy infants. The partial pressure of oxygen in the blood flowing from the placenta to fetus is 25–30 mmHg. As a result, the oxygen saturation is 45–50% and results in a relatively low oxygen content. In order to meet the oxygen requirements of the fetus, either cardiac output can be increased or the red cell mass is increased. Under normal conditions, the relative hypoxia is sensed by the liver, which produces erythropoietin (EPO) in the fetus. EPO stimulates the production of RBCs, leading to a higher hemoglobin, HCT and oxygen-carrying capacity. The result is a normal oxygen content in the blood oxygenated in the placenta and adequate oxygen delivery to the tissues without compromise of cardiac performance. When there is a pathology that prohibits a sustained increase in red mass, cardiac output will increase up to the point of heart failure. Following birth, the partial pressure of oxygen increases as does oxygen saturation and arterial oxygen content. Fetal concentrations of EPO increase with gestational age. The fetus at term will have a concentration of 17–18 mU/ml. The increased arterial oxygen content and tissue delivery following birth results in a decrease in EPO production; blood concentration falls to 9 mU/ml. As a result, RBC production decreases as reflected by a decrease in the reticulocyte count (newborn at birth = 6–8% to 1–2%). HCT and hemoglobin concentrations decrease until the arterial oxygen content and tissue oxygen delivery decrease to a level resulting in relative tissue hypoxia. This is referred to as a physiologic anemia of the newborn. This anemia, which occurs at 8 weeks of life in the term infant, results in increased EPO production and a rise in the reticulocyte count, hemoglobin and HCT, assuming that there is adequate iron as well as a good state of general nutrition. In the preterm infant, anemia occurs at about 5 weeks of age as a result of similar post-natal conditions in addition to growing blood volume, iatrogenic blood loss and decreased RBC survival time.

Anemia in the newborn period (defined as a HCT < 2SD of the norm for gestational age) may originate during fetal life and up to the first days and weeks of life. Multiple genetic, immunologic, infectious, pregnancy and metabolic factors may play a role in anemia, although there is generally one predominate factor in a particular infant. The assessment of anemia requires a family and pregnancy history, a physical examination as well as laboratory evaluation that is pertinent to the clinical situation. Similarly, therapy is dependent on the cause of the anemia and condition of the fetus or the newborn.

The first determination to be made is whether the infant is truly anemic. This should be based on gestational age norms. (see Table 2). The cause and symptoms of anemia, will determine therapy. Anemia in the newborn can be categorized in several ways:

1. Congenital Infection
2. Hemolysis
3. Failure of Production
4. Blood Loss
    a. Acute
    b. Chronic
5. Failure of Production

History is essential in determining the cause of the anemia. Start with the maternal history which will help determine such important factors as blood type, blood dyscrasia and exposure to toxin or infection. Family history will reveal such problems as thalassemias, G6PD and other pertinent genetic information. Pregnancy history will help ascertain infectious and toxic exposures, bleeding, trauma, change in fetal movement (severe anemia is associated with decreased or absent fetal movement), or other complications such as twinning and placentation.

Physical examination of the newborn and assessment of the placenta will also give etiological insight as well as appropriate therapy. The following are examples of physical findings that are either diagnostic or help determine the cause of the anemia:

1. Congenital anomalies:
   a. Blueberry muffin spots – infection such as congenital rubella
   b. Petechiae – infection such as CMV
   c. Hemangioma – cavernous hemangioma
2. Hepatosplenomegaly suggests chronic anemia:
   a. Hemolytic disease
   b. Congenital infection
   c. Blood loss
3. Occult signs of blood loss such as subgaleal hemorrhage
4. Others signs of congestive heart failure
5. Placental abnormalities:
   a. Abnormal cord insertion
   b. Signs of abruption
   c. Abnormal vessels

Laboratory investigation should include a CBC with reticulocyte count and morphology, maternal and newborn blood type, Coombs test (direct and indirect) and serum bilirubin concentration. The CBC alone can be extremely helpful. Figure 1 is a flowchart in which the information from the CBC, Coombs test and blood smear can point toward the diagnosis.

Perinatal conditions associated with anemia in the newborn

1. Infection

Perinatal infections leading to anemia are generally viral infections of the mother that are passed transplacentally to the fetus. A history of infection in the mother, supported with appropriate serology, PCR or the finding of hydrops fetalis, is often the first clue to fetal anemia due to infection. In the past, syphilis was a common infectious cause of marrow suppression

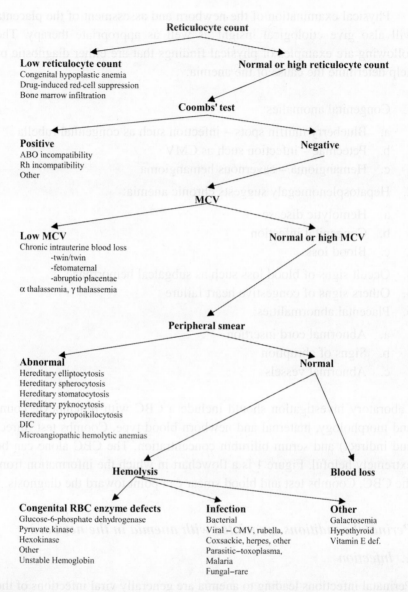

Figure 1. Diagnostic approach to anemia based on CBC and Coomb's test. Used with permission. De Alarcon PA, Johnson MC and Werner EJ. (2005) Erythropoiesis, red cells and the approach to anemia. In *Neonatal Hematology,* de Alarcon P and Werner E (eds), Cambridge University Press, NY, p. 52.

and anemia. Currently, Parvovirus B19 is the most common cause, especially in the second trimester. Parvovirus infection causes suppression of the bone marrow so that red cell production stops at the point of pronormoblasts. The suppression is time-limited. Presentation in the fetus requires close surveillance, assessment of fetal hematocrit and transfusion to prevent hydrops. If anemia is still an issue at birth, transfusion and close follow-up is appropriate therapy. The bone marrow generally recovers in several weeks to months. Fetal loss is 5%. Other viral infections associated with red cell suppression in the fetus and newborn include:

a. Cytomegalovirus
b. HIV
c. Adenovirus
d. EBV
e. Rubella

2. Hemolysis

RBC incompatibility (alloimune hemolysis)

a. Rh Erythroblastosis

The most common cause of hemolysis in the fetus and newborn is due to RBC destruction by maternal antibody. It is referred to as hemolytic disease of the newborn (HDN). The most common cause is Rh erythroblastosis which is due to a maternal response to the RhD antigen on the fetal RBC. This entity was elucidated beginning in the late 1930's at a time when the mortality rate for the fetus/newborn was 50%. The RhD antigen is a polypeptide attached to the surface of the RBC. The polypeptide is a product of the RHD RHCe, RHD RhcE, RHD Rhce or RHDRHCE alleles. Those individuals who do not have such proteins on their RBC are lacking the genetic code for the protein (RHD-negative). Hemolysis occurs when the mother is RHD-negative and the fetus is RHD-positive. During the pregnancy, fetal cells enter the maternal circulation and invoke an immune response with the production of IgM antibodies. Pregnancy complications such as antepartum hemorrhage, PIH, external version, caesarean section and manual removal of the placenta are associated with larger transfer of fetal RBCs into the maternal circulation. As IgM antibodies do not cross the placenta, less than 1% of fetuses are affected in the first pregnancy, although up to 15% of the mothers are affected. With subsequent pregnancies in which there is RhD incompatibility, IgG antibody is maternally produced as a result of repeat immunologic response, crossing the placenta and resulting in fetal RBC destruction. IgG antibodies may start to cross the placenta at as early as 15 weeks gestation, but it is not until 22 weeks that there is clinically significant transfer. The fetal concentration of maternally derived antibodies continues to increase with gestation. Fifty percent of these subsequent pregnancies will result in infants who will not require intervention while 25% will require fetal transfusion to prevent hydrops due to anemia and 25% will require exchange transfusion to correct anemia and prevent hyperbilirubinemia and kernicterus. However, other antigens including RhC, Rhc, RhE and Kell, are becoming more common etiologic causes of HDN due to transfusions and exposure to blood through other sources. Use of anti-D immunoglobulin prophylaxis and treatment has reduced the incidence of maternal sensitization and hemolytic disease due to Rh incompatibility to 1–2%. The dosing is dependent on the knowledge of the volume of fetal cells that have entered the maternal circulation using the Kleihauer–Betke test or flow cytometry.

b. ABO incompatibility
The ABO antigens were the first discovered antigens and are carbohydrate molecules. Individuals who have A antigen have the gene for A transferase. The A allele encodes a glycosyltransferase that bonds α-N-acetylgalactosamine to the H antigen, producing the A antigen. Those with the B antigen have the gene for B-transferase which bonds α-D-galactose to the H antigen, creating the B antigen. Those who are AB have an allele that codes for each carbohydrate. Individuals with Type O blood have a deletion that results in lack of production of any carbohydrate antigen in the ABO system. Antibodies to the A and B antigen are produced in early life due to exposure and sensitization to environmental substances such as food, bacteria and viruses. Thus initial exposure during

the pregnancy results in IgG antibodies that interact with the fetal RBC, leading to hemolysis. ABO incompatibility affects 3% of all deliveries.

The degree of hemolysis will vary with antibody concentration, antigen concentration on the RBC and other binding sites in the fetus for the antibody. AB, Duffy and Kidd antigens are expressed on RBC and non-erythroid tissue, while only erythroid and myeloid cells express RhD, Kell and MN Ss antigens. This combination of factors (maternal antibody production, placental transfer and antigen density on the RBC) will determine the degree of hemolysis observed in the fetus and newborn. Rh incompatibility is generally associated with a more brisk hemolytic reaction and is likely to cause significant anemia and hyperbilirubinemia in the fetus and newborn. This contrasts with ABO incompatibility which rarely causes anemia in the fetus or newborn and the hyperbilirubinemia is generally milder.

Management of anemia due to hemolytic disease of the newborn

Management is determined by the degree of hemolysis and anemia. Critical information includes blood type of father of the current pregnancy, maternal antibody titers, fetal ultrasound, amniotic fluid spectrophotometry and fetal blood sampling. Assessment begins at a time of fetal viability. The degree of anemia in the fetus is best assessed by measurement of fetal blood flow velocity in the middle cerebral artery (MCA). Fetal transfusion is undertaken to maintain the hematocrit and prevent hydrops. Fetal transfusion can also reverse hydrops if it has begun to develop. Timing of delivery is based on risk of intrauterine transfusion and risks of preterm delivery. If the fetus is doing poorly, then delivery will occur earlier. If transfusion therapy is maintaining the fetus, then getting the pregnancy to a gestation age when risks of prematurity decrease is optimal (see Fig. 2). At birth, an assessment of the degree on anemia and hemolysis is assessed by a CBC, Coomb's test and bilirubin concentration. Treatment is guided by the results. In the absence of anemia at birth, phototherapy is very effective in treating hyperbilirubinemia. However, for the newborn with severe anemia with or without hydrops, an exchange transfusion is effective in normalizing the hematocrit, maintain a normal blood volume and removing maternal antibody. Exchange

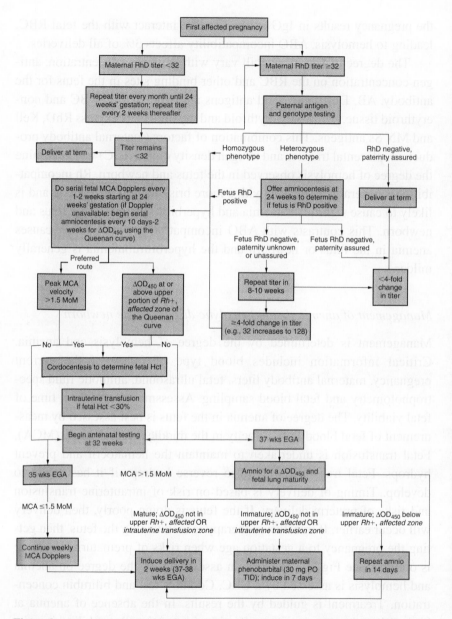

Figure 2. Management of the RhD sensitized pregnant woman. Adapted from Moise KJ. (2008) Management of rhesus alloimmunization in pregnancy. *Obstet Gynecol* **112**: 164–176. Used with permission.

transfusion is also used later in the course to treat hyperbilirubinemia not effectively controlled with phototherapy in the prevention of kernicterus. Infants who do not require an exchange transfusion in the nursery must be followed every 1–2 weeks until 4 months of age for late anemia that could result in congestive heart failure due to persistence of maternal antibody and ongoing hemolysis.

c. Immune disease of the mother

Autoimmune diseases of the mother may result in neonatal hemolysis. Such diseases as lupus may be associated with IgG antibody that may cross the placenta and cause RBC destruction in the newborn. The pathogenesis, clinical course and treatment are similar to that of RhD incompatibility.

d. Other causes of hemolysis

Hemolysis in the newborn, when not secondary to alloimmune disease (see HDN) or infection, is the result of chromosomal abnormities that result in defects of the cell membrane, hemoglobin or oxidative injury. The following is a discussion of those that present in the newborn period.

The RBC of the newborn has a shorter lifespan. Susceptibility of hemoglobin F to oxidative stress has been speculated. However, true anemia due to hemolysis generally is due to defects in cell metabolism that normally protects the RBC from oxidative injury and defects in the production of normal hemoglobin. The triad of presenting signs and symptoms includes anemia, reticulocytosis and hyperbilirubinemia. The normal hematocrit in the term newborn is 50–55% if the clamping of the umbilical cord is delayed at birth. The reticulocyte count is 3–7%. Lastly, the peripheral smear of the blood should be examined for cells with abnormal physical structure.

i.   Vitamin E deficiency

This is primarily a problem of the preterm infant who has low levels of Vitamin E at birth. Failure to provide Vitamin E, an antioxidant, places the infant at risk for anemia due to hemolysis of oxidative injury. Usual supplementation is 25 U/day.

ii. RBC membrane disorders

The cell membrane of the RBC is composed of a phospholipid bilayer that is interspersed by a protein layer that penetrates the lipid layer. The third component is a protein layer that helps to form the cytoskeleton of the cell. There are two common hereditary disorders seen in the newborn: spherocytosis and elliptocytosis.

a. Sphereocytosis: This is generally an autosomal dominant trait although up to 25% of diagnosed newborns will have had a new mutation. In addition, another 25% will be the result of an autosomal recessive form. The membrane defect is due to an abnormality in the cytoskeleton of the cell membrane resulting in the abnormal shape and predisposing to destruction in the spleen. The severity in the fetus and the newborn ranges from severe anemia and hydrops to a hemolytic anemia that does not become apparent until the first month of life. The diagnosis is suggested by the CBC, the abnormal morphology on blood smear and hyperbilirubinemia. An osmotic fragility test helps to confirm the diagnosis. Management in the newborn is primarily directed towards treatment of hyperbilirubinemia and correction of anemia by transfusion.

b. Elliptocytosis: It is the result of an autosomal dominant transmission of DNA that codes for an abnormal cytoskeleton. The abnormal shape and fragility of the cell make it subject to hemolysis. There are a number of genetic variants. It is those infants who are homozygotes or compound heterozygotes who will have severe hemolysis and anemia. The blood smear may have poikilocytosis, micro-elleiptocytes and red cell fragmentation. Treatment is symptomatic. A related entity is hereditary pyropoikilocytosis, an autosomally transmitted disorder of the cytoskeleton. Similarly, treatment is symptomatic and symptoms improve with age.

iii. RBC enzyme disorders

The two most common disorders in the newborn are glucose-6-phosphate dehydrogenase deficiency (G6PD) and pyruvate kinase deficiency (PK).

Glucose is the primary substrate for the RBC, generating energy (via the Embden Meyerhof pathway) and antioxidant protection (via the hexose monophosphate pathway).

a. Glucose-6-phosphase dehydrogenase deficiency (G6PD):
This is a sex-linked disorder with a higher incidence in those of Mediterranean, African or Chinese origin. There are a number of mutations responsible for the enzyme deficiency. All of them lead to inadequate amounts of glutathione, an important antioxidant. In the face of increased oxidants as seen with infection and the administration of certain drugs, the globin becomes denatured and precipitates, forming Heinz bodies. The Heinz bodies attach to the cell membrane, resulting in abnormal structure and destruction via hemolysis. The diagnosis is suggested by the blood smear and confirmed by an assay for the G6PD enzyme. Treatment is symptomatic and the disease is best treated by avoidance of offending medications and environmental factors. In the newborn, the primary issue is the treatment of hyperbilirubinemia and the prevention of kernicterus.

b. Pyruvate kinase deficiency:
This enzyme deficiency results in RBC energy compromise, as it is one of two sources of ATP available for the energy needs of the RBC. While less frequent than G6PD, it has a high frequency in the Amish of Pennsylvania. There are multiple mutations responsible for the enzyme deficiency. Hemolysis may occur in the fetus; however, it is primarily a newborn disease presenting with a non-immune hemolytic anemia and severe hyperbilirubinemia. Diagnosis is made by an assay for the enzyme. Treatment is symptomatic as with G6PD.

c. Other enzyme deficiencies with similar clinical presentations and consequences include glucose phosphate isomerase deficiency, phosphoglycerate kinase deficiency and phosphofructokinase deficiency, among others.

iv. Hemoglobinopathies
The thalassemias are the only hemoglobinopathies of consequence in the fetus and newborn. α-thalassemia affects the fetus and newborn

Table 3. The α-thalassemias. Adapted from Glader B and Allen G. *Neonatal Hemolysis in Neonatal Hematology*, de Alarcon P and Werner E (eds.), Cambridge University Press, NY, 2005, p. 43.

Genotype	Phenotype	Clinical expression
(α α / α α)	Normal	Normal hemoglobin and HCT
(- α / α α)	Silent carrier	Normal hemoglobin and HCT
(- - / α α)	α-thalassemia trait	Mild anemia
(- - / - α)	Hemoglobin H disease	Moderate hemolytic anemia
(- - /- -)	Homozygous α-thalassemia	Severe anemia/hydrops

while the *β*-thalassemia is not of consequence until the infant is several months of age.

There are two genes that code for the alpha globulin on each set of alleles of chromosome 16 for a total of four genes. α-thalassemia refers to one or more gene deletions and the corresponding abnormality in globin formation. The four possible genotypes are categorized with corresponding phenotypes in Table 3.

The *"silent carrier"* results from the pairing of a normal parent and a carrier while the *α-thalassemia trait* is the result of two parents who are both carriers or one who is normal and one who has the trait. A carrier parent and one with trait will produce a child with *Hemoglobin H disease* while the pairing of either trait/trait or H/H or trait/H have a high likelihood of a fetus with *homozygous α-thalassemia*. The newborn with the trait will have a microcytic anemia at birth and an increased Bart's hemoglobin (gamma-chain tetramer). There is no need for treatment and they are normal in adult life. Infants with H disease, commonly seen in southeast Asia, will be anemic with up to 30% Bart's hemoglobin over time, as there is conversion from production of gamma chains to beta chains and significant H hemoglobin. The hemolytic anemia is exacerbated by exposure to oxidants (as seen in G6PD) and infection. Homozygous α-thalassemia is not compatible with life. The fetus may survive for some time due to the production of abnormal hemoglobins and persistence of embryonic hemoglobins. The fetus commonly develops hydrops and is stillborn, and those who are born alive die shortly after birth. Genetic counseling of parents with alpha-thalassemia is important for reproductive planning as well as monitoring of the pregnancy.

3. Blood loss

Acute blood loss in the newborn period is uncommon. It may be observed in the preterm infant with an acute infection, IVH or from the umbilicus or umbilical catheter or other central line. Acute blood loss in the term infant is seen in subgaleal hemorrhaging, intracranial hemorrhaging or abdominal accidents associated with intestinal abnormalities (e.g. malrotation with volvulus, intussusception).

Blood loss in the fetus may be either an acute or chronic condition. Acute conditions include the following:

a. Cord hematoma
b. Ruptured cord
c. Placental laceration
d. Placental abruption
e. Fetomaternal hemorrhage
f. Twin-to-Twin Transfusion

Chronic conditions include the following:

a. Aberrant placental vessels
b. Placental chorangioma
c. Velamentous insertion
d. Communication placental vessels
e. Twin-to-Twin Transfusion
f. Cavernous hemangioma

As noted before, the management of the fetus will be based on the gestation age, fetal condition and acuity.

Blood loss in the newborn may be associated with surgery, central lines and phlebotomy. Management is dependent on the acuity or chronicity and clinical condition of the newborn as reviewed below.

4. Failure of production

While infection is a more common cause of RBC production failure, it is generally self-limited as discussed in the prior section. Genetic causes of marrow failure are less common, are less amenable to successful long term therapy and carry greater morbidity and mortality.

The evaluation of an anemic infant suspected to have bone marrow failure starts with a CBC with careful inspection of the smear. This is followed by examination of the bone marrow aspiration and biopsy. Cells should be processed using cytogenetic and chromosomal fragility tests, flow cytometry and genotyping. Therapy and prognosis will be dependent on the final diagnosis.

Below are some of the more common entities:

- Blackfan Diamond Anemia

  While often thought of as pure red cell failure, other cell lines may be affected, including neutrophils and platelets. In addition to marrow failure, there are associated skeletal abnormalities that aid in the diagnosis. The genetic defect tends to be associated with a new sporadic mutation. The defect has been linked to mutations on chromosomes 19, 8 and X. The mechanism for erythroid failure has yet to be determined. Presentation may occur at birth but many do not present until several weeks or months after birth with anemia and lack of reticulocytosis. The majority are initially responsive to corticosteroid therapy, but ultimately become dependent on chronic transfusion. Iron overload is a common morbidity. Bone marrow transplantation appears to be the only permanent solution and is highly successful.

- Fanconi's Anemia

  This appears to be an autosomal recessive disease. Several different abnormal proteins have been associated with the phenotype and have been mapped to several different chromosomal sites. The clinical presentation is classically a triad of boney abnormities, growth failure and café au lait spots. However, these features are inconsistent. Other associated features include hypogonadism and malformation of the GI, GU and CNS. It is these abnormalities that lead to the diagnosis as red cell aplasia frequently does not occur until later in the first decade of life. Other myeloid cell lines may be involved. The cells are very sensitive to alkylating agents and radiation that is used to treat leukemias and solid tumors that commonly occur in these patients. As such, toxicity of treatment to prepare the patient for bone marrow therapy may be fatal and the success rate for transport is poor. Androgen and hematopoietic therapy may provide short-term success. These patients have a high occurrence of other malignancies.

Other causes of RBC production failure include the following:

Pearson Syndrome
Cartilage-hair hypoplasia
Shwachman–Diamond Syndrome
Reticular dysgenesis
Congenial dyserythropoietic anemia
Sideroblastic anemia

5. *Principles of management of anemia in the fetus and newborn*

Management of anemia is dependent upon the etiology and condition of the newborn. Management of specific conditions has been given. However, the following principles may be applied in most situations as they are based upon basic physiology with the goal of maintaining blood volume and oxygen-carrying capacity.

- Acute blood loss, fetal or newborn:
  Examples include fetomaternal hemorrhage, subgaleal hemorrhage and NEC. Transfuse packed red cells. Volume is dependent on estimated loss. Goal is to normalize HR, BP and hematocrit. The initial hematocrit may give some estimation of the volume of the blood loss. Following acute blood loss, it may take several hours for equilibration to occur and observe the new hematocrit. The observed hematocrit compared to the expected hematocrit will give an estimate of the volume of blood lost.
- Prenatal chronic blood loss or anemia (e.g. TTTS, HDN):
  While the red cell mass is low, accounting for the anemia, the blood volume is normal. Simple transfusion may lead to volume overload,

especially if there is evidence of heart failure as in hydrops. The preferred method to normalize the hematocrit is via a partial exchange
transfusion utilizing packed red cells. This will correct the anemia and
oxygen-carrying capacity while maintaining the blood volume.

• Postnatal chronic anemia:
    The most common reason for this condition is the combination of
    phlebotomy in the preterm infant. During the period of convales-
    cence, appropriate nutrition, vitamins and iron will lead to a normal
    erythropoietic response over time. Transfusion is only needed if the
    infant has decompensation (CHF, tachycardia) prior to the expected
    response to the anemia. Similarly, transfusion may be reserved in ane-
    mia due to hemoglobinopathies, HDN or enzyme defects unless there
    is decompensation due to the degree of anemia or an acute episode of
    hemolysis that exacerbates the chronic compensated anemia.

Polycythemia

Polycythemia is defined as a hematocrit ≥65% on a blood sample from a
central large blood vessel as blood from other sources, such as a capillary
blood sample, will over estimate the true hematocrit. Polycythemia occurs
in 1–5% of term infants. The viscosity of newborn blood is primarily
determined by the RBC concentration and increases exponentially when
the hematocrit is greater than 65%. The *in vivo* viscosity also increases as
the size of the blood vessel decreases. However, there is an abrupt fall
in blood viscosity in the capillary bed where it becomes similar to the
viscosity of the plasma or water.

Primary mechanisms leading to polycythemia

1. Chronic fetal hypoxia:
    This leads to an increase in fetal erythropoietin production and
    increased RBC mass. The increased hematocrit compensates for the
    low oxygen saturation of the hemoglobin, resulting in normalization
    of the arterial oxygen content of the blood. Blood volume is normal.
    This is observed in the setting of maternal diabetes, PIH, fetal hyper-
    thyroidism and maternal smoking.

2. Acute fetal hypoxia:
    This results in a shift of blood volume from the placenta to the fetus due to vasodilatation in the fetus in response to the hypoxia. The affected infant will be polycythemic and have an increased blood volume at the time of birth.
3. Delayed cord clamping and stripping of the umbilical cord:
    This results in a hypervolemic polycythemia. Delayed cord clamping will increase the HCT by 15% (HCT 50% → 65%).
4. Genetic syndromes:
    Polycythemia occurs with increased frequency in Beckwith–Weiderman syndrome as well as in Trisomy 13, 18 and 21. The mechanism is unknown.

Physiologic alterations

Understanding the known physiologic changes due to polycythemia will lead to a clear understanding of the changes in organ function and clinical findings. Blood viscosity and arterial oxygen content (CaO_2) increase while the plasma volume is reduced.

1. Brain:
    Brain blood flow is decreased. This is a normal physiologic response to the increased CaO_2 of the blood, not hyperviscosity. Brain oxygenation and metabolism is normal.
2. Heart and lungs:
    Cardiac output is decreased. However the increased CaO_2 of the blood results in normal systemic oxygen delivery. Pulmonary blood flow is decreased due to hyperviscosity and increased pulmonary vascular resistance. This results in hypoxia and a picture of PPHN.
3. GI:
    Intestinal blood flow is decreased as is oxygen extraction and uptake.
4. Renal:
    Renal blood flow is normal, but plasma blood flow is decreased and results in decreased GFR.
5. Metabolic:
    Hypoglycemia is observed and is likely related to decreased plasma volume and flow and increased tissue extraction of glucose.

Clinical features

The infant may have a ruddy appearance. Other symptoms associated with polycythemia include lethargy, tachypnea, jitteriness, poor feeding and vomiting. Oliguria, hypoglycemia and hypocalcemia are also observed.

1. Brain:
   Short–term symptoms such as jitteriness, lethargy and poor feeding generally resolve within days. However, infants are at-risk for neurodevelopmental delays. Brain injury appears to be related to prenatal and perinatal events that are associated with polycythemia.
2. Heart and lungs:
   Respiratory distress and hypoxia are due to increased pulmonary vascular resistance and shunting of blood flow.
3. Feeding intolerance and NEC:
   It is not clear whether these symptoms are due to perinatal factors such as hypoxia or partial exchange transfusion (PET) used to treat polycythemia. However, the elevated hematocrit does not appear to be the underlying cause.
4. Renal dysfunction:
   This is due to the low GFR as discussed above.
5. Hypoglycemia:
   This occurs in 12–40% of infants.

Treatment

Partial exchange transfusion with either saline or a 5% albumin solution will lower the hematocrit and normalize the viscosity of the blood. The use of saline is cost-effective and avoids complications associated with blood products. The exchange volume is calculated as follows:

$$\text{Blood volume of infant} \times \frac{(\text{observed HCT} - \text{desired HCT})}{(\text{observed HCT})}$$

Blood volume of the term infant = 80–90 ml/k
Desired HCT = 50–55%

In many areas of the world, infants with polycythemia are routinely treated with PET if they are "symptomatic" and their HCT ≥ 65% or "asymptomatic" with a HCT ≥ 70%. This approach is not consistent with our current knowledge of polycythemia and the efficacy of PET. Below is a concise review of the PET treatment by organ system:

1. CNS function:
   Based on multiple studies and two meta-analyses including a Cochrane review, there is no evidence that a PET will improve the neurodevelopmental outcome of infants with polycythemia.
2. Cardiopulmonary:
   PET will normalize pulmonary vascular resistance and blood flow in those infants with respiratory distress and hypoxia due to polycythemia.
3. GI:
   PET will not relieve feeding problems or prevent NEC.
4. Hypoglycemia:
   Hypoglycemia resistance to feeding or intravenous glucose infusion and not due to some other metabolic derangement may be successfully treated with PET which will increase the plasma volume and glucose delivery to the various organs.
5. Renal:
   PET will increase the plasma volume and GFR with improvement of urine output.

As such, only those infants with symptoms known to be reversed by PET should be treated. Current evidence does support the routine treatment.

Thrombocytopenia and Platelet Disorders

Platelets originate from the burst-forming unit-megakaryocyte (BFU-Mk). Under the influence of thrombopoietin, there is differentiation to the megakaryocyte. Psuedopodes develop with the formation of proplatelets which are then released. Due to their size and blood flow, the platelets tend to flow in the periphery of blood vessels, giving them proximity to areas of injury. Within the cell are granules that contain factors necessary for activation of the platelet and allow clot formation in conjunction with fibrinogen.

Platelet counts increase with gestational age. At 28 weeks gestation, the mean is 280,000/microliter and 325,000/microliter by term. Thrombocytopenia, defined as a platelet count less than 150,000/microliter, is commonly found in "sick" infants admitted to an NICU (up to 22%). For many, the underlying cause is not clear. However, it is common to find an elevated platelet-associated IgG (PAIgG) in many of the infants although there is no antibody found in the mother.

There are rare intrinsic disorders of platelet function. The most common cause in clinical practice is the administration of COX inhibitors to the infant. Examples include indomethacin or ibuprofen for closure of the ductus arteriosus or indomethacin for prevention of intraventricular hemorrhage.

Maternal diseases associated with maternal and neonatal thrombocytopenia include the following:

Chronic Hypertension
Pregnancy Induced Hypertension (PIH)
HELLP syndrome
Infection
TTP
ITP
Hemolytic-Uremic Syndrome

It has been postulated that the thrombocytopenia observed in infants born to affected mothers is immune-mediated as noted above. These entities, as well as other causes of thrombocytopenia in the fetus and newborn, are reviewed below. Figure 3 provides a diagnostic approach to the infant with thrombocytopenia.

• Maternal Hypertension and Pregnancy Induced Hypertension (PIH): In maternal hypertension, there appears to be a relationship between the maternal platelet count and newborn platelet count, suggesting an immune mechanism. A similar mechanism has been postulated for the

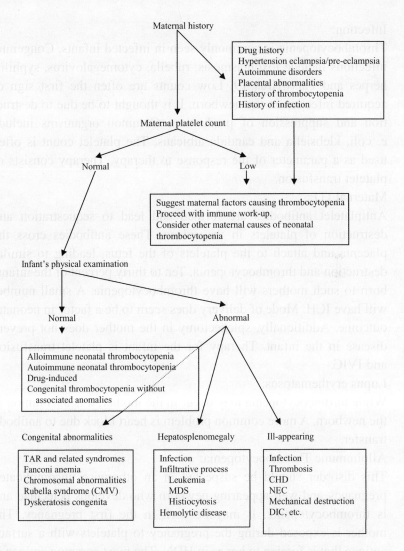

Figure 3. Diagnostic paradigm for the infant with thrombocytopenia. Used with permission. De Alarcon PA. (2005) Newborn platelet disorders. In *Neonatal Hematology*, de Alarcon P and Werner E (eds), Cambridge University Press, NY, p. 229.

thrombocytopenia seen in infants born to mothers with PIH. The incidence is between 10–20%. It is more common in the preterm infant. The thrombocytopenia generally resolves without therapy in the first week of life.

- Infection:
  Thrombocytopenia is commonly seen in infected infants. Congenital infections include toxoplasmosis, rubella, cytomegalovirus, syphilis, herpes and Parvovirus 19. Low counts are often the first sign of acquired infection in the newborn. It is thought to be due to destruction and suppression of production. Common organisms include e. coli, klebsiella and candida albicans. The platelet count is often used as a parameter of the response to therapy. Therapy consists of platelet transfusion.

- Maternal ITP:
  Antiplatelet antibodies are formed and lead to sequestration and destruction of platelets in the spleen. These antibodies cross the placenta and attach to the platelets of the fetus, leading to similar destruction and thrombocytopenia. Ten to thirty percent of the infants born to such mothers will have thrombocytopenia. A small number will have ICH. Mode of delivery does seem to be a factor in neonatal outcome. Additionally, splenectomy in the mother does not prevent disease in the infant. Therapy for the infant is platelet transfusion and IVIG.

- Lupus erythematosus:
  While thrombocytopenia may occur in the mother, it is uncommon in the newborn. A more common problem is heart block due to antibody transfer.

- Alloimmune Thrombocytopenia:
  This disorder should be suspected in an otherwise uncomplicated pregnancy and well-appearing newborn who develops petechiae and is thrombocytopenic. It may be seen in the first pregnancy. The mother is exposed during the pregnancy to platelets with a surface antigen that is foreign to her as in HDN. The most common antigen is PLA-1, although other platelet antigens have been involved. The mother produces IgG antibodies against the antigen on the fetal platelets. The incidence is 1–2/1000 births, although maternal sensitization is twice as common. It represents 10% of thrombocytopenic newborns. Diagnosis is established by testing the mother's serum for the platelet antibody. Confirmation is provided by testing the platelet type of mother and father as well as testing the infant. Initial therapy

consists of transfusing the infant with compatible platelets. If not available, random platelets may be used and generally result in a good response. This is followed by infusion of IVIG (1 mg/k/d × 2 days). The thrombocytopenia resolves in 1–2 weeks. The most concerning complication is intracranial hemorrhage which occurs in 10% of infants. The hemorrhage is a prenatal event in 25–50% of infants. All affected newborns should have a cranial ultrasound or other appropriate brain imaging. Alloimmune thrombocytopenia will occur in the majority of subsequent pregnancies to a similar degree or worse. Prenatal therapy should always be provided in subsequent pregnancies as there is no way to predict the severity of the disease in the subsequent pregnancy. Treatment generally begins at 13–16 weeks gestation and consists of weekly IVIG therapy plus prednisone.

- Genetic:
  There are a number of chromosomal anomalies associated with thrombocytopenia. They include Thrombocytopenia-Absent Radius syndrome (TAR), amegakaryocytic thrombocytopenia, and Wiskott–Aldrich syndrome, as well as other rate entities.

- Other causes:
  Include Kasabach–Merritt syndrome, hypoxia, ECMO therapy and exchange transfusion.

Therapy

Platelet transfusion for thrombocytopenia is dictated by the etiology, natural course of the disease and other complicating medical and surgical conditions. Clinical bleeding generally does not occur until the platelet count is less than 20,000. However, patients may be transfused at higher levels if there is an active destruction of platelets as in sepsis or alloimmune thrombocytopenia, or if there is anticipation of an invasive procedure.

References

1. de Alarcon P, Werner E (eds). (2005) *Neonatal Hematology* Cambridge University Press, NY, pp. 40–57, 58–67, 68–90, 91–131, 132– 187–253.

2. Bhutani VK, Johnson L, Sivieri EM. (1999) Predictive ability of a predischarge hour-specific serum bilirubin for subsequent significant hyperbilirubinemia in healthy term and near-term newborns. *Pediatrics.* Jan; **103**(1): 6–14.

3. Orkin SH, Nathan DG, Ginsburg D *et al.* (eds). (2009) *Nathan and Oski's Hematology of Infancy and Childhood*, 7th edition. Saunders Elsevier, Philadelphia, PA, pp. 21–66, 67–102, 275–306, 455–466, 839–910, 1015–1108, 1379–1398, 1463–1486, 1771.

4. Martin RJ, Fanaroff AA, Walsh MC (eds). *Fanaroff and Martin's Neonatal-Perinatal Medicine: Diseases of the Fetus and Infant.* 8th edition. Mosby Elsevier, Philadelphia, PA, pp. 367–374.

5. Sarkar S, Rosenkrantz TS. (2008) Neonatal polycythemia and hyperviscosity. *Seminars in Fetal and Neonatal Medicine* **13**: 248–255.

6. Vera EV, Gonzalez–Quintero VH. (2009) Thrombocytopenia in Pregnancy. eMedicine.

7. Bussei JB, Sola–Visner M. (2009) Current approaches to the evaluation and management of the fetus and neonate with immune thrombocytopenia. *Seminars in Perinatology* **33**: 35–42.

8. Creasy RK, Resnik R, Iams JD (eds). (2009) *Creasy and Resnik's Maternal-Fetal Medicine*, Saunders Elsevier, Philadelphia, PA, pp. 477–504, 739–796, 825–854, 869–884.

9. Robertson J, Shilkofski N (eds). (2005) *The Harriet Lane Handbook*, 17th Edition, Elsevier Mosby, Philadelphia, PA, p. 337.

Chapter 12

Fluid and Electrolyte Management of Very Low Birth Weight Infants

Stephen Baumgart

Introduction

This chapter discusses three problems in achieving fluid and electrolyte balance in the extremely low birth weight infant (ELBW), and for the very low birth weight (VLBW) infant (birth weights: <1,000 and 1,000–1,500 grams, respectively). The principles for attaining fluid balance in each group represent the same physiology at different phases of fetal development. The first of these problems is a poor epidermal barrier. In ELBW babies, thin, gelatinous skin promotes rapid transcutaneous evaporation, resulting in severe dehydration. Immature skin also provides a poor barrier to the invasion of infections. A second area of concern is the formation of pulmonary edema from aggressive fluid volume replacement. The tendency of ELBW lung physiology biases the retention of water in the pulmonary interstitium (pulmonary edema) that has been implicated in the pathogenesis of RDS, PDA and congestive heart failure, resulting in an historical controversy of fluid restriction (dry) versus fluid replenishment (wet) in the development of chronic lung disease in both VLBW and ELBW babies. Also controversial is the use of diuretics and steroids for the treatment of pulmonary edema associated with acute lung illnesses.

Finally, a relatively new area of concern is the neurodevelopmental outcome of those infants manifesting severe electrolyte imbalances early in life, particularly in those who develop hyponatremia, or hypernatremia.

Poor Epidermal Barrier

Immature barrier function and body water composition

The *tiny baby* (ELBW, <1,000 grams birth weight) experiences large transepidermal water losses immediately upon birth.[1,2] In proportion, these infants have more extracellular water (with a relatively high saline content in equilibrium with the plasma[3]) from which water evaporates, leaving sodium behind.[4,5] During fetal life, more than 85% of body mass may be comprised of water, two-thirds of which resides in the extracellular space. By term, water comprises 75% of body mass, with approximately half in the extracellular and intracellular spaces. Contributing to the problem of dehydration, the ELBW neonate has a geometrically larger skin surface area exposed for evaporation than in more mature infants and adults,[6] having over six times the skin surface area exposed per kilogram of body weight, with at least three times the mass of water content available for evaporation.[5,6]

Transcutaneous insensible water loss

In 1981, we proposed a geometric model (Fig. 1) for estimating insensible water loss (IWL) in extremely low birth weight infants, using a metabolic balance for the continuous measurement of body weight loss (*insensible weight loss IWL*) over a 1–3 hour period.[1,7] IWL estimates in ELBW babies ≤700 grams were as high as 7.0 mL/kg/hr (170 mL/kg/day). These findings were exactly reproduced by Hammerlund and Sedin in 1983,[2] using transcutaneous evaporimetry (transcutaneous epidermal water loss or TEWL), reporting similar estimations of transcutaneous evaporation 50–60 grams/M^2/hr, or approximately 170–200 mL/kg/day in the first 1–3 days of life.[2]

We also reported a series of extremely low birth weight infants, who despite fluid replenishment as much as 250 mL/kg/day, developed

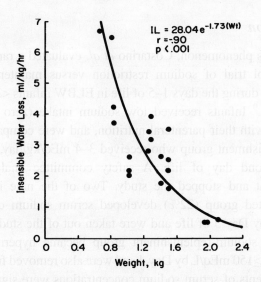

Figure 1. 1981, concept of a geometric model for estimating *insensible water loss* in extremely low birth weight infants, using a metabolic balance for the continuous measurement of body weight loss.(with permission, J.B. Lippincott Co. from Baumgart S, Langman CB, Sosulski R, Fox WW, Polin RA. (1982) Fluid, electrolyte and glucose maintenance in the very low birthweight infant. *Clin Pediatr* **21**:199–206.[1]

hypernatremic serum sodium concentrations by Day 3 of life, with values averaging 155 mEq/L, peaking in the smallest babies at serum sodium near 180 mEq/L.[1] These observations led to our first description of the pathogenesis of the development of hypernatremia, hyperglycemia, hyperosmolarity and a hyperkalemic state.[8] Large free water loss through evaporation is balanced by clinicians by increasing the rates of fluid replacement. These influxes contribute to an immense sodium load presented to an immature kidney. Added to this applied sodium load, the large salt reservoir in the extracellular space was dehydrated and the low GFR of the ELBW kidney led to salt retention. Immature renal tubules with poor concentrating ability tended to waste additional free water, and, an osmolar diuresis may also occur. The result was that in 48–72 hours, a hyperosmolar, hypernatremic state develops. This state contributes to the development of life-threatening hyperkalemia as well.

Salt restriction

To prevent this phenomenon, Costarino *et al.* evaluated a randomized and blinded control trial of sodium restriction versus maintenance sodium administration during the days 1–5 of life in ELBW infants <28 weeks gestation at birth.[9] Infants received low sodium intake (zero mEq sodium replacement) with their parenteral nutrition, and were compared to a high sodium replenishment group who received 3–4 mEq/kg/day, administered from the second day of life. A safety committee analyzed data at half-enrollment and stopped the study. Two of the nine infants in the sodium-restricted group (22%) developed serum sodium concentrations ≤130 mEq/L by Day 5 of life and were taken out of the study. One fourth (25%) of the sodium-replenishment group became hypernatremic with serum sodium ≥150 mEq/L by Day 4 and were also removed from the study. Daily assessments of serum sodium concentrations were significantly and consistently higher in the sodium supplemented infants after Day 1 of life.[9]

Sodium intake ranged between 4–6 mEq/kg/day in the sodium-supplemented maintenance group.[9] Infants in the restricted group nevertheless received 1 to $1\frac{3}{4}$ mEq/kg/day of inadvertent sodium additives with sodium heparin, sodium ampicillin and sodium citrated blood products. It was impossible to eliminate sodium intake entirely. Sodium output in the urine of these ELBW babies remained the same for the first three days of the study, but began to increase after Day 4 in infants in the sodium-supplemented group. Calculated sodium balance was nearly zero in the sodium-supplemented group where sodium intake nearly matched urinary sodium excretion, but remained markedly negative in the sodium-restricted group by as much as 6 mEq/kg/day net sodium loss, as the extracellular compartment natriurised.

Fluid intakes prescribed independently of the study by the physicians (blinded to group assignment) were similar in both groups of babies, ranging between 90 and 130 mL/kg/day during the first three days of life. However, after three days, fluid volume exceeded 130 mL/kg/day in the sodium-supplemented infants and was significantly higher than the salt-restricted babies who only received approximately 90 mL/kg/day. Infants in the sodium-supplemented group were prescribed increasing amounts of fluid to compensate for their rising serum sodium. Conversely, infants in the sodium-restricted group required relative fluid restrictions.

Also of interest is that urine output was fixed throughout the study in both groups, at between 2–4 mL/kg/hr (or about 50–100 mL/kg/day), and was not dependent on either the volume of fluid administered, or the amount of salt intake. There was a trend towards infants developing bronchopulmonary dysplasia in the high sodium/high fluid intake group: 7 of 7 infants versus 4 of 8 infants in the low sodium/low fluid intake group, P = 0.08. However, this safety analysis was underpowered.

Hartnoll et al.[10] observed that sodium supplementation after preterm birth does not affect the rate of transition in pulmonary arterial pressure. Therefore, increased oxygen requirement in ELBW infants is more likely to be a direct consequence of persistent fluid volume expansion (rather than contraction) of the extracellular compartment contributing to pulmonary interstitial fluid resulting from sodium intake. This adds further weight to this author's view that the timing of routine sodium supplementation should be delayed until the onset of postnatal extracellular volume contraction, marked clinically by weight loss.

Hyperkalemia without renal failure in ELBW infants

Gruskay et al. first reported non-oliguric hyperkalemia in ELBW infants.[11] These authors measured renal functions in ELBW infants, some of whom developed serum potassium concentrations ≥6.8 mEq/L, a level identified by Usher to increase the occurrence of life-threatening cardiac arrhythmias.[12] Peak serum potassium averaged 8.0 ± 0.3 mEq/L in the hyperkalemic babies and all eight infants developed electrocardiographic abnormalities requiring treatment.

Renal functions for these two groups of babies demonstrated similar serum creatinine and glomerular filtration. Urine sodium concentrations exceeding 140 mEq/L and fractional excretion of sodium nearly 15% in the hyperkalemic group, compared to only 5% in the normokalemic infants, were observed. Potassium excess is normally secreted from the distal renal tubule. Hyperkalemic infants' revealed significantly less urine potassium secretion than normal infants. These findings suggest an immaturity in renal tubular response to aldosterone.

Stefano *et al.* reported a similar investigation in 12 ELBW infants developing non-oliguric hyperkalemia; compared to 27 ELBW babies of whom remained normokalemic.[13] In addition to urine and renal function studies, these authors reported erythrocyte Na^+/K^+ ATP'ase activity which was significantly higher in normokalemic infants, suggesting that the cellular maturation of this enzyme was immature in the hyperkalemic babies and contributed towards the exudation of potassium from the intracellular space. Cell leakage of potassium is facilitated by high serum sodium, when extracellular sodium leaks into cells and competitively exceeds the Na^+/K^+ ATP'ase pump capacity to exclude sodium from the intracellular compartment. We conclude that hyperkalemia is due to an intracellular-to-extracellular potassium shift with diminished Na^+/K^+ ATP'ase, and that glomerular-tubular imbalance in the kidney may not explain the development of hyperkalemia in ELBW babies. Subsequent observational studies by Lorenz, and others have confirmed this finding.[14]

Reducing transcutaneous evaporation

An alternative strategy for preventing these electrolyte disturbances is to reduce the large transepidermal water loss. Several techniques have been proposed to accomplish this, and include:

(1) Incubator humidification,
(2) "swamping" babies in mist either within incubators or within plastic body chambers,
(3) application of petroleum-based ointments used on the skin as an emollient,
(4) polyvinyl chloride plastic blankets or body bags, and
(5) non-occlusive semi-adherent polyurethane artificial skins.

TEWL gradually lessens, as spontaneous keratinization of the epidermis develops over 1–4 weeks.[15]

Environmental humidification

Incubator humidification for premature babies recommended by the American Academy of Pediatrics and the American College of Obstetricians guidelines,[16] are 40–50% saturated relative humidity.

Completely saturated environments for "swamping" babies at 80–100% relative humidity leads to "rain-out" or "swamp-like" condensation of water on the interior surfaces of incubators or other plastic covers, raising a concern for water-borne infections particularly inside incubators already warmed to near body temperature.

Harpin and Rutter used 80–90% humidified incubators for 33 very low birth weight (VLBW) infants and compared them to 29 historical controls nurtured dry.[17] All infants were less than 30 weeks gestation and were studied for two weeks after birth. Two infants developed Pseudomonas sepsis in the humidified group of which one died; one developed Pseudomonas in the dry group who also died. These authors concluded that saturated humidification may be associated with water-borne nosocomial infection.

Gaylord studied 70 infants in dry incubators as historical controls for 85 babies nursed in humidified incubators.[18] Despite similar fluid balance, dry incubator babies were significantly more likely to develop hypernatremia, hyperkalemia, azotemia, oliguria and to receive more fluid volume replacements; whereas babies in humidified incubators didn't have these problems, but had more gram-negative isolates (62%) recovered from surface cultures. Therefore, humidity should be employed cautiously, not exceeding 80% relative humidity during incubator care. "Swamping" infants either within incubators, or under radiant warmers, is not recommended. Any visible water (even mist), is condensation, which promotes bacterial and fungal growth.

Using sophisticated humidification monitoring and control systems now incorporated into modern incubators is also suggested. The Giraffe Omnibed™ General Electric Co. employs a novel servo-regulated humidifier that can be set to humidify the enclosed-incubator condition to the desired *relative humidity* between 70–80%, optimal to avoid excessive insensible water loss and electrolyte disturbances in extremely low birth weight premature neonates in the first week of life when incubated conventionally dry.[19]

Skin emollients

Rutter and Hull applied paraffin oil to premature infants every 4–6 hours, reducing transepidermal water loss, but not significantly altering fluid balance over the first week of life.[20] Nopper et al. rediscovered this technique, conducting a randomized trial in 16 infants, using Aquaphor®, a preservative-free ointment to prevent skin dessication, bacterial colonization and sepsis.[21] In 2000, Campbell and Baker reported an increasing occurrence of candidiasis in their nurseries after the introduction of Aquaphor® use.[22] In a multi-center Vermont Oxford trial, an increase in coagulase-negative staphylococcal sepsis was observed in babies who were treated with Aquaphor®.[23] Because of concern for infection, we no longer use this technique in our nurseries.

Plastic shields

Alternatively, we have reported the use of a single layer of Saran® polyvinyl chloride to reduce insensible water loss during the first few days of life by more than half in low birth weight babies under open radiant warmer beds during the first 24–72 hours of life. There have been no studies to evaluate the occurrence of infection with use of these plastic "blankets."[24] Knauth et al. alternatively suggested the use of a semi-permeable polyurethane plastic, non-occlusive skin barrier (Tegaderm® or OpSite®).[25] Knauth evaluated transcutaneous evaporation using these materials and produced a two-thirds reduction in transcutaneous water loss in a series of premature babies. However, after removal on the fifth day, evaporation increased, with exfoliation of developing keratin underneath this adhesive barrier.

Porat and others published the use of polyurethane dressings covering low birth weight infants completely in a customized body suit. They demonstrated significant reductions in: hypernatremia, excessive fluid volume intake, weight loss, bronchopulmonary dysplasia and mortality with the use of polyurethane barriers during the first two weeks of life.[26]

Donahue conducted a randomized trial of this technique in 61 babies, but did not reveal changes in fluid volume requirements, although improved skin integrity was suggested by these authors.[27] A consistent effect in reducing electrolyte disturbances has not been demonstrated. Humidification and emollient ointments may increase the risk of infection. Some randomized data exist, none of which supports their use. Alternatively, standard incubation at moderate humidity between

40–60%, with or without a plastic barrier, remains a popular practice in our nurseries.

Hybrid incubator–radiant warmer design

A more promising new development in commercial convection-warmed incubator and radiant warming technology is a hybrid design, combining two separate warming modes into one device. The U.S. manufacturer currently marketing such a device is the General Electric, Ohmeda corporation, (Giraffe Omnibed™). In the incubator mode, movable plastic walls enclose the premature infant providing servo-controlled air warming and the overhead radiant warmer is incorporated into the roof of this design pod, but remains off during incubator mode. In the radiant warmer mode, the plastic walls are retracted and the radiant warmer rises to an appropriate height on a motorized pylon, rapidly firing-up to seamlessly maintain servo-controlled skin temperature during the performance of infant care procedures. The infant is not moved during the transition and no plastic barrier is interposed between the infant and the radiant heater when on. The humidification system on the Giraffe is sophisticated and has already been described.[19]

Pulmonary Edema Formation

Fluid replenishment volume, when administered aggressively, may result in increased lung water and contribute to the pathogenesis of bronchopulmonary dysplasia.[28–35] High fluid intakes (>100–140 mL/kg/day) have been associated with the development of clinically significant PDA and congestive heart failure.[31] Excessive fluid intake may also contribute to the pathogenesis of BPD.[28,29,32,34] Increased pulsatility and diastolic run-off with a clinically significant PDA may contribute to the development of necrotizing enterocolitis[35] and IVH or intraventricular hemorrhage.[36]

Perhaps the root cause of this problem is the premature infant's markedly immature renal and pulmonary development. At 25 weeks, the fetal kidney has a thin cortex that has fewer, less well-developed juxtamedullary nephrons and lacks robust cortical nephrons. The result of diminutive anatomy is less glomerular filtration of any fluid volume or salt excess. We can only imagine the severe functional limitations present in the kidneys of an extremely low birth weight infant between 400–1,000 grams, although the few data available suggest glomerular filtration is a single digit measurement with slightly higher than normal serum creatinine concentration prevalent at about 1.6–1.8 mg/dL.[37]

Prevention of Iatrogenic fluid overload

Bell and Acarregui recently performed a meta-analysis of four randomized controlled trials Table 1.[38] Of the studies reported, fluid intakes ranged from as low as 50 mL/kg/day, to as high as 200 mL/kg/day routinely. All four were conducted primarily in VLBW populations and only two of the studies demonstrated significant differences in the occurrences of PDA, congestive heart failure, BPD, NEC or death in the high fluid

Table 1. Meta-analysis of four studies evaluating high versus low fluid volume intake strategies for maintenance therapy in very low birth weight infants. PDA, congestive heart failure (CHF), and necrotizing enterocolitis (NEC) was significantly more common with high fluid volumes administered. Adapted from Bell EF, Acarregui MJ: (2001) *Cochrane Database of Systematic Reviews* **3**:CD000503.[38]

	Study design	Weights and gestations	High/low fluid volume limits	Outcomes
Bell, *et al.* (1980) New Engl J Med 302: 598–604[31]	170 sequential matched pairs, 30 days	1.41 kg 31 weeks	122/169 mL/kg/day	PDA, CHF, NEC in high fluid group
Von Stackhauser, *et al.* (1980) Klin Pediatr 192: 539–46[32]	56 random pairs, 3 days	1.9/2.0 kg 34.6/34.2 weeks	60/150 mL/kg/day	No differences
Lorenz, *et al.* (1982) J Pediatr 101: 423–32[33]	88 random matched pairs, 5 days	1.20 kg 29 weeks	60–85 mL/kg/day 80–140 mL/kg/day	No differences
Tammela, *et al.* (1992) Acta Paediatr 81: 207–12[34]	100 random pairs, 28 days	1.30 kg 31 weeks	50–150 mL/kg/day 80–200 mL/kg/day	Death, BPD in high fluid group

groups. The meta-analysis of all randomized data, however, favored low fluid volume infusions, revealing that PDA with congestive heart failure and necrotizing enterocolitis were more frequently observed in the high fluid administration groups; death was significantly higher as well.

Finally, Oh *et al.* reported a cohort of 1,382 ELBW who were followed prospectively to characterize their daily fluid volume intakes (parenteral and enteral, net intake mL/kg/day, Fig. 2.) and percent of birth weight loss daily over the first ten days of life. These data were analyzed retrospectively for their association with the occurrence of death or BPD.[30] Multivariate logistic regression demonstrated that higher fluid intake volumes with weight retention over the first ten days of life were significantly associated with higher risk of death or BPD. Wide ranges of daily fluid volume prescriptions (41–389 mL/kg/day) were observed in this network study, with average group differences of as little as 7–24 mL/kg/day.

We concluded from these published data that careful fluid volume restriction reduces death, PDA and necrotizing enterocolitis in VLBW

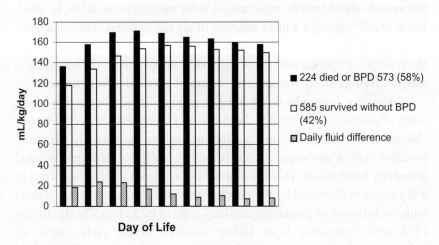

Figure 2. Multivariate logistic regression demonstrated that higher fluid intake volumes with weight retention over the first 10 days of life were significantly associated with higher risk of death or BPD. (Adapted with permission from Elsevier, Inc. from Oh W, Poindexter BB, Perritt R *et al.* (2005) Association between fluid intake and weight loss during the first ten days of life and risk of bronchopulmonary dysplasia in extremely low birth weight infants. *J Pediatr* **147**: 786–790.[30]

babies and may also be prudent for the ELBW population; there is also a trend towards less chronic lung disease in infants from both birth weight categories. However, we cannot readily extrapolate a fluid restriction strategy to the treatment of extremely low birth weight babies during the first 3–5 days of life because of the risk for dehydration with severe electrolyte disturbances. Randomized trials of either artificial epidermal barriers, with or without free water restriction to avoid weight retention and to allow body water and sodium contraction over the first week after birth are warranted.

Diuretic therapy

In 2001, Brion and Sol conducted a meta-analysis describing six randomized controlled trials for the use of furosemide in treating lung edema in acute RDS.[39] Oxygenation was only transiently improved with furosemide. However, furosemide is also a vasodilator and was associated with the development of symptomatic PDA in RDS babies. Moreover, in some cases, significant hypovolemia developed, requiring excess fluid administration to recover blood pressure. Brion concluded that furosemide should not be recommended for treating acute RDS. In 2002, Brion et al.[40] reported a meta-analysis of six randomized controlled trials for the combination of spironolactone and thiazide diuretics given for three weeks or longer, with some success in the treatment of chronic lung disease. Neither study was done in the era of prenatal steroid therapy.

Regarding lung edema, in a 1990 review, Bland summarized lung water physiology.[41] Prenatally, the pulmonary epithelium actively secretes chloride ions with water in an exocrine fashion; postnatally, the lung switches into a dry organ, with an active Na^+/K^+ exchange-mediated absorbing mechanism. This transitional change from a secretory organ to a dry organ is disrupted by the development of RDS in premature infants with the hallmark of producing capillary leak, or by a clinically significant PDA with congestive heart failure involved in the pathogenesis of pulmonary edema.

Corticosteroid therapy

Helve reported the use of postnatal steroids on the epithelial sodium channel and described mRNA expression as diminished in very low birth weight babies with RDS, comparing them to normal term control infants.[42] All five RDS subjects' mothers had received prenatal beta-methasone. Subsequently, when four subjects were given dexamethasone for the treatment of BPD after one month of age, increased sodium channel mRNA expression was observed, suggesting a potential role for postnatal steroids in reabsorption of lung edema and diminishing lung water.

In the only study of water and sodium homeostasis in ELBW babies exposed to prenatal steroids, Omar and Lorenz reported prenatal corticosteroid effects on development in extremely low birth weight infants ranging from 565 to 865 grams.[43] Higher urine output was observed during the first two days of life in babies receiving prenatal steroids when compared to controls.

It is the opinion of this author that results of studies on corticosteroids and fluid balance remain highly speculative at this time, and unfortunately, no routine recommendations for therapy should be made.

Electrolyte Imbalances and Neurodevelopment

Hyponatremia

Bhatty *et al.* have examined the effects of fluid and electrolyte imbalance on neurodevelopment in surviving ELBW prematures <1,000 grams.[44] Significant hyponatremia: (serum sodium concentration <125 mEq/L) was observed in 35 babies during the first weeks of life and were compared retrospectively to 43 non-hyponatremic birth weight-matched control infants using multivariate regression. The hyponatremic group babies were more critically ill — *all* subsequently developed BPD, had longer ventilator and oxygen courses, with longer hospital stays. More severe IVHs (grades 3 and 4) occurred in 23% of the hyponatremic subjects, but only 5% of the normonatremic controls. Similarly, significant retinopathy (grades 3 and 4) was more prevalent in hyponatremic subjects.

In a neurodevelopmental clinic follow-up, Bhatty observed a higher occurrence of spastic cerebral palsy in infants who had developed hyponatremia, more hypotonia and an increased occurrence of sensory-neural hearing loss, as well as behavioral problems reported by parents later in childhood. The authors suggested an association between recovery from hyponatremia and neurodevelopmental problems developing in the ELBW population.

When looking at the recovery from hyponatremia, the 11 infants with more rapid correction of serum sodium concentrations (by more than 10 mEq/L in 24 hours), experienced the worst neurodevelopmental outcomes later on. The authors conclude that rapid correction of hyponatremia, particularly within the first 24 hours of onset of serum sodium concentration <125 mEq/L, may be associated with adverse neurodevelopmental sequelae and that the calculated sodium correction should proceed at no more than 0.4 mEq/L/hour, or at most, 10 mEq/L/day. We presently avoid entirely the use of 3% hypertonic saline acutely for correction of hyponatremia in ELBW or VLBW neonates.

Several other studies associate hyponatremia and neurodevelopmental problems. In a matched case-control study, Leslie showed a significant sensory-neural hearing deficits in extremely low birth weight babies under 28 weeks gestation and 1,000 grams at birth.[45] In this study, hyponatremia was also diagnosed at a sodium concentration <125 mEq/L. Murphy reported 134 case controls for 59 very low birth weight babies developing cerebral palsy and associated cerebral palsy with hyponatremia.[46] Ertl and Sulyok matched 22 sensory-neural hearing loss babies to 25 case-controls for multivariate analysis, and found an association between hearing impairment and hyponatremia specifically.[47]

Hypernatremia

In contrast (and despite the frequent observation of hypernatremia in extremely low birth weight babies already described), the data associating hypernatremia with central nervous system disruptions have not been as closely examined. Simmons and Battaglia suggested restricting hypertonic sodium bicarbonate use, associating hypernatremia with significant intraventricular hemorrhages.[48]

We certainly have seen more severe hypernatremia in the extremely low birth weight population with serum sodium concentrations ranging from >150 to as high as 180 mEq/L.[50] Existing developmental follow-up data for this population, should probably be examined.

Areas for Investigation and Suggestions for Clinical Management

Epidermal barrier augmentation seems to be a first rational step in these investigations to avoid the disruption of fluid and electrolyte balance in the first place. Materials for promoting a temporary artificial skin barrier that is neutral to infection are more elusive than we might have imagined. Using more modern delivery tools, incubator humidification is also desirable.

Manipulations of both sodium and free water volume intake are also warranted. Testing specified wet versus dry net volume intakes seems to be a rather dogmatic approach. A more accurate and precise definition of fluid balance is needed. Currently, serum sodium concentration is used to evaluate whether ELBW babies need more or less water replenishment. The trouble with this approach is that serum sodium concentration must be perturbed before we can adjust fluid intake to offset changing losses.

Clinical trials of diuretics and steroids should be performed before prescribing these therapies routinely. In the area of neurodevelopmental outcomes, hyponatremia, water restriction and sodium supplementation are hot topics for investigation, given the numerous associations with sensory-neural hearing loss and cerebral palsy reviewed here. Randomized controlled trials for routine sodium replacement versus restriction therapy may now be warranted.

Final Thoughts

"Maintenance" fluid therapy is probably not an easy recipe to concoct. Fluid volumes administered to ELBW patients should be adjusted frequently, at least two or three times daily, depending on our periodic assessments of hydration and balance (intake and outputs both for water volume and weight change and net sodium intake and excretion). We should try to anticipate and to avoid both extremes of under- and over-hydration in ELBW babies by anticipating their physiological progress as demonstrated in a hypothetical 600 gram patient in Fig. 3.[50] On day one of life the primary problem is the tremendously high TEWL. We

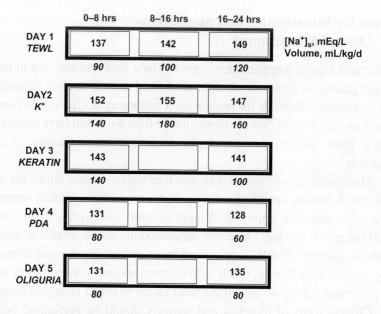

Figure 3. On the first day of life, the primary problem is tremendously high TEWL. We recommend checking serum electrolytes every eight hours during the first day or two of life, and adjusting an electrolyte-free solution upwards in 10–20 mL increments every 6–8 hours, depending on the rate of rise in the measured serum sodium concentration. The key to this strategy is checking electrolytes frequently, because once the serum sodium rises, you're already behind. By day two, the problem of hyperkalemia emerges — volume replacement maximizes, as serum sodium concentration peaks, and sodium leaks into the cells displacing potassium outwards from the intracellular compartment. Then on day three, TEWL begins to diminish in response to incubator care with humidification. Serum sodium suddenly decreases. We anticipate this change by diminishing water volume *immediately* when we first see serum sodium concentration falls, thus anticipating fluid overload and the risk for promoting a hemodynamically significant PDA by day four of life. The occurrence of iatrogenic hyponatremia is most often observed at this time and may be associated with patent ductus physiology,[49] and is best addressed by aggressive water volume restriction to as little as 60 mL/kg/day, minimizing the *rate* of sodium correction and avoiding entirely the use of hypertonic salt infusions. Oliguria observed while treating for PDA and hyponatremia should not be addressed by liberalizing fluid volume administration or giving saline bolus, nor by the use of furosemide which may actually dilate the PDA. Maintenance fluid restriction should be continued while the PDA is addressed definitively either with Indocin, or surgical ligation. (Adapted with permission Cambridge University Press, Cambridge, UK from Sridhar S, Baumgart S. (2006) Hay WW, Thureen PY (eds.), Water and electrolyte balance in newborn infants. In: *Neonatal Nutrition and Metabolism*, 2nd edition).[58,59]

recommend checking serum electrolytes every 8 hours during the first day or two of life and adjusting an electrolyte-free solution upwards or downwards in 10–20 mL increments every 6–8 hours, depending on the rate of rise in the measured serum sodium concentration (a ± 5 mEq/dL change suggests a direction of acceleration or deceleration for serum sodium concentrations). The key to this strategy is checking electrolytes more frequently, because once the serum sodium rises, you are already behind in water volume administration, as shown by this figure. By day 2, the problem of hyperkalemia often emerges — volume replacement maximizes, as serum sodium concentration peaks, and sodium leaks into the cells displacing potassium outwards from the intracellular compartment. On day 3, TEWL begins to diminish as keratin deposition occurs, or in response to incubator care with additional humidification. At this juncture, the serum sodium concentration may suddenly decrease. We should anticipate this change by diminishing water volume *immediately* when we first see the serum sodium concentrations fall, thus anticipating fluid overload and the risk for promoting a hemodynamically significant PDA. The occurrence of iatrogenic hyponatremia is most often observed at this time and may be associated with ductal physiology,[51] and is best addressed by aggressive water volume restriction to as little as 60 mL/kg/day, minimizing the rate of sodium correction and entirely avoiding the use of hypertonic salt infusions. Oliguria observed while treating PDA with fluid restriction and hyponatremia should not be treated by liberalizing fluid volume or bolus saline administration, nor by the use of furosemide which may actually dilate the PDA.[39] Rather, fluid restriction should be maintained while the PDA is addressed definitively either with Indocin or by early surgical ligation.

Monitoring changes in body weight is also an important means of assuring appropriate fluid balance. As a reflection of transitional physiologic contraction of extracellular fluid compartment, the VLBW weight infants experience a 2–3% per kg per day weight loss [about 15 grams/day from a 500 gram ELBW baby — any weight gain would be abnormal], during the first three days.[52] The body weight loss stabilizes during the fourth and fifth day of life suggesting completion of the transitional ECF contraction. The weight gain at 2–3% per kg per day from day 6 onwards is a reflection of anabolic phase of infants' metabolic status. It is very useful to plot the daily weight changes on the postnatal weight grid in infants as published by Shafer et al.[53]

A parting shot at PDA management

Much of this discussion regarding fluids and electrolyte imbalances in ELBW premature infants is around the prevention of a clinically significant patent ductus arteriosus. In a recent and controversial opinion paper, Laughon et al. questioned the significance of a PDA and how it can and should be managed.[54] The ductus before birth is essential to maintain systemic circulation in the fetus by delivering oxygenated blood to vital organs while bypassing the lungs. After birth at term, the ductus closes functionally (if not anatomically) within three days. In the ever-troublesome VLBW premature newborn at <30 weeks gestation, and in the ELBW population, at least two-thirds of infants have PDA's that do not close during the first week of life and, incidentally, this is the group with serious pulmonary disease and high pulmonary vascular resistance to shunting left-to-right. The importance of diagnosis of a clinically significant PDA (i.e. pulmonary congestion with predominantly left-to-right blood flow through the ductus and directed towards the sick lung) is raised by these authors. Echocardiography invariably demonstrates an anatomically patent ductus in these critically ill babies with refractory respiratory distress. However, identifying the significance of this finding when screening for a ductus with echocardiography routinely on day 4 of life, as suggested above, requires examining the patient, not just for the presence, nor just for echogenic evidence of an otherwise normal structure, but for bounding pulses, a hyperactive precordium and a widened pulse pressure. Doppler evidence of a significant left-to-right ductal shunt is often vaguely represented as "bi-directional" on an echocardiogram and deleterious effects of diastolic flow velocities seem exaggerated. Failure to improve oxygenation leads to frustration when asking, "What more can we do?" Therefore, treating the ductus aggressively seems prudent, even though a markedly premature lung morphology and fluid physiology and pulmonary inflammation may remain the true culprits producing premature lung water congestive disease. Surgical ligation is the gold standard for premature ductal closure.

Although 40% of observed murmurs remain asymptomatic, the majority of symptomatic murmurs become asymptomatic with fluid restriction alone (a strong recommendation for a "dry" approach to parenteral fluid prescription during the first week of life in ELBW infants).[30] Surgery is not without risks for a hemodynamically unstable patient: bleeding, pneumothorax, vocal cord paralysis, grades 3–4 retinopathy and infection have all been associated with PDA surgical ligation. Each institution treating these size babies might be advised to monitor these complications rates.

Indomethacin medical therapy is used to avoid surgery in patients not responding to fluid restriction within 48 hours. In the landmark multicenter collaborative trial authored by Gersony in 1983, over 3,500 infants with significant PDA's failing fluid restriction received indomethacin for one or two courses by two weeks postnatal age (with 79% closure), before offered surgery (35%).[55] There were no differences in mortality or duration of mechanical ventilation or hospital stay; nor IVH or NEC in medical vs surgical treatment groups. At the end of the study however, all ductuses were closed. Other landmark studies of indomethacin therapy have followed (e.g. prophylactic treatment for all vulnerable premature infants to prevent PDA and intraventricular hemorrhages, or only for those with asymptomatic PDA's having echocardiographic evidence of a ductus on screening), but amelioration of final adverse outcomes remains wanting as neurodevelopmental delays persist, as does chronic lung disease at ≥36 weeks post-conceptional age.[56,57]

Conclusion/speculation

If judicious fluid and electrolyte balance is achievable in ELBW babies, neither indomethacin nor surgery may be required.

References

1. Baumgart S, Langman CB, Sosulski R *et al.* (1982) Fluid, electrolyte and glucose maintenance in the very low birthweight infant. *Clin Pediatr* **21**: 199–206.

2. Hammarlund K, Sedin G. (1983) Transepidermal water loss in newborn infants. VIII. Relation to gestational age and post-natal age in appropriate and small for gestational age infants. *Acta Paediatr Scand* **72**: 721.

3. Michel CC. (1984) Renkin Eu and Michel CC (eds.), Fluid movements through capillary walls. Chapter 9 In: Handbook of Physiology, Section II Vol II. Bethesda: American Physiologic Society.

4. Costarino AT, Baumgart S. (1986) Modern fluid and electrolyte management of the critically ill premature infant. *Ped Clin No Amer* **33**: 153–178.

5. Friis-Hansen B. (1961) Body water compartments in children. *Pediatrics* **28**: 169–181.

6. Haycock GB, Schwartz GJ, Wisotsky DH. (1978) Geometric method for measuring body surface areas: A height-weight formula validated in infants, children and adults. *J Pediatr* **93**: 62–66.

7. Baumgart S, Engle WD, Fox WW *et al.* (1981) Radiant warmer power and body size as determinants of insensible water loss in the critically ill neonate. *Pediatr Res* **15**: 1495–1499.

8. Baumgart S. (1983) Burg F, Polin RA (eds.), Fluid and electrolyte therapy in the premature infant: Case management. In, Workbook in Practical Neonatology. WB Saunders, Philadelphia, pp. 25–39.

9. Costarino AT, Gruskay JA, Corcoran L *et al.* (1992) Sodium restriction vs daily maintenance replacement in very low birthweight premature neonates, a randomized and blinded therapeutic trial. *J Pediatr* **120**: 99–106.

10. Hartnoll G, Betremieux P, Modi N. (2000) Randomized controlled trial of postnatal sodium supplementation on body composition in 25 to 30 week gestational age infants. *Arch Dis Child Fetal Neonatal Ed* **82**(1): F24–F28.

11. Gruskay J, Costarino AT, Polin RA *et al.* (1988) Non-oliguric hyperkalemia in the premature infant less than 1000 grams. *J Pediatr* **113**: 381–386.

12. Usher RH. (1959) The respiratory distress syndrome of prematurity. I. Change in potassium in the serum and the electrocardiogram and effects of therapy. *Pediatrics* **24**: 562.

13. Stefano JL, Norman ME, Morales MC *et al.* (1993) Decreased erythrocyte Na+, K+ ATPase activity associated with cellular potassium loss in extremely low birth weight infants with nonoliguric hyperkalemia. *J Pediatr* **122**: 276–284.

14. Lorenz, JM, Kleinman LI. (1989) Nonoliguric hyperkalemia in preterm neonates (Letter). *J Pediatr* **114**: 507.

15. Kalia Yn, Nonato LB, Lund CH *et al.* (1998) Development of skin barrier function in premature infants. *J Investig Derm* **111**: 320–326.

16. American Academy of Pediatrics and American College of Obstetricians and Gynecologists. (1988) *Guidelines for perinatal care*, 2nd ed. Elk Grove Village, IL 278.

17. Harpin VA, Rutter N. (1985) Humidification of incubators. *Arch Dis Child* **60**: 219.

18. Gaylord MS, Wright K, Lorch K *et al.* (2001) Improved fluid management utilizing humidified incubators in extremely low birth weight infants. *J Perinatol* **21**: 438–443.

19. Lynam L, Biagotti L, BS (2002) Testing for bacterial colonization in a Giraffe humidification system. *Neonatal Intensive Care* **15**: 2.

20. Rutter N, Hull D. (1981) Reduction of skin water loss in the newborn. I. Effect of applying topical agents. *Arch Dis Child* **56**: 669.

21. Nopper AJ, Horii KA, Sookdeo-Drost S *et al.* (1996) Topical ointment therapy benefits premature infants. *J Pediatr* **128**: 660.

22. Campbell JR, Zaccaria E, Baker CJ. (2000) Systemic candidiasis in extremely low birth weight infants receiving topical petrolatum ointment for skin care: A case-control study. *Pediatrics* **105**: 1041–1045.

23. Edwards WH, Conner JM, Soll RF. (2004) Vermont Oxford Network Neonatal Skin Care Study Group. The effect of prophylactic ointment therapy on nosocomial sepsis rates and skin integrity in infants with birth weights of 501–1000 g. *Pediatrics* **113**: 1195–1203.

24. Baumgart S. (1984) Reduction of oxygen consumption, insensible water loss and radiant heat demand with use of a plastic blanket for low birthweight infants under radiant warmers. *Pediatrics* **74**: 1022–1028.

25. Knauth A, Gordin M, McNelis W *et al.* (1989) A semipermeable polyurethane membrane as an artificial skin in the premature neonate. *Pediatrics* **83**: 945–950.

26. Porat R, Brodsky N. (1993) Effect of Tegederm use on outcome of extremely low birth weight (ELBW) infants. *Pediatr Res* **33**: 231(A).

27. Donahue ML, Phelps DL, Richter SE *et al.* (1996) A semipermeable skin dressing for extremely low birth weight infants. *Journal of Perinatology.* **16**(1): 20–26.

28. Palta M, Babbert D, Weinstein MR *et al.* (1991) Multivariate assessment of traditional risk factors for chronic lung disease in very low birth weight neonates. *J Pediatr* **119**: 285–292.

29. Van Marter LJ, Pagano M, Allred EN et al. (1992) Rate of bronchopulmonary dysplasia as a function of neonatal intensive care practices. J Pediatr 120: 938–946.

30. Oh W, Poindexter BB, Perritt R et al. for the Neonatal Research Network (2005) Association between fluid intake and weight loss during the first ten days of life and risk of bronchopulmonary dysplasia in extremely low birth weight infants. J Pediatr 147: 786–790.

31. Bell EF, Warburton D, Stonestreet BS et al. (1980) Effect of fluid administration on the development of symptomatic patent ductus arteriosus and congestive heart failure in premature infants. N Engl J Med 302: 598–604.

32. von Stockhausen HB, Struve M. (1980) Die Auswirkungen einer stark unterschiedlichen parenteral en Flussigkeitszufuhr bei Fruh- und Neugeborenen in den ersten drei Lebenstagen. Klin Padiatr 192: 539–546.

33. Lorenz JM, Kleinman LI, Kotagal UR et al. (1982) Water balance in very low-birth weight infants: Relationship to water and sodium intake and effect on outcome. J Pediatr 101: 423–432.

34. Tammela OKT, Koivisto ME. (1992) Fluid restriction for preventing bronchopulmonary dysplasia? Reduced fluid intake during the first weeks of life improves the outcome of low-birth-weight infants. Acta Paediatr 81: 207–212.

35. Bell EF, Warburton D, Stonestreet BS et al. (1979) High volume fluid intake predisposes premature infants to necrotizing enterocolitis. Lancet 2: 90.

36. Perlman JM, McMenamin JB, Volpe JJ. (1983) Fluctuating cerebral blood flow velocity in respiratory distress syndrome: Relationship to the development of intraventricular hemorrhage. N Egl J Med 309: 209–213.

37. Stonestreet BS, Oh W. (1978) Plasma creatinine levels in low-birth-weight infants during the first three months of life. Pediatrics 61: 788–789.

38. Bell EF, Acarregui MJ. (2001) Restricted versus liberal water intake for preventing morbidity and mortality in preterm infants. Cochrane Database of Systematic Reviews 3: CD000503.

39. Brion LP, Sol RF. (2001) Diuretics for respiratory distress syndrome in preterm infants. 2: CD001454; PMID: 10796265.

40. Brion LP, Primhak RA, Ambrosio-Perez I. (2002) Diuretics acting on the distal renal tubule for preterm infants with (or developing) chronic lung disease. Cochrane Database of Systematic Reviews 3: CD001817; PMID:10908511.

41. Bland RD. (1990) Lung epithelial ion transport and fluid movement during the perinatal period. *Am J Physiol* **259**: L30–L37.

42. Helve O, Pitkanen OM, Andersson S *et al.* (2004) Low expression of human epithelial sodium channel in airway epithelium of preterm infants with respiratory distress. *Pediatrics* **113**: 1267–1272.

43. Omar SA, Decristofaro JD, Agarwal BI *et al.* (1999) Effects of prenatal steroids on water and sodium homeostasis in extremely low birth weight Neonates. *Pediatrics* **104**: 482–488.

44. Bhatty SB, Tsirka A, Quinn PB *et al.* (1997) Rapid correction of hyponatremia in extremely low birth weight (ELBW) premature neonates is associated with long term developmental delay. *Pediatr Res* **41**: 140A and Privileged Communication, Dr. DeCristofaro.

45. Leslie GI, Kalaw MB, Bowen JR *et al.* (1995) Risk factors for sensorineural hearing loss in extremely premature infants. *J Paediatr Child Health* 312–316.

46. Murphy DJ, Hope PL, Johnson A. (1997) Neonatal risk factors for cerebral palsy in very preterm babies: Case-control study. *BMJ* **314**: 404–408.

47. Ertl T, Hadzsiev K, Vincze O *et al.* (2001) Hyponatremia and sensorineural hearing loss in preterm infants. *Biology of the Neonate* **79**: 109–112.

48. Simmons MA, Adcock EW 3rd, Bard H *et al.* (1974) Hypernatremia and intracranial hemorrhage in neonates. *New Engl J Med* **291**: 6–10.

49. Lupton BA, Roland EH, Whitfield MF *et al.* (1990) Serum sodium concentration and intraventricular hemorrhage in premature infants. *Am J Dis Child* **144**: 1019–1021.

50. Baumgart S. (2006) Burg FD, lnglefinger JR, Polin RA, Gershon AA (eds.), Water and electrolyte balance in low birth weight infants. In, Current Pediatric Therapy, 18th Edition, Elsevier Science, USA, Philadelphia, PA, pp 85–88.

51. Gupta J, Sridhar S, Baumgart S, *et al.* (2002) Hyponatremia in extremely low birth weight (ELBW) infants may precede the development of a significant patent ductus arteriosus (PDA) in the first week of life. *Pediatric Res* **51**: 387A.

52. Stonestreet BS, Bell EF, Warburton D *et al.* (1983) Renal response in low-birth-weight neonates. Results of prolonged intake of two different amounts of fluid and sodium. *Am J Dis Child* **137**: 215–219.

53. Shaffer SG, Quimico CL, Anderson JV *et al.* (1987) Postnatal weight changes in low birth weight infants. *Pediatrics* **187**: 702–705.

54. Laughon MM, Simmons MA, Bose CL. (2004) Patency of the ductus arteriosus in the premature infant: Is it pathologic? Should it be treated? *Curr Opin Pediatr*, **16**: 146–151.

55. Gersony WM, Peckham GJ, Ellison RC, *et al.* (1983) Effects of indomethacin in premature infants with patent ductus arteriosus: Results of a national collaborative study. *J Pediatr* **102**: 895–906.

56. Fowlie P, Davis PG. (2005) Prophylactic intravenous indomethacin for preventing mortality and morbidity in preterm infants. *Cochrane Database of Systematic Reviews*, ISSN 1464–780X.

57. Cooke L, Steer P, Woodgate P. (2005) Indomethacin for asymptomatic patent ductus arteriosus in preterm infants. *Cochrane Database of Systematic Reviews*, ISSN 1464–780X.

58. Sridhar S, Baumgart S. (2006) Hay WW, Thureen PJ (eds.), Water and electrolyte balance in newborn infants. In Neonatal Nutrition and Metabolism, 2nd Edition, Cambridge University Press, 2006.

59. Baumgart S. (2008) Oh W, Guignard JP, Baumgart S, Polin RA consulting (eds.), Acute problems with prematurity: Balancing fluid volume and electrolyte replacements in very low birth weight (VLBW) and extremely low birth weight (ELBW) neonates. In *Nephrology and Fluid/Electrolyte Physiology: Neonatology Questions and Controversies*, Saunders, Elsevier, Philadelphia, PA, pp. 161–183.

Chapter

Nutritional Support of the High-Risk Infant

Jae H. Kim and Richard J. Schanler

Introduction

The high-risk infant (HRI) faces one of the greatest nutritional challenges during life because of the incredible postnatal rate of growth required to mimic normal fetal development. Thus, intense support is needed to prevent and correct these deficits and promote appropriate growth. This chapter describes the nutritional needs and goals for the HRI, the latter term will be used interchangeably with very low birth weight (VLBW) infants (birthweight <1500 g) and both parenteral and enteral nutritional needs will be addressed (Table 1).

Goals for Nutrient Intakes

While the nutritional reference standard for the term newborn is the exclusively breastfed infant, a similar standard is not available for HRIs. Instead, the reference standard for the HRI is the estimated intrauterine rate of growth and nutrient accretion rate at corresponding stages during the last trimester of pregnancy.[1,2] To determine the advisable intake needed for a particular nutrient, we need to use the factorial approach.[3] This method includes a summation of the quantity of the nutrient deposited and an estimate of nutrient losses (Table 2).

Table 1. Parenteral and enteral fluid, energy and nutrient intakes for stable, growing very low birth weight premature infants.[63]

Component, units	Unit/kg/day (except as noted)	
	Parenteral	Enteral
Water, ml	120–160	135–190
Energy, kcal	90–100	110–130
Protein, g	3.2–3.8	3.4–4.2
Fat, g	3–4	5.3–7.2
Carbohydrate, g	9.7–15	7–17
Linoleic Acid, mg	340–800	600–1440
Vitamin D, IU	40–160	150–400
Vitamin E, IU	2.8–3.5	6–12
Vitamin K, μg	10	8–10
Thiamin (vitamin B_1), μg	200–350	180–240
Riboflavin (vitamin B_2), μg	150–200	250–360
Pyridoxine (vitamin B_6), μg	150–200	150–210
Vitamin B_{12}, μg	0.3	0.3
Niacin, mg	4–6.8	3.6–4.8
Folic Acid, μg	56	25–50
Sodium, mg	69–115	69–115
Potassium, mg	78–117	78–117

(Continued)

Table 1. (*Continued*)

Component, units	Unit/kg/day (except as noted)	
	Parenteral	Enteral
Chloride, mg	107–249	107–249
Calcium, mg	60–80	100–220
Phosphorus, mg	45–60	60–140
Magnesium, mg	4.3–7.2	7.9–15
Iron, μg	100–200	2000–4000
Zinc, μg	400	1000–3000
Copper, μg	20	120–150
Chromium, μg	0.05–0.3	0.1–2.25
Manganese, μg	1	0.7–7.5
Selenium, μg	1.5–4.5	1.3–4.5
Carnitine, mg	~3	~3

LEGEND FOR TABLE 1:

Vitamin K, 0.5–1.0 mg given at birth

The following conversion factors are used:

Ca 40 mg = 1 mmol = 2 mEq

P 31 mg = 1 mmol

Mg 24 mg = 1 mmol = 2 mEq

Na 23 mg = 1 mmol = 1 mEq

K 39 mg = 1 mmol = 1 mEq

Cl 35 mg = 1 mmol = 1 mEq

Vitamin A 1 μg retinol = 3.33 IU vitamin A = 6 μg carotene = 1.83 μg retinyl palmitate = 1 retinol equivalent (RE)

Vitamin E 1 mg tocopherol = 1 IU vitamin E

Vitamin D 1 μg vitamin D (cholecalciferol) = 40 IU vitamin D (cholecalciferol)

Niacin 1 mg niacin equivalent (NE) = 60 mg tryptophan

Table 2. Computation of net enteral and/or parenteral nutrient need for calcium based on the factorial approach.[3]

Net fetal Ca deposition	= 105 mg/kg/day
Postnatal urinary losses	= 5 mg/kg/day
Postnatal cutaneous losses	= 2 mg/kg/day
Subtotal (parenteral need)	= 112 mg/kg/day
Net absorption (%)	= 50%
Total (enteral need)	= 224 mg/kg/day

Parenteral Nutrition (PN)

The early provision of parenteral nutrition (PN) is essential for the HRI who is born with limited nutrient stores, who may have increased energy expenditure and severity of illness, and because of their immaturity, are often precluded from enteral feedings immediately after birth. Thus, a regimen of PN is initiated, consisting of intravenous glucose, amino acids, lipids, electrolytes, vitamins and trace minerals.

Enteral Nutrition

The transition of nutrient delivery from parenteral to enteral source involves several important changes. The first is the change in the nutrient retention of specific nutrients as there are processes of digestion and absorption that interact between the nutrients delivered enterally and the nutrients finally received in the circulation. Other important factors to consider with enteral feeding are the added energy required for digestion by the gastrointestinal tract and when infants are establishing enteral feeding. Fortunately, the enteral route enables a greater amount of total nutrient delivery compared with the parenteral route that is often limited by physicochemical issues such as solubility.

There are numerous arguments in favor of using human milk instead of formula milk. Intestinal permeability is increased in premature infants compared to term infants. An increased intestinal permeability may make the immature gut more susceptible to the development of necrotizing enterocolitis. A human milk diet has been shown to decrease the intestinal permeability in infants less than 32 weeks gestation.[4] Tolerance of feedings seems to be improved with human milk as full enteral feeding was achieved sooner when premature infants were fed human milk versus formula.[4] Thus, for extremely HRIs who are ill, trophic feeding of small volumes (10 to 20 ml/kg/day) may be initiated in the first few days after birth and continue for approximately 3–7 days before advancement of feeding.[5]

Water

Preterm infants are particularly susceptible to fluid losses because of their large body surface area in relation to weight, increased body water and increased skin permeability. Fluid requirements of the preterm infant are dependent on both measurable losses in stool and urine as well as insensible water losses (IWL) through respiratory tract and skin. IWL decreases with increasing birth weight and gestational age and decreases over the first two weeks as skin becomes less permissive to water loss. Fluid needs depend on history, gestational age, postnatal age, clinical assessment of hydration, urine specific gravity, presence or absence of patent ductus arteriosus and increases in fluid loss associated with therapy.

Energy

The daily energy need for the growing HRI, as measured by indirect calorimetry, has been summarized.[5,6] The range in resting energy expenditure increases with postnatal and less with gestational age, with a range between 33 and 81 kcal/kg/day. Initially, when nourished parenterally, the HRI has less fecal energy loss, generally fewer episodes of cold stress, and somewhat less activity so that the actual energy needs for growth are lowered to approximately 80 to 100 kcal/kg/day. On the other extreme, in infants with bronchopulmonary dysplasia, the resting energy expenditure rises significantly because of greater energy expenditure, activity, and possibly fecal energy losses. Such infants may require as much as 150 kcal/kg/day to achieve appropriate weight gain. To ultimately meet *in utero* growth and postnatal demands, the smallest HRIs need to grow in body weight at a rate of approximately 21 grams/kg/day.

The high growth rate of the HRI requires optimum amounts of both energy and protein since protein accretion can only be achieved when resting energy demands are met. Therefore, energy supply from non-protein components (carbohydrate and fat) need to be carefully administered. Daily monitoring of the intakes for all energy sources in PN is essential to ensure a relatively balanced distribution of calories derived from glucose and fat.

Carbohydrate

The HRI requires a high glucose infusion rate (approximately 5–8 mg/kg/min vs 3–5 mg/kg/min in term infants) to meet their needs because of their diminished stores, higher energy expenditure, and relatively greater brain to body weight ratio. As their clinical condition may preclude enteral nutrition directly after birth, PN can provide adequate glucose to prevent hypoglycemia. The smallest HRI, however, may develop hyperglycemia because of ineffective insulin secretion and end-organ sensitivity, decreased intracellular transporters, elevated catecholamines and glucocorticoids, or as a response to a high glucose infusion rate. The use of insulin has some theoretical benefits but practically the use of insulin has been more problematic than beneficial with no measurable anabolic effect, additional lactic acidosis and infusion difficulties with adherence of insulin to infusion tubing.[7,8] As the smallest HRIs have been shown to manifest gluconeogenesis, early administration of amino acids and lipids, that are substrates for gluconeogenesis, enables lower glucose infusion rates to be achieved.[9]

The primary carbohydrate in human milk is lactose (90–95%) but this is followed closely by oligosaccharides (5–10%). Because of earlier concerns regarding lactose utilization by premature infants and high osmolality of the milk, preterm formulas contain about half of their carbohydrate as corn syrup solids (glucose polymers).[10] Human milk oligosaccharides are small sugars that resist digestion in the GI tract and are the classic prebiotic agents because they stimulate the growth of beneficial probiotic bacteria in the GI tract.[11] These sugars may vary in chain length from 3–40 sugar molecules and number more than 150 unique structural forms. These sugars are important factors that stimulate the more favorable colonic flora in human milk fed infants compared to formula-fed infants.

Protein

Intravenous amino acids

Accurate amino acid requirements for the preterm infant remain incompletely understood. For the HRI, several amino acids including arginine, cysteine, glutamine, glycine, histidine, taurine and tyrosine may be conditionally essential amino acids.[12] Limiting amounts of a specific amino acid can result in inadequate protein synthesis in favor of excess oxidation of the remaining amino acids.[13] Intravenous administration of amino acids is complicated by the variability of content profiles among the representative preparations. For example, tyrosine and cysteine are not present in all preparations, principally because of difficulties in solubility. Taurine and glutamic acid are not present in all solutions.[12] Glutathione is the major intracellular antioxidant whose primary function is to protect the cell against free-radical damage. Cysteine serves as a key precursor of glutathione, but since cysteine hydrochloride (HCl) is not stable in water, it must be added to PN solutions daily.[14] A collateral benefit with the addition of cysteine HCl to PN solutions is the lowering of pH that increases the solubility of calcium and phosphorus.[15] Glutamine is an important amino acid for cell growth, specifically intestinal epithelial growth, has a role in immune function and is a precursor in glutathione synthesis. However, benefits of supplemental parenteral glutamine have not been shown with respect to growth, protein synthesis, or host defense. Selection of an amino acid solution should contain the greatest quantity of essential amino acids targeted to meet the needs of the HRI.[16]

Early initiation of amino acids

Provision of the maximum tolerable amount of energy and protein within the first few weeks of life is key to minimizing the accrued energy and protein deficit that incurs in all VLBW infants within weeks of birth.[17] The use of a combined glucose and amino acid source for PN through a central vein should be initiated soon after birth to minimize the acute metabolic stress faced by the newborn due to an abrupt cessation of parenteral nutrients from the placenta.[18] Early infusion of a stock amino acid and dextrose solution helps bridge the nutrient gap between birth and the first complete PN order, thereby avoiding any lapse in macronutrient delivery. Early PN delivery counteracts the negative nitrogen balance attributed to a constant urinary nitrogen loss, equivalent to a loss of protein of 1 g/kg/day[19] by effectively increasing the serum concentration of essential amino acids, and the rate of protein synthesis.[20,21] An amino acid intake of 3 g/kg/day was associated with a significantly more positive nitrogen balance and greater plasma insulin concentrations without significant effects on BUN or glucose concentrations when started as early as 24 hours after birth in extremely LBW infants.[22] To match *in utero* growth, the smallest preterm infants need at least 4 gm/kg/day.[6,23] Long-term follow-up studies of extremely LBW infants given early amino acid infusions compared to late initiation of PN demonstrate significant benefits to growth at 36 weeks postmenstrual age along with sustained positive effects on head growth up to 18 months.[24]

Protein needs

The quantity and quality of protein needed for premature infants have been investigated.[25,26] Protein needs should be considered in conjunction with energy need as protein synthesis consumes energy. If energy intake is inadequate, protein synthesis may be depressed and amino acid oxidation increase.[27] Protein retention, or balance, generally is a function of protein intake if energy intake is adequate.[28] The appropriate intake of protein for HRI infants has been defined further from evaluations of weight gain, nitrogen retention and serum biochemical indicators of protein nutritional status.[29,30] An assumption is also made that about 78% of enteral protein is absorbed by the GI tract. Research has shown that protein intakes of approximately 3.5–4.0 g/kg/day at 120 kcal/kg/day seem appropriate for the otherwise healthy HRI infant.[29,30] Whey-dominant protein formulations are well-absorbed and the provision of hydrolyzed protein formulations, usually casein-derived, for the otherwise healthy premature infant, are not indicated. Infants demonstrating bovine milk protein intolerance are the exception to this and benefit from breastmilk or a milk containing extensively hydrolyzed protein or free amino acids.

Human milk protein composition

Mature human milk contains 70% whey and 30% casein whereas bovine milk contains an inverse ratio, 18% whey and 82% casein. The whey fraction of milk consists of easily digestible soluble proteins which is more suitable for the preterm infant. Human milk, then whey-dominant bovine milk, in that order, promote more rapid gastric emptying than casein-dominant milk.[31] The major human whey protein is α-lactalbumin, a nutritional protein for the infant and a component of mammary gland lactose synthesis. Lactoferrin, lysozyme and secretory immunoglobulin A (sIgA) are specific human whey proteins that are particularly resistant to hydrolysis and as such, line the gastrointestinal (GI) tract to play a primary role in host defense.[32] In the first few weeks after birth, the protein content of milk from mothers who deliver premature infants (preterm milk) is greater than term milk.[33]

Human milk, whether preterm or term, does not contain enough protein to meet the high growth needs of the premature infant. The lowest plasma concentrations of amino acids, albumin, and urea nitrogen, and the slowest rates of weight gain, were found in the human milk-fed premature infants.[26,34] For example, the protein contents of mature human milk and fortified human milk are 1.0 and 2.4 g/dL, respectively, and preterm formula is 2.4 g/dL. Growth rates and serum protein and urea nitrogen concentrations in premature infants increase when human milk is fortified with protein to achieve a protein intake of at least 3.5 g/kg/day.[30] The protein content of human milk is highest at birth and rapidly declines in the first few weeks to reach the more stable level observed in mature human milk (Table 3). Furthermore, the mother-to-mother variability in protein expression is not well understood. Therefore, to meet protein needs, the human milk-fed premature infant needs a protein supplement (Table 3). This range of protein intake is adequate, assuming that no protein deficit has arisen as a result of a prolonged or deficient parenteral nutrition phase. For this reason, greater intakes of protein may be necessary for premature infants to allow for catch-up protein nutritional

Table 3. Nutrient composition of human milk and selected fortified human milk.[63]

	Human milk (1 week)	Mature preterm human milk (1 month)	Mature preterm human milk + Human milk fortifier
Volume, ml	100	100	100
Energy, kcal	67	69	83
Protein, g	2.4	1.5	2.5–2.6
Whey/Casein (%)	70/30	70/30	70/30
Fat, g	3.8	3.6	4.0–4.6
MCT (%)	2	2	11–17
Carbohydrate, g	6.1	6.7	7.1–8.5
Lactose (%)	100	100	80–85
Calcium, mg	25	29	119–146
Phosphorus, mg	14	9.3	59–76
Magnesium, mg	3.1	2.4	3.4–9.4
Sodium, mEq (mmol)	2.2	0.9	1.6
Potassium, mEq (mmol)	1.8	1.3	2–2.9
Chloride, mEq (mmol)	2.6	1.5	1.9–2.6
Zinc, μg	500	215	935–1215
Copper, μg	80	51	95–221
Vitamin A, IU	560	227	847–1177
Vitamin D, IU	4	1.2	122–151
Vitamin E, mg	1.0	0.3	3.5–4.9

Enfamil Human Milk Fortifier (Mead Johnson Nutritionals, Evansville, IN)
Similac Human Milk Fortifier (Abbott Nutrition, Columbus, OH)
4 packets + 100 ml Mature Preterm Human Milk.

support. Thus, intakes of approximately 4.0 g/kg/day, with adequate intakes of energy and minerals, often are indicated.

Lipids

Lipids are the largest, most important source of energy as well as the sole source of essential fatty acids (EFA). The two primary EFA, linoleic acid (18:2ω6) and linolenic acid (18:3ω3), cannot be synthesized and thus need to be provided to prevent EFA deficiency, characterized by dermatitis, thrombocytopenia, infection and failure to thrive. Only small amounts of essential fatty acid (~4% of total calories or 0.5 g/kg/day) are required to prevent essential fatty acid deficiency. Intravenous lipid emulsions given along with the PN regimen in the first few days will prevent essential fatty acid deficiency,[35] provide needed energy for tissue healing and growth and equalize the distribution of non-protein calories (Table 1). A review of early use of intravenous lipid identified no adverse effects on growth, lung disease, or overall morbidity when compared with later use of intravenous lipid infusion.[36]

HRIs should receive 20% solution over other lipid concentrations due to improved tolerance, lower levels of serum triglycerides, cholesterol and phospholipids.[37] Twenty-four hour continuous lipid infusions is preferable to intermittent infusions as the latter is associated with higher serum triglyceride concentrations.[38] Plasma triglyceride concentrations should be used to monitor lipid tolerance. A triglyceride concentration greater than approximately 200 mg/dL should lead to a downward adjustment of the infusion rate. The use of intravenous lipids have raised past concerns regarding the worsening of pulmonary function and the potential for oxidant toxicity, but studies do not indicate an increased risk.[36]

Soybean-based lipid emulsions may be pro-inflammatory, immunosuppressive, procoagulatory and may reduce bile flow, thereby contributing to liver injury.[39] Newer intravenous fat emulsions containing fish oil or olive oil with a concurrent reduction in soybean lipids appear promising, but are not readily available in the US and other countries. Further research in these new areas is warranted.

EFAs are present in surplus quantities in human milk and infant formula. Premature infants do not synthesize enough long-chain polyunsaturated fatty acids (LCPUFA) from the EFA on their own and therefore require human milk or formula supplemented with LCPUFA (all current premature formulas). These fatty acids, which include docosahexaenoic acid (DHA) and arachidonic acid (ARA), are components of phospholipids found in brain, retina and red blood cell membranes. They have been associated with body growth, vision and cognition as well as being integral parts of prostaglandin metabolism. Wide variations are seen in the amounts of DHA in human milk worldwide that depend largely on fish consumption.[40] Follow-up studies of supplemented formula-fed preterm infants suggest improvements in visual acuity and short-term neurodevelopmental measures compared with unsupplemented infants, but of similar magnitude to infants fed human milk.

Human milk lipid composition

The human mammary gland packages milk fat in large, membrane-bound fat globules of varying size. The lipid system in human milk is structured in a way that facilitates fat digestion and absorption. There is an organized human milk fat globule containing an outer protein coat and an inner lipid core that is made up of 98% triglycerides.[41] The pattern of fatty acids (high in palmitic 16:0, oleic 18:1, linoleic 18:2ω6 and linolenic 18:3ω3), their distribution on the triglyceride molecule (16:0 at the 2-position of the molecule) and the presence of bile salt-stimulated lipase characterize the lipid system in human milk.[42] Because the lipase is heat-labile, the superior fat absorption from human milk is reported only when unprocessed milk is fed.

The most variable nutrient component in human milk is fat, the major energy source, comprising nearly 50% of the calories. The fat content of human milk varies among women, changes during the day, rises slightly during lactation and increases dramatically within a single milk expression.[43] While the variability in total fat content is unrelated to maternal dietary fat intake, the fatty acid profile of maternal dietary intake is very much mirrored in the types of fatty acids found in their milk.[44]

Without homogenization, fresh human milk will quickly separate into lipid and aqueous fractions within minutes. Furthermore, the separated fat may adhere to collection containers, feeding tubes and syringes. This is a major source of lost energy for the premature infant. Minimizing the number of times milk is transferred between different containers from pumping to delivery of the milk will help minimize nutrient loss. The greatest losses of fat occur from continuous milk infusion systems. Care should be taken when using the continuous milk infusion system to ensure the inclusion of only a short length of tubing. Milk infusion systems that use a syringe and small infusion pump, where the syringe is oriented upright, will allow more complete delivery of fat.[45]

Hindmilk

The variability in the fat content of human milk may be made advantageous for the premature infant. Most milk transfer during a feeding occurs in 10–15 minutes, but continued serial milk expressions yield a low volume with a high fat content (hindmilk) than the earlier foremilk. The fat content of hindmilk may be two to threefold greater than that of foremilk.[33] The additional fat, and therefore energy intake from hindmilk, has been shown to improve the body weight gain in premature infants.[46] Separating out a hindmilk fraction is only practical if mothers' milk production is greater than that needed by her infant. The use of hindmilk fortified with a milk fortifier can be recommended for premature infants whose rate of weight gain is low (below 20 g/kg/day).

Medium-chain fatty acids

The proportion of MCFA (carbon length 6:0 to 12:0) is below 12% of total fatty acids in human milk, but approaches 50% in preterm formulas (Table 4).[3] MCFA are non-essential fatty acids. MCFA are absorbed passively, to a greater extent than long-chain fatty acids (LCFA), and in older studies have been associated with improved growth and mineral absorption. However, no differences in nitrogen retention, weight gain, energy digestibility, expenditure and storage were found in contemporary studies of premature infants fed formulas with MCFA at 46% versus 4%.[47] Thus, there are no compelling data to use the high proportion of MCFA found in preterm formulas.

Minerals

Calcium and phosphorus

Calcium (Ca) and phosphorus (P) are fundamental components of skeletal bone matrix accounting for 99% and 85%, respectively. Most transplacental transfer of Ca occurs in the last trimester. The HRI is prone to several clinical conditions that cause or result in abnormalities in mineral metabolism, e.g. hypocalcemia, hyperphosphatemia and hypermagnesemia. Postnatally, serum Ca declines over the first several days due to a blunted parathyroid hormone response and elevated calcitonin

Table 4. Nutrient composition of fortified human milk, preterm formula, post-discharge formula, and term formula.

	Fortified human milk	Preterm formula	Post discharge formula	Term formula
Volume, ml	100	100	100	100
Energy, kcal	83	81	73	67
Protein, g	2.5–2.6	2.4	2.0–2.1	1.4–1.5
Whey/Casein (%)	70/30	60/40	60/40, 50/50	100/0, 60/40, 48/52
Protein calories (%)	12	12	11	8–9
Fat, g	4.0–4.6	4.1–4.4	3.9–4.1	3.4–3.7
MCT (%)	11–17	40–50	20–25	0
Fat calories (%)	43–50	44–47	47–49	46–49
Carbohydrate, g	7.1–8.5	8.4–9.0	7.5–7.6	7.3–7.5
Lactose (%)	80–85	40–50	40–50	70–100
CHO calories (%)	34–41	41–44	40–42	43–45
Calcium, mg	119–146	134–146	78–88	43–53
Phosphorus, mg	59–76	65–81	46–48	24–29
Magnesium, mg	3.4–9.4	7.3–9.7	5.9–6.7	4.0–5.4
Sodium, mEq (mmol)	1.6	1.5–2.0	1.1	0.7–0.8
K, mEq (mmol)	2.0–2.9	2.0–2.7	2.0–2.7	1.8–1.9
Chloride, mEq (mmol)	1.9–2.6	1.9–2.0	1.6	1.2
Zinc, μg	935–1215	1200	913	500–670
Copper, μg	95–221	100–200	88	50–61
Vitamin A, IU	847–1177	1000	329–342	200
Vitamin D, IU	122–151	120–194	52–58	40
Vitamin E, mg	3.5–4.9	3.2–5.1	2.7–2.9	1.0–1.3
Osmolality, mOsm/L	325–385	280–300	250–260	250–300
Potential renal solute load, mOsm	22–23	22–23	18.1–18.7	12.7–13.1

FHM: Enfamil Human Milk Fortifier (Mead Johnson Nutritionals, Evansville, IN) and Similac Human Milk Fortifier (Abbott Nutrition, Columbus, OH), 4 packets + 100 ml Mature Preterm Human Milk.

Preterm: Similac Special Care Advance with iron (Ross) and Enfamil Lipil Premature Formula with iron (Mead Johnson)

Post-Discharge: NeoSure Advance (Ross) and EnfaCare Lipil (Mead Johnson)

Term: Enfamil Lipil with iron (Mead Johnson), Good Start Supreme (Nestle), Similac Advance with iron (Ross) levels. Thus, intravenous Ca must be provided in the early postnatal period to prevent hypocalcemia. Because there is a transient period of oliguria and renal insufficiency, postnatal serum P values occasionally may be elevated in some HRIs. Ca and P deficiency also result in hypercalciuria and, in combination with the use of diuretics, may result in nephrocalcinosis. Therefore, P must be provided in parenteral nutrition solutions.

Another important consideration in the provision of adequate minerals is the physical limitation of the solubility of Ca and P in solution. Careful attention to pH, temperature, amino acid concentration and source must be given so as to provide a recommendation for the appropriate quantity of Ca and P in PN.[48] Ultimately, PN solutions cannot match the Ca and P needs of the HRI and will lead to some mineral deficits until they establish enteral feeding.

Ca and P must be provided together for optimal bone deposition; without P, bone Ca deposition is blunted and hypercalcemia and hypophosphatemia will occur. The optimal molar ratio of Ca to P in PN for HRIs is generally Ca/P >1:1 as lower ratios result in elevated urinary P and serum P concentrations, suggestive of inadequate P utilization because of inadequate Ca intake.[49,50,51]

The goal for premature infant nutrition is to achieve a bone mineralization pattern similar to the fetus and to avoid osteopenia and fractures. This requires an equivalent influx of Ca and P in the blood from parenteral and enteral sources. Preterm human milk contains approximately 250 mg/L and 140 mg/L, of Ca and P respectively.[52] In contrast, the Ca and P content of enteral products designed for premature infants in the United States is significantly greater (Table 4). In human milk, Ca and P exist in ionized and complexed forms that are easily absorbed whereas the salts in commercial formulas are relatively insoluble. Thus, in the design of commercial formulas, greater quantities of these minerals are added to compensate for their poorer bioavailability.

Skeletal radiographs may reveal poor bone mineralization, rickets, and fractures in the premature infant fed unsupplemented-human milk.[53] The supplementation of human milk with both Ca and P, improves the net retention of both minerals, as well as bone mineral content.[54] A linear relationship exists between Ca (or P) intake and net retention in enterally-fed premature infants. Premature infants receiving unfortified human milk or term or specialized (non-preterm) formulas never achieve intrauterine accretion rates for Ca and P. Intakes of Ca and P of approximately 200 and 100 mg/kg/day, respectively, can be achieved with the use of specialized human milk fortifiers and preterm formulas, thus making it possible to meet intrauterine estimates (Tables 3,4). Several factors affect the absorption of Ca and P, including postnatal age and intake of Ca, P, lactose, fat and vitamin D. Vitamin D, however, is responsible for only a small component of Ca absorption in premature infants.[55]

Magnesium

Magnesium (Mg) is an essential component of bone mass that contains approximately 60% of the body's magnesium. Hypermagnesemia in HRI infants is not an uncommon finding following maternal Mg therapy. However, once serum Mg concentrations normalize, parenteral Mg should be provided. The absorption of Mg is significantly greater in unfortified human milk (73%) compared with formula (48%).[56] However, net Mg retention in premature infants fed either unfortified human milk or premature formula meets intrauterine estimates. Therefore, Mg supplements are not needed for premature infants.[57]

Iron

The iron needs of the premature infant are determined by birth weight, initial hemoglobin, rate of growth, and magnitude of iron loss and/or transfused blood.[58] The concentration of iron in human milk declines through lactation, from approximately 0.6 mg/L at 2 weeks to 0.3 mg/L after 5 months of lactation.[59] The absorption of Fe is affected adversely by blood transfusion.[60] Premature infants fed human milk are in negative Fe balance that, if not transfused, corrects with Fe supplements. Iron absorption also appears to be facilitated by a modest degree of anemia.[61] The provision of small doses of Fe at 2 mg/kg/day beginning two weeks postnatally has been demonstrated, in the absence of blood transfusions, to prevent the development of Fe deficiency at 3 months postnatal age. When recombinant erythropoietin for the treatment of anemia of prematurity is used, higher doses of Fe are needed, in the range of 6 mg/kg/day, to support the more rapid rate of erythropoiesis. Generally, ferrous sulfate (2–4 mg/kg/day) is given to human milk-fed premature infants beginning soon after the achievement of complete enteral feedings. Formula-fed premature infants should receive iron-fortified formula from the onset of milk feeding.

Trace Elements

Zinc

Zinc (Zn) participates in a multitude of ways with different enzymes in catalytic, structural and regulatory roles.[62] Its importance is clear with growth arrest when inadequate amounts of zinc are supplied.[19] The classical signs of zinc deficiency include an erythematous skin rash involving perioral, perineal, and facial areas, as well as the extremities.[58] A very low serum alkaline phosphatase activity, a zinc-dependent enzyme, is suggestive of deficiency. The major excretory route is via the GI tract and so infants with large GI fluid losses may become zinc deficient. Unfortified or pasteurized human milk (0.7 mg/kg/day) does not contain sufficient zinc for the premature infant. Therefore, enteral zinc supplementation is required.

Copper

Copper (Cu) has primarily a catalytic role in the body for oxidases to reduce molecular oxygen. One key enzyme is superoxide dismutase, a critical enzyme in antioxidant defense. Parenteral intake also has been suggested using serial balance studies.[19,50] Symptoms of copper deficiency include osteopenia, neutropenia and hypochromic anemia. Copper status is difficult to define with serum indices. Copper needs are increased in cases of excess biliary losses and in patients with jejunostomies. Conversely, impaired biliary secretion may lead to an accumulation of Cu. Therefore, it is advised that Cu intakes be reduced in patients with impaired biliary excretion, such as in cholestatic syndromes. To prevent copper deficiency in infants with cholestasis, some clinicians provide parenteral copper once or twice per week. Enteral copper supplementation is required to meet the needs of the growing preterm infant.

Selenium

Selenium (Se) is a component of glutathione peroxidase and its absence from long-term PN solutions results in a deficiency of the element. A review of parenteral Se intakes suggests that intakes of 1.5–7 μg/kg/day were associated with significant reductions in neonatal sepsis compared with no Se in PN.

Manganese

Recommendations for manganese (Mn) intakes are not clearly defined.[50] Inadvertent Mn intake occurs due to minute amounts of Mn found in the environment and materials such as IV tubing. As a result, it is difficult to manifest symptoms of manganese deficiency even with no supplementation. Therefore infants who are developing cholestasis should be taken off Mn until their cholestasis resolves since Mn excretion is limited in these infants.

Chromium

Chromium (Cr) needs may be associated with insulin activity at the receptor level.[50] Cr deficiency, therefore, may result in impaired glucose tolerance. High doses of Cr may accumulate in the body.

Vitamins

Fat-soluble vitamins

The fat-soluble vitamins, A, D, and E, are stored in the body and large doses may result in toxicity. Vitamin K, while fat-soluble, is not readily stored in the liver until 2–3 months of age.[63] An initial dose of vitamin K at birth is an essential part of care for the premature infant to prevent spontaneous hemorrhage. The stores of vitamin D of the premature infant at birth reflect maternal vitamin D stores. There is increasing awareness that a significant number of pregnant mothers are relatively deficient in vitamin D even in latitudes with more direct sun exposure.[64] Attempts to measure maternal and infant levels of 25-OH vitamin D are not routine neonatal practice but are incresingly becoming available due to inaccessibility to accurate lab measurements. Enteral vitamin D supplementation is included in human milk fortifiers and preterm formulas so no additional dosing is required.

Vitamin A

Vitamin A has diverse functions, being essential for vision, growth, reproduction, cell differentiation and immunocompetency.[50,63] Plasma vitamin A concentrations in HRI infants receiving PN are low. Infants developing bronchopulmonary dysplasia (BPD) reported have lower plasma vitamin A concentrations at 4, 14, 21 and 28 days of age compared with infants not developing BPD.[65] Randomized controlled trials of vitamin A supplementation in HRI infants susceptible to BPD have been reported. A meta-analysis suggests that supplementation with vitamin A is associated with a modest reduction in oxygen requirement at 36 weeks postmenstrual age with a trend toward a reduction in retinopathy of prematurity. Guidelines should be adopted and parenteral preparations reformulated to provide intakes that approximate 500 μg/kg/day for vitamin A, initiated within the first 12 hours after birth.

Vitamin E

In humans, vitamin E functions as a biological antioxidant or free-radical scavenger that prevents the naturally occurring peroxidation of polyunsaturated fatty acids, components of the lipid layer of cell membranes.[63] Early use of PN containing multivitamins and within the intravenous lipids will optimally raise plasma vitamin E levels. Pharmacologic doses of vitamin E have been shown to have a modest impact on severe (Stage 3, plus disease) retinopathy of prematurity (ROP) with half the incidence (2.4%) seen in the supplemented group compared with controls (5.7%). Insufficient evidence exists for vitamin E supplementation for the reduction in severity of BPD but older studies showed that early (within 12 hours of birth) vitamin E delivery could reduce the incidence and severity of IVH. Guidelines for PN preparations should target approximately 3 mg/kg/day for vitamin E starting soon after birth.

Water-soluble vitamins

Water-soluble vitamins, thiamin, riboflavin, niacin, vitamin B_6, folate, vitamin B_{12}, pantothenic acid, biotin and vitamin C, are not stored in the body and excess intakes are excreted in the urine or bile (vitamin B_{12}). The intake of water-soluble vitamins, therefore, should be at frequent intervals to avoid deficiency states. Current parenteral formulations generally provide more water-soluble vitamins than are needed by HRI infants. Supplementary vitamins are provided in human milk fortifiers and in preterm formulas. There is no indication for additional multivitamin supplements for infants receiving adequate intakes of fortified human milk, preterm formula, or enriched formula. Once the premature infant transitions to unfortified human milk or standard formula, a multivitamin supplement should be added. The supplemental vitamins should be continued until the infant is consuming 300 kcal/day or weighs more than 2.5 kg.

References

1. Ziegler EE, O'Donnell AM, Nelson SE *et al.* (1976) Body composition of the reference fetus. *Growth* **40**: 329–341.
2. Ellis KJ, Shypailo RJ, Schanler RJ. (1993) Body elemental composition of the neonate: New reference data. *Am J Hum Biol* **5**: 323–330.
3. Klein CJ. (2002) Nutrient requirements for preterm infant formulas. *J Nutr* **132**: 1395S–1577S.
4. Taylor SN, Basile LA, Ebeling M *et al.* (2009) Intestinal permeability in preterm infants by feeding type: Mother's milk versus formula. *Breastfeed Med* **4**: 11–15.
5. Schanler RJ, Shulman RJ, Lau C *et al.* (1999) Feeding strategies for premature infants: Randomized trial of gastrointestinal priming and tube-feeding method. *Pediatrics* **103**: 434–439.

6. Bauer J, Werner C, Gerss J. (2009) Metabolic rate analysis of healthy preterm and full-term infants during the first weeks of life. *Am J Clin Nutr*: [Epub ahead of print].

7. Poindexter BB, Karn CA, Denne SC. (1998) Exogenous insulin reduces proteolysis and protein synthesis in extremely low birth weight infants. *J Pediatr* **132**: 948–953.

8. Collins JW, Jr., Hoppe M, Brown K *et al.* (1991) A controlled trial of insulin infusion and parenteral nutrition in extremely low birth weight infants with glucose intolerance. *J Pediatr* **118**: 921–927.

9. Sunehag AL, Haymond MW, Schanler RJ *et al.* (1999) Gluconeogenesis in very low birth weight infants receiving total parenteral nutrition. *Diabetes* **48**: 791–800.

10. Ziegler EE, Fomon SJ. (1983) Lactose enhances mineral absorption in infancy. *J Pediatr Gastroenterol Nutr* **2**: 288–294.

11. Bode L. (2006) Recent advances on structure, metabolism and function of human milk oligosaccharides. *J Nutr* **136**: 2127–2130.

12. Mitton SG. (1994) Amino acids and lipid in total parenteral nutrition for the newborn. *J Pediatr Gastroenterol Nutr* **18**: 25–31.

13. Elango R, Ball RO, Pencharz PB. (2008) Indicator amino acid oxidation: Concept and application. *J Nutr* **138**: 243–246.

14. Vina J, Vento M, Garcia-Sala F *et al.* (1995) L-cysteine and glutathione metabolism are impaired in premature infants due to cystathionase deficiency. *Am J Clin Nutr* **61**: 1067–1069.

15. Dunham B, Marcuard S, Khazanie PG *et al.* (1991) The solubility of calcium and phosphorus in neonatal total parenteral nutrition solutions. *JPEN J Parenter Enteral Nutr* **15**: 608–611.

16. Heird WC, Dell RB, Helms RA *et al.* (1987) Amino acid mixture designed to maintain normal plasma amino acid patterns in infants and children requiring parenteral nutrition. *Pediatrics* **80**: 401–408.

17. Embleton NE, Pang N, Cooke RJ. (2001) Postnatal malnutrition and growth retardation: An inevitable consequence of current recommendations in preterm infants? *Pediatrics* **107**: 270–273.

18. Van Goudoever JB, Colen T, Wattimena JL *et al.* (1995) Immediate commencement of amino acid supplementation in preterm infants: Effect on serum amino acid concentrations and protein kinetics on the first day of life. *J Pediatr* **127**: 458–465.

19. Schanler RJ, Shulman RJ, Prestridge LL. (1994) Parenteral nutrient needs of very low birth weight infants. *J Pediatr* **125**: 961–968.

20. van Lingen RA, van Goudoever JB, Luijendijk IH *et al.* (1992) Effects of early amino acid administration during total parenteral nutrition on protein metabolism in pre-term infants. *Clin Sci (Lond)* **82**: 199–203.

21. Rivera A, Jr., Bell EF, Bier DM. (1993) Effect of intravenous amino acids on protein metabolism of preterm infants during the first three days of life. *Pediatr Res* **33**: 106–111.

22. Thureen PJ, Melara D, Fennessey PV *et al.* (2003) Effect of low versus high intravenous amino acid intake on very low birth weight infants in the early neonatal period. *Pediatr Res* **53**: 24–32.

23. Hay WW, Jr. (2008) Strategies for feeding the preterm infant. *Neonatology* **94**: 245–254.

24. Poindexter BB, Langer JC, Dusick AM *et al.* (2006) Early provision of parenteral amino acids in extremely low birth weight infants: Relation to growth and neurodevelopmental outcome. *J Pediatr* **148**: 300–305.

25. Gaull GE, Rassin DK, Raiha NC *et al.* (1977) Milk protein quantity and quality in low-birth-weight infants. III. Effects on sulfur amino acids in plasma and urine. *J Pediatr* **90**: 348–355.

26. Raiha NC, Heinonen K, Rassin DK *et al.* (1976) Milk protein quantity and quality in low-birthweight infants: I. Metabolic responses and effects on growth. *Pediatrics* **57**: 659–684.

27. Groh-Wargo S, Jacobs J, Auestad N *et al.* (2005) Body composition in preterm infants who are fed long-chain polyunsaturated fatty acids: A prospective, randomized, controlled trial. *Pediatr Res* **57**: 712–718.

28. Zlotkin SH, Bryan MH, Anderson GH. (1981) Intravenous nitrogen and energy intakes required to duplicate *in utero* nitrogen accretion in prematurely born human infants. *J Pediatr* **99**: 115–120.

29. Kashyap S, Forsyth M, Zucker C *et al.* (1986) Effects of varying protein and energy intakes on growth and metabolic response in low birth weight infants. *J Pediatr* **108**: 955–963.

30. Polberger SK, Axelsson IA, Raiha NC. (1989) Growth of very low birth weight infants on varying amounts of human milk protein. *Pediatr Res* **25**: 414–419.

31. Billeaud C, Guillet J, Sandler B. (1990) Gastric emptying in infants with or without gastro-oesophageal reflux according to the type of milk. *Eur J Clin Nutr* **44**: 577–583.

32. Schanler RJ, Goldblum RM, Garza C *et al.* (1986) Enhanced fecal excretion of selected immune factors in very low birth weight infants fed fortified human milk. *Pediatr Res* **20**: 711–715.

33. Saarela T, Kokkonen J, Koivisto M. (2005) Macronutrient and energy contents of human milk fractions during the first six months of lactation. *Acta Paediatr* **94**: 1176–1181.

34. Kashyap S, Schulze KF, Forsyth M *et al.* (1988) Growth, nutrient retention and metabolic response in low birth weight infants fed varying intakes of protein and energy. *J Pediatr* **113**: 713-721.

35. Gutcher GR, Farrell PM. (1991) Intravenous infusion of lipid for the prevention of essential fatty acid deficiency in premature infants. *Am J Clin Nutr* **54**: 1024–1028.

36. Simmer K, Rao SC. (2005) Early introduction of lipids to parenterally-fed preterm infants. *Cochrane Database Syst Rev*: CD005256.

37. Haumont D, Richelle M, Deckelbaum RJ *et al.* (1992) Effect of liposomal content of lipid emulsions on plasma lipid concentrations in low birth weight infants receiving parenteral nutrition. *J Pediatr* **121**: 759–763.

38. Kao LC, Cheng MH, Warburton D. (1984) Triglycerides, free fatty acids, free fatty acids/albumin molar ratio and cholesterol levels in serum of neonates receiving long-term lipid infusions: Controlled trial of continuous and intermittent regimens. *J Pediatr* **104**: 429–435.

39. Gura KM, Duggan CP, Collier SB *et al.* (2006) Reversal of parenteral nutrition-associated liver disease in two infants with short bowel syndrome using parenteral fish oil: Implications for future management. *Pediatrics* **118**: e197–e201.

40. Lauritzen L, Jorgensen MH, Hansen HS *et al.* (2002) Fluctuations in human milk long-chain PUFA levels in relation to dietary fish intake. *Lipids* **37**: 237–244.

41. Hamosh M. (1998) Protective function of proteins and lipids in human milk. *Biol Neonate* **74**: 163–176.

42. Jensen RG, Jensen GL. (1992) Specialty lipids for infant nutrition. I. Milks and formulas. *J Pediatr Gastroenterol Nutr* **15**: 232–245.

43. Neville MC, Keller RP, Seacat J *et al.* (1984) Studies on human lactation. I. Within-feed and between-breast variation in selected components of human milk. *Am J Clin Nutr* **40**: 635–646.

44. Jensen RG. (1999) Lipids in human milk. *Lipids* **34**: 1243–1271.

45. Greer FR, McCormick A, Loker J. (1984) Changes in fat concentration of human milk during delivery by intermittent bolus and continuous mechanical pump infusion. *J Pediatr* **105**: 745–749.

46. Valentine CJ, Hurst NM, Schanler RJ. (1994) Hindmilk improves weight gain in low-birth-weight infants fed human milk. *J Pediatr Gastroenterol Nutr* **18**: 474–477.

47. Whyte RK, Campbell D, Stanhope R *et al.* (1986) Energy balance in low birth weight infants fed formula of high or low medium-chain triglyceride content. *J Pediatr* **108**: 964–971.

48. Pelegano JF, Rowe JC, Carey DE *et al.* (1989) Simultaneous infusion of calcium and phosphorus in parenteral nutrition for premature infants: Use of physiologic calcium/phosphorus ratio. *J Pediatr* **114**: 115–119.

49. Koo WW. (1992) Parenteral nutrition-related bone disease. *JPEN J Parenter Enteral Nutr* **16**: 386–394.

50. Greene HL, Hambidge KM, Schanler R *et al.* (1988) Guidelines for the use of vitamins, trace elements, calcium, magnesium, and phosphorus in infants and children receiving total parenteral nutrition: Report of the Subcommittee on Pediatric Parenteral Nutrient Requirements from the Committee on Clinical Practice Issues of the American Society for Clinical Nutrition. *Am J Clin Nutr* **48**: 1324–1342.

51. Prestridge LL, Schanler RJ, Shulman RJ *et al.* (1993) Effect of parenteral calcium and phosphorus therapy on mineral retention and bone mineral content in very low birth weight infants. *J Pediatr* **122**: 761–768.

52. Butte NF, Garza C, Johnson CA *et al.* (1984) Longitudinal changes in milk composition of mothers delivering preterm and term infants. *Early Hum Dev* **9**: 153–162.

53. Koo WW, Sherman R, Succop P *et al.* (1988) Sequential bone mineral content in small preterm infants with and without fractures and rickets. *J Bone Miner Res* **3**: 193–197.

54. Horsman A, Ryan SW, Congdon PJ *et al.* (1989) Bone mineral accretion rate and calcium intake in preterm infants. *Arch Dis Child* **64**: 910–918.

55. Bronner F, Salle BL, Putet G *et al.* (1992) Net calcium absorption in premature infants: Results of 103 metabolic balance studies. *Am J Clin Nutr* **56**: 1037–1044.

56. Schanler RJ, Rifka M. (1994) Calcium, phosphorus and magnesium needs for the low-birth-weight infant. *Acta Paediatr Suppl* **405**: 111–116.

57. Schanler RJ, Abrams SA. (1995) Postnatal attainment of intrauterine macromineral accretion rates in low birth weight infants fed fortified human milk. *J Pediatr* **126**: 441–447.

58. Groh-Wargo S, Thompson M, Hovasi J. (2000) *Nutritional Care for High-Risk Newborns*. Precept Press Inc Chicago, Illinois.

59. Siimes MA, Vuori E, Kuitunen P. (1979) Breast milk iron — a declining concentration during the course of lactation. *Acta Paediatr Scand* **68**: 29–31.

60. Dauncey MJ, Davies CG, Shaw JC *et al.* (1978) The effect of iron supplements and blood transfusion on iron absorption by low birthweight infants fed pasteurized human breast milk. *Pediatr Res* **12**: 899–904.

61. Moody GJ, Schanler RJ, Abrams SA. (1999) Utilization of supplemental iron by premature infants fed fortified human milk. *Acta Paediatr* **88**: 763–767.

62. Cousins RJ. (1996) In: Zinc Filer LJ, Ziegler EE (eds.), *Present Knowledge in Nutrition*, 7th ed. Washington, DC: International Life Science Institute — Nutrition Foundation. pp. 293–306.

63. Tsang RC. (2005) Tsang RC, Uauy R, Koletzko B. (eds.) *et al. Nutrition of the Preterm Infant: Scientific Basis and Practice Guidelines*: Digital Educational Publishing, Inc. 427 p.

64. Hollis BW, Wagner CL. (2004) Assessment of dietary vitamin D requirements during pregnancy and lactation. *Am J Clin Nutr* **79**: 717–726.

65. Shenai JP, Chytil F, Stahlman MT. (1985) Vitamin A status of neonates with bronchopulmonary dysplasia. *Pediatr Res* **19**: 185–188.

Chapter  14

Neonatal Hypocalcemia and Neonatal Hypercalcemia

Ran Namgung and Reginald C. Tsang

Introduction

Disturbances in mineral homeostasis, common in the neonatal period, may be altered responses to normal physiological transition from intrauterine environment to neonatal independence. Hypocalcemia or hypercalcemia may result from pathological intrauterine conditions, fetal immaturity, birth stress, or genetic defects. Diagnosis and management of neonatal hypocalcemia and hypercalcemia require specific knowledge of the unique perinatal, clinical and biochemical features of newborn mineral metabolism. In this chapter, we review calcium (Ca) metabolism with emphasis on neonatal transition, followed by discussion of causes and management strategies of mineral disturbances in the neonatal period.

Perinatal Mineral Metabolism

The homeostasis of Ca in blood is maintained primarily through interaction of three hormones — parathyroid hormone (PTH), 1,25-dihydroxyvitamin D [1,25(OH)$_2$D] and calcitonin (CT) — which direct intestinal Ca absorption, Ca excretion and transfer of Ca stores from bone.

317

Parathyroid hormone

PTH is a blood Ca-elevating hormone. Secretion of PTH by the parathyroid glands is regulated by circulating Ca ion concentrations sensed by Ca-sensing receptors (CaSR) in the parathyroids. An increase in serum Ca inhibits PTH secretion; a decrease in serum Ca stimulates PTH secretion.[1] The CaSR plays key roles in maintenance of a narrow range (4.4–5.2 mg/dL; 1.1–1.3 mM/L) of extracellular ionized Ca concentration (Ca^{2+}). The CaSR is expressed also in other target tissues for PTH involved in Ca homeostasis, such as kidney and bone, to sense alterations in Ca^{2+} and to respond with changes directed at normalizing blood Ca^{2+} concentration.[2] Genetic mutations of the *CASR* gene, on the long arm of chromosome 3, result in either activation or suppression: The CaSR is reset, so that either higher or lower than normal blood Ca^{2+} is sensed by the receptor as "normal." Inactivating mutations (loss-of-function) of the CaSR cause hypercalcemia (hyperparathyroidism), whereas activating mutations (gain-of-function) cause a hypocalcemic syndrome of varying severity (hypoparathyroidism).[3–5]

PTH acts directly on bone, stimulating resorption, thereby releasing Ca and phosphorus (P) into circulation. PTH acts directly on kidneys to increase urinary P excretion and decrease urinary Ca excretion. PTH indirectly enhances intestinal absorption of Ca, through effects on synthesis of $1,25(OH)_2D$. Thus, the net actions of PTH increase serum Ca concentrations.

Active transport of Ca is facilitated by CaSR that "sense" extracellular Ca levels. Placental CaSRs regulate maternal-fetal Ca transport, up to 150 mg of Ca/kg of fetal weight/day in the third trimester, when approximately 80% of fetal Ca accumulation and bone mineralization occur.[6] Thus, the fetus develops in a relatively hypercalcemic state (about 1 mg/dL higher Ca concentrations than maternal levels): cord PTH levels are low, presumably suppressed by hypercalcemia.[7]

At birth, abrupt termination of the maternal-to-fetal Ca supply occurs. To maintain serum Ca homeostasis, an increase of 16–20% in Ca flux from bone to extracellular space is required, pending sufficient exogenous intake of Ca. Ca intake over the first hours to days does not normally match fetal Ca delivery rate, setting the stage for rapid, dramatic decline in serum Ca concentrations. In term infants, for the first 24 to 48 hours, serum Ca concentration declines to 7.5–8.5 mg/dL (1.9–2.1 mM/L) nadir. Thereafter, Ca concentrations progressively rise to mean values of older children and adults by one week.[8] In preterm infants, serum Ca concentration decreases to even lower nadirs at 24 to 36 hours; this hypocalcemia is usually not associated with tetany or decreased cardiac contractility,[9,10] and rises at about six days to values exceeding cord blood concentration.[8]

In normal term infants, when serum Ca concentrations fall after birth, PTH concentrations increase appropriately (twofold to fivefold increase during the first 48 hours) and remain elevated for several days. The PTH secretion in term infants appears substantial, and negatively correlates with Ca levels. Term neonates also show an appropriate calcemic response when challenged with PTH. However, in extremely preterm infants, even with significant hypocalcemia as a stimulus, PTH remains low for the first two days of life. During this time, a transient hypocalcemia exists, which typically resolves within the first week and often requires no treatment.[9–11]

Vitamin D

Vitamin D is necessary for maintenance of normal Ca and P homeostasis. 1,25(OH)$_2$D is the major hormone affecting active intestinal Ca and P absorption. Production of 1,25(OH)$_2$D by renal proximal tubule is enhanced by hypocalcemia, hypophosphatemia and PTH and appears tightly regulated.[12] 1,25(OH)$_2$D is required for effective PTH stimulation of bone resorption and acts on kidney to conserve Ca and P. The overall result of this hormone is to increase serum Ca and P concentrations.

Insufficiency of infant vitamin D arises from maternal vitamin D deficiency (sunshine deprivation coupled with insufficient dietary vitamin D intake), reduced production of vitamin D or its active metabolites caused by liver or renal disease, congenital deficiency of renal 1-α-hydroxylase and 1,25(OH)$_2$D resistance. Deficiency of vitamin D or its metabolites predominantly causes decreased intestinal Ca absorption and renal Ca reabsorption and neonatal hypocalcemia.[13–15]

Newborn stores of vitamin D are usually adequate unless there is significant maternal vitamin D deficiency. The majority of vitamin D for newborn infants usually comes from maternal and dietary sources. Levels of 25-hydroxyvitamin D (25OHD), the major marker of vitamin D status, change with gestational age and are lower in preterm than in term infants. However, conversion of 25-OHD to $1,25(OH)_2D$ occurs normally in premature infants.[16]

In normal term infants, serum $1,25(OH)_2D$ concentrations are low at birth but increase to adult normal ranges by 24 hours of life, possibly reflecting the need for optimum intestinal Ca and P absorption.[17] In preterm infants, serum $1,25(OH)_2D$ concentrations at birth are comparable to reference values for healthy children and adults, increase significantly during the first few days of life and are far above reference values between 3 and 12 weeks of life.[18] Cord serum $1,25(OH)_2D$ concentrations are lower in small for gestational age infants compared with appropriate for gestational age infants, possibly reflecting decreased $1,25(OH)_2D$ production from reduced uteroplacental blood flow.[19]

Calcitonin

CT is a Ca^{2+}-lowering hormone produced by parafollicular cells of the thyroid, which, acts as the physiologic antagonist to PTH. The secretion of CT is under direct control of blood Ca.[20] Elevation in Ca^{2+} stimulates CaSR and lowers Ca^{2+} by enhancing CT secretion; and a decrease in Ca^{2+} causes a decrease in CT concentrations. Once secreted, CT has a circulatory half-life of 2 to 15 minutes. CT inhibits osteoclast-mediated bone resorption (decreasing Ca and P released from bone) and secondarily increases renal Ca and P excretion (at high doses). The net consequence of CT decreases serum concentrations of Ca and P.[20]

Chronic fetal hypercalcemia leads to higher CT levels in the fetus and newborn than those in the mother.[21] Cord serum CT concentrations decrease with increasing gestational age. Infants < 32 weeks' gestation have CT concentration nearly three times higher than term cord serum CT concentrations.[22]

After birth, serum CT concentrations further increase in both preterm and term infants, peaking at 24 to 48 hours, followed by decline to childhood values by one month.[21–23] The physiologic importance of this increase in serum CT is unclear, but may relate to counteracting PTH bone resorptive action.

Neonatal Hypocalcemia

Definition

Hypocalcemia is generally defined as serum total Ca concentration below 8.0 mg/dL (<2 mM/L) in term and 7 mg/dL (<1.75 mM/L) in preterm infants, or ionized Ca concentration below 3.0–4.4 mg/dL (<0.75–1.1 mM/L). Based on onset, hypocalcemia has been classified as early or late. Early neonatal hypocalcemia typically occurs during the first few days, with the lowest Ca concentrations at 24 to 48 hours, whereas late hypocalcemia occurs toward the end of the first week.

Etiology

Early-onset neonatal hypocalcemia is most commonly associated with prematurity, birth asphyxia, maternal insulin-dependent diabetes, gestational exposure to anticonvulsant and maternal hyperparathyroidism. Late-onset hypocalcemia, which is less frequent than early-onset, is most commonly associated with administration of relatively high P-containing diets, disturbed maternal vitamin D metabolism, intestinal malabsorption of Ca, hypomagnesemia and hypoparathyroidism.

Pathophysiology

Early neonatal hypocalcemia represents exaggeration of the normal fall in serum Ca concentration that occurs during the first 24 to 48 hours. Early hypocalcemia occurs from inability to compensate for the sudden loss of placental Ca supply at birth, through insufficient release of PTH by immature parathyroid glands[9] or inadequate responsiveness of the renal tubular cells to PTH. Preterm infants may or may not exhibit the surge in PTH secretion of term infants at birth and restricted oral Ca intake may aggravate the problem; end-organ resistance to $1,25(OH)_2D$ and an exaggerated rise in CT secretion may also contribute to hypocalcemia.[9,22] In asphyxiated infants, decreased Ca intake as a result of delayed feedings, increased endogenous P load, bicarbonate alkali therapy and increased serum CT concentration may contribute to early hypocalcemia. Hypocalcemia in infants of insulin-dependent diabetic mothers appears related to magnesium (Mg) insufficiency and consequent impaired PTH secretion. Transient neonatal hypoparathyroidism occurs in infants exposed to maternal hypercalcemia *in utero*. Intrauterine hypercalcemia suppresses fetal parathyroid activity and apparently impairs responsiveness of the parathyroid to hypocalcemia after birth.[24]

Late hypocalcemia commonly results from dietary Ca and P imbalance, and rarely from maternal hypercalcemia. Infants receiving cow-milk-derived formulas have lower serum ionized Ca and higher serum P in the first week of life, compared to breast-fed infants, related to the higher absolute P amount of formula[25] or limited P excretion from low glomerular filtration rate in the newborn. P-containing enemas have resulted in P overload and hypocalcemia. Late neonatal hypocalcemia may be due to relative resistance of the immature kidney to PTH, leading to renal retention of P and hypocalcemia: biochemical features resemble those of pseudohypoparathyroidism (defects in the *GNAS1* gene) but with normal nephrogenous cyclic AMP responses to PTH.[26,27]

Congenital hypoparathyroidism is the most significant cause of late-onset hypocalcemia that has to be treated early in life. Congenital hypoparathyroidism also occurs as part of the DiGeorge triad of hypoparathyroidism, T-cell incompetence from partial or absent thymus and conotruncal heart defects or aortic arch abnormalities.

Isolated hypoparathyroidism includes genetic defects that impair PTH synthesis (i.e. *PTH* gene defects) or secretion (i.e. *CASR* gene defects), or parathyroid gland development (i.e. *GCMB* gene defects). Gain-of-function (activating) mutations in the *CASR* gene encoding the CaSR are the most common cause of mild isolated hypoparathyroidism (autosomal dominant hypocalcemia), associated with inappropriately low or low-normal levels of serum PTH and relative hypercalciuria.[2–5] By contrast, mutations in the *GCMB* gene (loss of this transcription factor) result in developmental failure of the parathyroids during embryogenesis (i.e. parathyroid agenesis).[28] Defects in the *PTH* gene are uncommon causes of hypoparathyroidism.[29]

Clinical presentation

The neonate with hypocalcemia may be asymptomatic; the less mature the infant, the more subtle and varied the clinical manifestations. The main clinical signs are jitteriness, tremors, twitching, exaggerated startle responses or seizures (generalized or focal). Frank convulsions are seen more commonly with late hypocalcemia. Infants also may be lethargic, feed poorly, vomit and have abdominal distension. Apnea, cyanosis, tachypnea, tachycardia, vomiting, or heart failure may also be seen. The classic signs of peripheral hyperexcitability of motor nerves (carpopedal spasm and laryngospasm) are uncommon in newborn infants.

Diagnosis

The diagnosis of hypocalcemia is based on the determination of serum ionized or total Ca. In addition to history and physical examination, certain data are useful when there is not a clear cause: serum P, Mg concentrations, glucose concentrations and serum pH. Electrocardiographic prolonged QTc (>0.40 sec) suggests hypocalcemia. Functional atrioventricular block from prolonged QTc (0.53 sec) interval is reported in hypocalcemic preterm infants[30,31]: QTc normalizes after Ca infusion, supporting QTc use to monitor response to Ca therapy.

When the infant is refractory to therapy or there are unusual findings in initial evaluation, additional data may be of value to diagnose less common causes of neonatal hypocalcemia (e.g. primary hypoparathyroidism, malabsorption and disorders of vitamin D metabolism). Other laboratory tests, including PTH, 25OHD and 1,25(OH)$_2$D are not usually needed unless neonatal hypocalcemia does not readily resolve with Ca therapy.

Differential diagnosis

Elevated P concentration (>8 mg/dL) may reflect P overload (high dietary P intake), renal insufficiency, or hypoparathyroidism. A serum Mg concentration of 0.8 mg/dL (0.3 mM/L) or less strongly supports primary hypomagnesemia. Urinary Ca excretion ≥4 mg/kg/day or urine Ca/creatinine ratio ≥ 0.2 (mg/mg) indicates hypercalciuria. Hypercalciuria, associated with hypocalcemia, supports a deficiency of PTH (hypoparathyroidism). Low serum 25-OHD concentration (< 11 ng/mL) indicates vitamin D deficiency. Normal to moderately elevated 1,25(OH)$_2$D concentrations are consistent with hypoparathyroidism. Absence of thymic shadows on chest radiograph and the presence of aorto-cardiac anormalies suggest the 22q11 syndrome (*CARCH22* or *DiGeorge sequence*).

Prolonged hypocalcemia should prompt the physician to investigate permanent causes, such as hypoparathyroidism. DNA analysis for mutations which cause these conditions may help confirm the diagnosis in the proband and relatives.[32]

Treatment approaches

The treatment of symptomatic hypocalcemia is through intravenous Ca supplementation, at doses of 30–75 mg elemental Ca/kg/day, titrated to clinical and biochemical response; the amount of Ca should be adjusted to maintain ionized Ca in the low-normal range, with frequent monitoring of serum ionized Ca. Clinical signs of hypocalcemia are usually reversed rapidly by correcting serum Ca concentrations, which helps confirm the diagnosis.

When there are seizures (serum Ca usually <6 mg/dL [1.5 mM/L]), emergency Ca therapy (1–2 mL of Ca gluconate 10% per kg; about 9–18 mg elemental Ca per kg) is given intravenously over 10 minutes; heart rate should be measured continuously during the infusion to prevent bradycardia, for which the infusion should be stopped temporarily; the infusion site should be watched for possible tissue injury from extravasation. Follow-up bolus or intermittent infusions of Ca salts should be avoided, if possible, because of wide excursions in serum Ca concentrations.

For less urgent purposes, or follow up after initial treatment for seizures, continuous intravenous Ca supplementation at 75 mg elemental Ca/kg/day is generally sufficient to restore normocalcemia. After normocalcemia is achieved, stepwise reduction of intravenous Ca may help to prevent rebound hypocalcemia; 75 mg/kg/day for the first day, half the dose the next day, half again, then discontinue. Alternatively, if infants can tolerate oral feeding, Ca gluconate can be given orally at the same doses (divided in four to six doses) after initial correction. Oral Ca-administration may not be practical in sick infants because oral Ca can stimulate bowel movements. All oral Ca preparations are hypertonic (high osmolar) and should be used with caution in infants who are at risk of necrotizing enterocolitis. Vitamin D metabolites are not recommended for clinical management of early hypocalcemia because of their variable response and potential side effects.

When there is persistent hypocalcemia, the serum Mg level should be measured because hypocalcemia generally cannot be corrected until hypomagnesemia is alleviated: Mg plays an important role in PTH secretion and action; chronic Mg deficiency causes impaired secretion of PTH and PTH resistance at target organs.[33] If hypocalcemia is associated with hypomagnesemia (serum Mg below 1.5 mg/dL [0.6 mM/L]), Mg sulfate 50% solution (500 mg or 4 mEq/mL), 0.1–0.2 mL/kg, IV or IM (may cause local tissue necrosis) should be given and repeated after 12 to 24 hours. Serum Mg should be obtained before each dose (one or two doses may resolve transient hypomagnesemia).

Because most causes of hypocalcemia in the neonate are transient, the duration of supplemental Ca therapy varies with the cause of hypocalcemia; commonly as little as 2–3 days for early hypocalcemia is needed. Ca supplementation is usually required for long periods in the case of hypocalcemia caused by malabsorption or hypoparathyroidism.

In asymptomatic neonates with hypocalcemia, opinions vary as to the need for therapy. Most hypocalcemia of this nature resolves spontaneously with time, but hypocalcemia has potential adverse effects on the cardiovascular and central nervous systems, so treatment may be needed.[10] For asymptomatic ill infants, or infants with severe hypocalcemia (serum total Ca < 6.0 mg/dL [1.5 mM/L] or ionized Ca < 3 mg/dL [0.75 mM/L]), therapy is usually required. Either intravenous or oral therapy as described above, can be given.

Because late hypocalcemia is usually symptomatic, there is little debate on treatment. The goals of therapy are to reduce P load and increase Ca absorption by using feedings with Ca/P ratio $\geq$ 4:1, such as use of low-P feedings (human milk or low-P formula), in conjunction with an oral Ca supplement. Phosphate binders are generally not necessary.

Treatment of hypoparathyroidism is directed at maintaining a plasma Ca level which prevents symptoms, without causing nephrocalcinosis. Hypoparathyroidism requires therapy with $1,25(OH)_2D$ (or 1 α-hydroxy-vitamin D_3, a synthetic analog) and life-long Ca supplementation. Infants with severe or persistent hypocalcemia may benefit from addition of $1,25(OH)_2D$, intravenously or orally, 50–100 ng/kg per day in two or three divided doses. Vitamin D deficiency should be treated with supplemental vitamin D (200–2000 IU/day).

Recombinant PTH (teriparatide®), successfully used in hypoparathyroid adults,[34,35] has been tried as an initial management of neonatal hypoparathyroidism. In infants with life-threatening seizures and persistent hypocalcemia despite aggressive management with high doses of 1,25(OH)$_2$D and Ca infusion, short-term use of teriparatide (5 μg subcutaneously) can raise Ca levels faster (in less than four hours) and more safely than other commonly used methods, which take a day or longer.[36] Use of recombinant PTH in pediatrics has been hampered by concern about long-term exposure and risk of osteosarcoma. Since Teriparatide® is a faster, safer and more physiologic means of correcting hypocalcemia due to hypoparathyroidism, further evaluation is required.

Prevention

In neonates at risk, early hypocalcemia can be prevented by oral or parenteral Ca supplementation (75 mg elemental Ca/kg/day). Early feeding and provision of Ca to the gut is important in preventing hypocalcemia. Use of continuous Ca infusion to maintain total Ca > 8.0 mg/dL (2 mM/L) and ionized Ca > 4.0 mg/dL (1 mM/L) may be helpful to prevent hypocalcemia in sick newborns with cardiovascular compromise requiring cardiotonic drugs or pressure support.

Maintenance of normal maternal vitamin D status by exogenous vitamin D supplement, may help maintain normal fetal vitamin D status and prevent late hypocalcemia in some neonates. To prevent hypocalcemia in very low birth weight infants, vitamin D metabolites have been attempted, but serum Ca was normalized only at pharmacologic doses of 1,25(OH)$_2$D.[16] In sick infants, judicious use of bicarbonate and avoidance of respiratory alkalosis from excessive mechanical ventilation may reduce the risk of symptomatic hypocalcemia.

Prognosis

In most cases, early hypocalcemia resolves spontaneously within the first week of life. In preterm infants, hypocalcemia is usually asymptomatic and temporary and gradually reverts to normal Ca after one to three days. Prolonged hypocalcemia caused by malabsorption or hypoparathyroidism requires therapy with $1,25(OH)_2D$ or synthetic analog, 1α-hydroxyvitamin D and Ca supplementation possibly for life. In infants with prolonged hypocalcemia, regular follow-up monitoring of serum Ca concentration and appropriate monitoring of underlying disease (e.g. PTH concentrations) are necessary. Some infants may have hypoparathyroidism that lasts for several years; these infants may still be at risk for "recurrence" of hypoparathyroidism and hypocalcemia, as late as adolescence.

Neonatal Hypercalcemia

Definition

Neonatal hypercalcemia is defined as a serum total Ca concentration above 11 mg/dL (2.75 mM/L) or an ionized Ca concentration above 5.6 mg/dL (1.4 mM/L).

Etiology

Hypercalcemia is uncommon in term infants, but relatively more common in preterm infants. The most common cause of hypercalcemia in infants is a relative deficiency in P supply and hypophosphatemia from inappropriate parenteral nutrition, with or without excessive Ca, or human milk feeding in preterm infants (low P content relative to preterm needs).[37] Iatrogenic hypercalcemia results from excessive Ca and/or vitamin D for hypocalcemia or during exchange blood transfusion. Chronic maternal exposure to excessive vitamin D or its metabolites, secondary to treatment of maternal hypocalcemic disorders, may result in hypercalcemia of mother and neonate. Chronic diuretic therapy with thiazides during pregnancy may lead to maternal, fetal and neonatal hypercalcemia.

Other rarer causes of hypercalcemia in the newborn include hyperparathyroidism (primary, or secondary to maternal hypoparathyroidism), and hypercalcemia associated with subcutaneous fat necrosis, idiopathic infantile hypercalcemia, severe infantile hypophosphatasia and Bartter syndrome variant. Primary hyperparathyroidism is rare in neonates and children.

Pathophysiology

The physiologic mechanisms that normally prevent hypercalcemia are inhibition of PTH and $1,25(OH)_2D$ synthesis. Elevated serum Ca concentration in pathologic conditions with PTH or vitamin D overactivity implies inappropriately increased Ca efflux into the extracellular fluid from bone, intestine, or kidney. Hypophosphatemia can increase circulating $1,25(OH)_2D$, with attendant increased intestinal Ca absorption and bone resorption; Ca cannot be deposited in bone in the absence of P and contributes to hypercalcemia. An increase in net Ca mobilization from the skeleton is most often the cause of hypercalcemia, although excessive intake via intestinal tract or parenteral alimentation can also result in hypercalcemia.[38]

Homozygous inactivating mutations of the CaSR, known to result from inheritance of two mutant alleles associated with the *CASR* gene on chromosome 3, produce severe hypercalcemia, termed "neonatal severe primary hyperparathyroidism (NSPHT)." Heterozygous inactivating mutations of the CaSR produce a "benign" hypercalcemia, termed "familial hypocalciuric hypercalcemia (FHH)," inherited as an autosomal dominant trait with high penetrance. Mutations in the Ca^{+2}-sensor lead to a dual defect in parathyroid cells (causing parathyroid hyperplasia) and renal tubules (causing hypocalciuria). Although FHH and NSHPT have been associated with mutations in the *CASR* gene at 3q13.3–21 in nearly all affected subjects, in some families the disorder has been linked to unknown genes present on the long or short arms of chromosome 19, suggesting genetic heterogeneity.[39]

Hypercalcemia associated with subcutaneous fat necrosis occurs usually in asphyxiated, large-for-gestational-age infants; possible mechanisms are increased prostaglandin-E activity, increased release of Ca from fat and tissues, and unregulated production of $1,25(OH)_2D$ from macrophages infiltrating fat necrotic lesions.

Idiopathic infantile hypercalcemia (which may be part of Williams syndrome) is associated with mutations in the elastin gene on the long arm of chromosome 7; there may be a vitamin D hyperresponsive state and a blunted CT response to Ca loading may contribute. Infantile hypophosphatasia is a rare autosomal recessive disorder, and may be lethal *in utero* or shortly after birth because of inadequate bony support of the thorax and skull. The Bartter variant related hypercalcemia is associated with polyhydramnios and prematurity; *in utero* hypercalcemia may result in fetal hypercalciuria and polyuria, leading to early delivery; increased serum 1,25(OH)$_2$D, normal serum PTH and increased urinary prostaglandin-E$_2$ are associated with the condition.

Clinical presentation

The clinical features of hypercalcemia are dependent on the underlying disorder, age and degree of hypercalcemia. Its onset may be at birth or delayed for weeks or months. Neonates with hypercalcemia may be asymptomatic or have serious clinical signs (especially in hyperparathyroidism) requiring urgent treatment. Infants with mild increases in serum Ca (11–13 mg/dL, 2.65–3.25 mM) often fail to manifest specific signs of hypercalcemia. Mild hypercalcemia may present as feeding difficulties or poor linear growth. Lack of signs in infants with hypercalcemia is particularly problematical since unrecognized hypercalcemia can result in significant morbidity or death.[40]

With a moderate-to-severe hypercalcemia, nonspecific signs, such as anorexia, vomiting and constipation (rarely diarrhea), polyuria and dehydration may occur. Infants with chronic hypercalcemia may present with failure to thrive (poor growth) as the principal problem. Severe hypercalcemia can affect the nervous system and cause lethargy, drowsiness or irritability to confusion, and seizure; in extreme cases, stupor and coma can ensue. Thus, timely recognition and treatment of hypercalcemia in infants is critical in determining the prognosis. In severely affected infants, hypertension, respiratory distress (due to hypotonia, demineralization and deformation of the rib cage), nephrocalcinosis (from long-standing hypercalcemia) and band keratopathy of the limbus of the eye (rare) may be present. Associated features, e.g. elfin faces, cardiac murmur, and mental retardation (in Williams syndrome) and bluish-red skin indurations (in subcutaneous fat necrosis) may be present on physical examination.

Diagnosis

Diagnosis may be made incidentally on a routine screening of chemistry tests. Initial diagnostic workup may include serum total Ca, ionized Ca, P, Mg, alkaline phosphatase, pH, total protein, creatinine, electrolytes, PTH and 25OHD concentrations; urine Ca, P, tubular reabsorption of P and cyclic AMP with renal function evaluation; chest x-ray, hand x-ray, abdominal ultrasound, ophthalmologic evaluation and electrocardiogram (i.e. shortened QT interval) to determine the effect of hypercalcemia.

The diagnosis of NSPHT is based on the presence of inappropriately normal or elevated PTH levels along with relative hypocalciuria in severe hypercalcemia (high Ca levels, 20–24 mg/dL [5–6 mM/L]). The hyperparathyroidism causes erosion of bone (particularly along the sub-periosteal margins of long bone and a "moth-eaten" appearance) which radiologically may be mistaken for rickets. In contrast to NSPHT, the infant with FHH usually remains asymptomatic; PTH is usually in the normal range, but inappropriately high for hypercalcemia; urine Ca excretion is low and nephrocalcinosis is not a problem. A family history of FHH or NSPHT in a sibling provides strong confirmation of the diagnosis. Care must be taken to distinguish these disorders from the transient neonatal hyperparathyroidism associated with maternal hypocalcemia (such as in maternal pseudohypoparathyroidism or renal tubular acidosis).[41–43]

DNA analysis for FHH and NSPHT is currently only available in a few laboratories, and requires molecular analysis of the entire *CASR* gene in a proband. Relatives of the proband may be studied for genetic abnormalities and serum Ca levels.[32]

Maternal Ca and vitamin D status during pregnancy may influence parathyroid function in the developing fetus and newborn. A maternal dietary and drug history (e.g. excessive vitamin A or D, thiazides) or history of possible mineral disturbances or polyhydramnios during pregnancy should be obtained. Family screening will depend on the primary diagnosis.[38]

Additional information concerning nephrocalcinosis from hypercalcemia, or soft tissue calcification (e.g. in basal ganglia) can be obtained by appropriate ultrasound or computed tomography analysis. If hyperparathyroidism is diagnosed (rarely), localization of parathyroid adenoma or hyperplasia by radionuclide scintigraphy may be useful.[32]

Differential diagnosis

Very elevated serum Ca level (>15 mg/dL [3.75 mM/L]) usually indicates primary hyperparathyroidism, or P depletion in very low birth weight infants. To differentiate hypercalcemia associated with parathyroid disorders from nonparathyroid conditions, the following measurements may help: serum P concentration (low in hyperparathyroidism, FHH and rickets of prematurity); percent renal tubular P reabsorption (usually lower than 85% in hyperparathyroidism, high in rickets of prematurity associated with hypophosphatemia); and serum PTH concentration (elevated in hyperparathyroidism). Very low urinary Ca/urinary creatinine ratio [U_{ca}/U_{cr}] in the face of hypercalcemia suggests FHH. Very low serum alkaline phosphatase concentration suggests hypophosphatasia. Serum 25OHD determination may be useful when vitamin D excess is suspected. Bone x-ray films will identify demineralization and/or osteolytic lesions (hyperparathyroidism) or osteosclerotic lesions (occasionally with vitamin D excess) consistent with the etiology of hypercalcemia.

Treatment approaches

Therapy of neonatal hypercalcemia consists of correction of specific underlying causes and removal of iatrogenic or external causes, for example, surgical removal of hyperparathyroid glands and stopping of excessive Ca or vitamin D intake. Treatment of neonatal hyperparathyroidism depends on severity of presentation. For mild asymptomatic hypercalcemia in a thriving infant, conservative management is appropriate. For a moderate-to-severe hypercalcemic infant, prompt investigation and more aggressive therapy is instituted; stopping excessive dietary Ca and vitamin D intake and maintenance of adequate hydration are mainstays of therapy. Enhancement of renal Ca excretion by loop-acting diuretics and inhibition of intestinal absorption or bone resorption may also be used.

For short-term treatment of acute hypercalcemic episodes (symptomatic or serum Ca > 14 mg/dL [3.5 mM/L]), expansion of the extracellular fluid with 10–20 mL of 0.9% sodium chloride per kg intravenously, followed by an intravenous injection of a potent loop diuretics (1 mg of furosemide/kg every 6 to 8 hours), may be effective by increasing urinary

Ca excretion. Fluid and electrolyte imbalance should be avoided with frequent monitoring of fluid balance and serum Ca, P, Mg, sodium, potassium and osmolarity; reduced glomerular filtration rate from dehydration can paradoxically worsen the hypercalcemia. In hypercalcemic patients with low serum P concentrations, P supplements of 0.5–1.0 mM (16–31 mg) of elemental P/kg/day in divided oral doses may normalize the serum P and lower serum Ca concentration; parenteral P, however, should be avoided in severely hypercalcemic patients (serum total Ca > 12 mg/dL [3 mM/L]) unless hypophosphatemia is severe (< 1.5 mg/dL), since extra skeletal calcification theoretically may occur.[37,44]

For restriction of dietary intakes of Ca and vitamin D, a low-Ca-low-vitamin D_3-infant formula, which contains trace amount of Ca (<10 mg/100 Kcal compared with standard formula, 78 mg/100 Kcal) and no vitamin D (also low iron), is available for the short-to-medium term management of hypercalcemia in infants. (CalciloXD, Ross Laboratories, Columbus, OH); iron supplement is usually needed. As the hypercalcemia resolves, the usual infant formula or human milk (approximately 10 mg of Ca/oz) can be mixed with the CalciloXD to increase Ca intake and close monitoring of serum and urine Ca is required to prevent rickets or hypocalcemia.

Adjuvant therapies in the acute phase of hypercalcemia are CT, glucocorticoids, bisphosphonate and dialysis. Minimal information is available on the use of hormonal and other drug therapy for neonatal hypercalcemia. Symptomatic infants with non-parathyroid dependent forms of hypercalcemia may require long-term medical treatment with CT or bisphosphonates. Short-term treatment with salmon CT (at a dose of 4–8 IU/kg every 6 to 12 hours, subcutaneously or intramuscularly), prednisone (1–2 mg/kg/day), or a combination may be useful. The hypocalcemic effect of CT (a potent inhibitor of bone resorption) may be transient and abates after a few days which is not ideal for chronic therapy; its effects may be prolonged with concomitant glucocorticoids, though there is limited experience in neonates.

High-dose glucocorticoids reduces the intestinal absorption of Ca and may decrease bone resorption; methylprednisolone (1–2 mg/kg/day, intravenously), hydrocortisone (10 mg/kg/day, intravenously) or their equivalent is effective, but is not recommended for long-term use because of many undesirable side effects. Although effective in several types of hypercalcemia, glucocorticoids are relatively ineffective in the treatment of hypercalcemia associated with primary hyperparathyroidism.

Bisphosphonate, an anti-bone resorptive agent, may be useful for the treatment of PTH-mediated hypercalcemia in children, or for hypercalcemia in subcutaneous fat necrosis of the newborn, though scant information is available. Infants with NSPHT and marked hypercalcemia should be managed aggressively. In the past, treatment consisted of urgent subtotal parathyroidectomy, but more recently, management options have extended to administration of intravenous bisphosphonates (pamidronate® 0.5–2.0 mg/kg).[45] In term infants with recessive NSPHT, pamidronate® therapy was effective in reversing severe hypercalcemia and parathyroidectomy can be delayed until the infant is clinically stable.[46] To control marked hypercalcemia in an extremely premature infant with NSPHT, pamidronate® (20 mg/m^2) was administered intravenously and serum Ca level was reduced significantly, by 7–28% with each dose and bone mineralization improved.[47] Bisphosphonate therapy seems safe in the short-term and effective in controlling hypercalcemia even in the very premature infant, allowing for planned surgery when feasible.

For severe and unremitting hypercalcemia, either hemodialysis (HD) using a suitable neonatal, acute dual-lumen HD catheter (Med Comp., Harleysville, Pa., USA) if the infant is hemodynamically stable, or peritoneal dialysis (PD) with a low-Ca dialysate (1.25 mM/L), may be helpful. To avoid iatrogenic mineral depletion in patients with normal renal function, supplemental P or Mg can be given either orally or intravenously for both HD or PD, or sodium phosphate can be added to the PD solution (should not exceed 0.75 mM). In PD, crystal formation in the bags should be inspected hourly and fresh solutions changed every 8 hours.

Prognosis

The need for prolonged treatment should be reassessed regularly, since some instances of neonatal hypercalcemia may resolve spontaneously. Virtually all cases of primary hyperparathyroidism require subtotal or total parathyroidectomy, since the hypercalcemia may be life-threatening and does not respond to medical management.

References

1. Blum JW, Fisher JA, Schwoerer D *et al.* (1974) Acute parathyroid hormone response: Sensitivity, relationship to hypocalcemia and rapidity. *Endocrinology* **95**: 753.

2. Bai M, Quinn S, Trivedi S *et al.* (1996) Expression and characterization of inactivating and activating mutations in the human Ca^{2+o}-sensing receptor. *J Biol Chem* **271**: 19537–19545.

3. Brown EM. (2007) The calcium-sensing receptor: Physiology, pathophysiology and CaR-based therapeutics. *Subcell Biochem* **45**: 139–167.

4. Egbuna OI, Brown EM. (2008) Hypercalcemic and hypocalcemic conditions due to calcium-sensing receptor mutations. *Best Practice & Research Clin Rheumatol* **22**: 129–148.

5. Pearce SH, Williamson C, Kifor O *et al.* (1996) A familial syndrome of hypocalcemia with hypercalciuria due to mutation in the calcium-sensing receptor. *N Engl J Med* **335**: 1115–1122.

6. Abrams SA. (2007) *In utero* physiology: Role in nutrient delivery and fetal development for calcium, phosphorus, and vitamin D. *Am J Clin Nutr* **85**(Suppl): 604S–607S.

7. Bass JK, Chan GM. (2006) Calcium nutrition and metabolism during infancy. *Nutrition* **22**: 1057–1066.

8. Wandrup J, Kroner J, Pryds O *et al.* (1988) Age-related reference values for ionized calcium in the first week of life in premature and full-term neonates. *Scand J Clin Lab Invest* **48**: 255–260.

9. Venkataraman PS, Blick KE, Fry HD *et al.* (1985) Postnatal changes in calcium-regulating hormones in very-low-birth-weight infants. *Am J Dis Child* **139**: 913–916.

10. Venkataraman PS, Wilson DA, Sheldon RE *et al.* (1985) Effect of hypocalcemia on cardiac function in very-low-birth-weight preterm neonates: Studies of blood ionized calcium, echocardiography, and cardiac effect of intravenous calcium therapy. *Pediatrics* **70**: 543–550.

11. Altirkawi K, Rozycki H. (2008) Hypocalcemia is common in the first 48 hours of life in ELBW infants. *J Perinat Med* **36**: 348–353.

12. Fraser DR. (1980) Regulation of the metabolism of vitamin D. *Physiol Rev* **60**: 551–613.

13. Myiya S, Sullivan SM, Allgrove J *et al.* (2008) Hypocalcemia and vitamin D deficiency: An important, but preventable, cause of life-threatening infant heart failure. *Heart* **94**: 581–584.

14. Camadoo L, Tibott R, Isaza F. (2007) Maternal vitamin D deficiency associated with neonatal hypocalcemic convulsions. *Nutrition Journal* **6**: 23–24.

15. Ashraf A, Mick G, Atchison J *et al.* (2006) Prevalence of hypovitaminosis D in early infantile hypocalcemia. *J Pediatr Endocrinol Metab* **19**: 1025–1031.

16. Chan GM, Tsang RC, Chen IW *et al.* (1978) The effect of 1,25(OH)$_2$ vitamin D$_3$ supplementation in premature infants. *J Pediatr* **93**: 91–96.

17. Steichen JJ, Tsang RC, Gratton TL *et al.* (1980) Vitamin D homeostasis in the perinatal period: 1,25-dihydroxyvitamin D in maternal, cord and neonatal blood. *N Engl J Med* **302**: 315–319.

18. Markestad T, Aksnes L, Finne PH *et al.* (1984) Plasma concentrations of vitamin D metabolites in premature infants. *Pediatr Res* **18**: 269–272.

19. Namgung R, Tsang RC, Specker BL *et al.* (1993) Reduced serum osteocalcin and 1,25-dihydroxyvitamin D concentrations and low bone mineral content in small for gestational age infants: Evidence of decreased bone formation rates. *J Pediatr* **122**: 269–275.

20. Austin LA, Heath H. (1981) Calcitonin: Physiology and pathophysiology. *N Engl J Med* **304**: 269.

21. Samaan NA, Anderson GD, Adam-Mayne ME. (1975) Immunoreactive calcitonin in the mother, neonate, child and adult. *Am J Obstet Gynecol* **121**: 622–625.

22. Venkataraman PS, Tsang RC, Chen IW *et al.* (1987) Pathogenesis of early neonatal hypocalcemia: Studies of serum calcitonin, gastrin and plasma glucagon. *J Pediatr* **110**: 599–603.

23. Hillman LS, Rojanasathit S, Slatopolsky E, Haddad JG. (1977) Serial measurements of serum calcium, magnesium, parathyroid hormone, calcitonin and 25-hydroxyvitamin D in premature and term infants during the first week of life. *Pediatr Res* **11**: 739–744.

24. Poomthavorn P, Ongphiphadhanakul B, Mahachoklertwattana P. (2008) Transient neonatal hypoparathyroidism in two siblings unmasking maternal normocalcemic hyperparathyroidism. *Eur J pediatr* **167**: 431–434.

25. Soecker BL, Tsang RC, Ho ML *et al.* (1991) Low serum calcium and high parathyroid hormone levels in neonates fed "humanized' cow's milk-based formula. *Am J Dis Child* **145**: 941–945.

26. Bastepe M, Juppner H. (2003) Pseudohypoparathyroidism and mechanisms of resistance toward multiple hormones molecular evidence to clinical presentation. *J Clin Endocrinol Metab* **88**: 4055–4058.

27. Lee CT, Tsai WY, Tung YC *et al.* (2008) Transient pseudohypoparathyroidism as a cause of late-onset hypocalcemia in neonates and infants. *J Formos Med Assoc* **107**: 806–810.

28. Ding CL, Buckingham B, Levine MA. (2001) Familial isolated hypoparathyroidism caused by a mutation in the gene for the transcription factor GCMB. *J Clin Invest* **108**: 1215–1220.

29. Sunthorbthepvarakul T, Cheresigaew S, Ngowngarmratana S. (1999) A novel mutation of the signal peptide of the preproparathyroid hormone gene associated with autosomal recessive familial isolated hypoparathyroidism. *J Clin Endocrinol Metab* **84**: 3792–3796.

30. Al-Wahab S, Munyard P. (2001) Functional atriventricular block in a preterm infant. *Arch Dis Child Fetal Neonatal Ed* **85**: F220–F221.

31. Stefanaki E, Koropuli M. (2005) Atrioventricular block in preterm infants caused by hypocalcemia: A case report and review of the literature. *Eur J Obstet Gynecol* **120**: 115–116.

32. Allgrove J. (2003) Disorders of calcium metabolism. *Current Pediatrics* **13**: 529–535.

33. Loughead JL, Mimouni F, Tsang RC *et al.* (1991) A role for Mg in neonatal parathyroid gland function. *J Am Coll Nutr* **10**: 123.

34. Angelopoulos NG, Goula A, Tolos G. (2007) Sporadic hypoparathyroidism treated with Teriparatide: A case report and literature review. *Exp Clin Endocrinol Diabetes* **115**: 50–54.

35. Puig-Domingo M, Diaz G, Nicolau J *et al.* (2008) Successful treatment of vitamin D unresponsive hypoparathyroidism with multipulse subcutaneous infusion of teriparatide. *Eur J Endocrinol* **159**: 653–657.

36. Newfiled RS. (2007) Recombinant PTH for initial management of neonatal hypocalcemia. *New Engl J Med* **356**: 1687.

37. Trindade CEP. (2005) Minerals in the nutrition of extremely low birth weight infants. *J Pediatr* (Rio J) **81**(Suppl. 1): S43–S51.

38. Hsu SC, Levine MA. (2004) Perinatal calcium metabolism: physiology and pathophysiology. *Semin Neonatol* **9**: 23–36.

39. Lloyd SE, Pannett AA, Dixon PH *et al.* (1999) Localization of familial benign hypercalcemia, Oklahoma varianr (FBHOk), to chromosome 19q13. *Am J Hum Genet* **64**: 189–195.

40. Ghirri P, Bottone U, Coccoli L *et al.* (1999) Symptomatic hypercalcemia in the first months of life: Calcium-regulating hormones and treatment. *J Endocrinol Invest* **22**: 349–353.

41. Savani RC, Mimouni F, Tsang RC. (1993) Maternal and neonatal hyperparathyroidism as a consequence of maternal renal tubular acidosis. *Pediatrics* **91**: 661–663.

42. Glass EJ, Barr DG. (1981) Transient neonatal hyperparathyroidism secondary to maternal pseudohypoparathyroidism. *Arch Dis Child* **56**: 565–568.

43. Rodriquez-Soriano J, Garcia-Fuentes M, Vallo A *et al.* (2000) Hypercalcemia in neonatal distal renal tubular acidosis. *Pediatr Nephrol* **14**: 354–355.

44. Singer FR. (1996) Medical management of nonparathyroid hypercalcemia and hypocalcemia. *Otolaryngol Clin North Am* **29**: 701–710.

45. Allgrove J. (2002) Use of bisphosphonates in children and adolescents. *J Pediatr Endocrinol Metab* **15**(Suppl. 3): 921–928.

46. Waller S, Kurzawinski T, Spitz L *et al.* (2004) Neonatal severe hyperparathyroidism: Genotype/phenotype correlation and the use of pamidronate as rescue therapy. *Eur J Pediatr* **163**: 589–594.

47. Fox L, Sadowsky J, Pringle KP *et al.* (2007) Neonatal hyperparathyroidism and pamidronate therapy in an extremely premature infant. *Pediatrics* **120**: e1350–e1354.

Chapter

15

Neonatal Jaundice

Thor Willy Ruud Hansen

Introduction

Jaundice is one of the most common problems which caregivers have to deal with in the neonatal period. Recognition of jaundice in the neonate goes back centuries. Eighteenth and nineteenth century medical texts and textbooks contain many suggestions for management, although few of these are likely to have been helpful and some may even have been harmful.

Kernicterus is a devastating complication of jaundice in the newborn infant and it is the reason why we make a point of clinically assessing infants for jaundice, measuring levels of bilirubin in blood or tissues and applying treatment when such levels become high. The clinical syndrome of chronic kernicterus consists of choreoathetosis, gaze paresis, sensorineural deafness, and occasional developmental delay. In infants with severe jaundice, acute bilirubin effects on the brain may manifest as mild, intermediate, and advanced bilirubin encephalopathy.[1] While mild acute bilirubin encephalopathy is generally reversible with treatment, the intermediate to advanced acute stages have largely been thought to be irreversible,[2] though recent data suggest that reversibility may be possible in some infants with aggressive and urgent treatment.[3,4]

Kernicterus appeared to have become rare following the introduction of effective treatment, but in the past two decades, a number of cases have been reported. The US-based Kernicterus Registry[5] has recorded more than 100 cases. Lack of attention to neonatal jaundice combined with early discharge from birthing units have been blamed for this apparent resurgence. Although not everyone agrees that there has indeed been an increase in the number of cases, there should be no disagreement that kernicterus should be preventable with proper attention to risk factors, parental education, and rapid institution of effective treatment. The purpose of this chapter is to provide the reader with an updated understanding of neonatal jaundice and its pathophysiology and management.

Diagnostic Process and Considerations

Presentation of neonatal jaundice

The diagnostic process typically begins with a recognition by the mother or care-givers that the infant's skin has a yellow hue, though detection by targeted screening is becoming more common and has been recommended in guidelines.[1,6] Jaundice in the neonate first becomes visible in the face and forehead. Pressure on the skin helps to reveal the underlying color. A total serum bilirubin level of 80–100 μmol/L (4.5–5.5 mg/dL) appears to be the minimum level at which dermal jaundice is perceived by the unaided eye. However, visual inspection is not reliable for assessing the degree of jaundice.

With time, jaundice moves further down the body.[7] This may be clinically useful because visible jaundice in the hands or feet suggests a significantly elevated bilirubin level which one should consider checking by appropriate tests. In most infants, yellow color is the only finding on physical examination, although infants who have pronounced jaundice may be drowsy.

So-called "physiologic jaundice" typically presents on the second or third day of life. When presentation occurs during the first 24 hours of life or later than day 3–4 of life, it is likely that factors in addition to those involved in normal physiology may contribute. Such infants merit closer evaluation. In the guidelines for management of neonatal jaundice, the American Academy of Pediatrics recommends that bilirubin levels be measured in all infants presenting with jaundice in the first 24 hours of life, either by transcutaneous measurement or by a blood test for total serum bilirubin.[1]

Assessing the jaundiced infant

When called upon to assess a newborn infant for jaundice, the physician should consider

(i) whether it is necessary to measure the bilirubin level;
(ii) whether treatment is indicated;
(iii) whether elements are present in the history or physical examination which suggest that non-physiological factors may contribute to jaundice (Table 1); and
(iv) if discharge is planned, what the infant's risk status is, and what the plans for follow-up should be.[1,6]

If an infant appears jaundiced by visual inspection, you should perform an objective measurement of the bilirubin level. Bilirubin can be measured non-invasively in the skin and this technique is commonly used as a screening instrument to decide whether there is a need to measure total serum bilirubin (TSB).[8] Traditionally bilirubin has been measured in blood or serum and all therapeutic guidelines refer to TSB values.

As there is a dynamic evolution of TSB levels in the neonatal period, indications for treatment not only refer to TSB, but relate the values to the infant's postnatal age. In addition, most therapeutic guidelines make allowances for immaturity/prematurity and disease states which may be present concurrently. Further details regarding treatment are discussed in the section on management of the jaundiced infant.

When an infant is about to be discharged, the AAP recommends a risk assessment as far as development of jaundice.[1] This may consist of a measurement of TcB or TSB, with plotting of the TcB/TSB value on a nomogram for hour-specific values. The nomogram recommended by the AAP is shown in Fig. 1.[9] An infant whose hour-specific bilirubin value is in the low-risk zone of the nomogram is at low-risk of developing severe jaundice after discharge.[9]

Additional risk assessment may include the factors listed in Table 2.[1] As will be noted, many of those risk factors are the same as those

Table 1.   Physical findings and elements in the case history which suggest a non-physiological contribution to neonatal jaundice and/or the need for increased vigilance.

Physical findings:

Pallor
Hepatosplenomegaly
Petecchiae
Large for gestation
Fracture(s) or bruising
Symptoms or signs of hypothyroidism
Symptoms or signs of metabolic disease (e.g. galactosemia)

History:

Maternal blood group O and/or Rhesus negative
Mother has isoimmune antibodies
DAT positive infant

Family history:

Older sibling with jaundice in the neonatal period, particularly
   if the jaundice required treatment
      Other family members with jaundice or known family history
         of Gilbert syndrome
Anemia, splenectomy, or bile stones in family members
      Known heredity for hemolytic disorders
      Liver disease

Pregnancy and delivery:

Maternal illness suggestive of viral or other infection
Maternal drug intake
Delayed cord clamping

Postnatal history:

Loss of stool color
Breast feeding
Greater than average weight loss
Prolonged total parental nutrition

associated with non-physiologic jaundice (Table 1). Absence of risk factors indicates a low risk of developing severe jaundice after discharge. Planning for discharge will be discussed in the section on management.

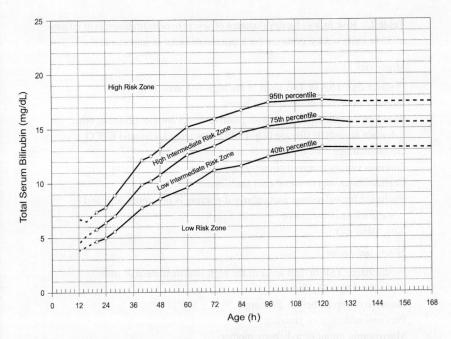

Figure 1. Risk designation of term and near-term well newborns based on their hour-specific serum bilirubin values. The high-risk zone is designated by the 95th percentile track. The intermediate-risk zone is subdivided to upper- and lower-risk zones by the 75th percentile track. The low-risk zone has been electively and statistically defined by the 40th percentile track. (Dotted extensions are based on <300 TSB values/epoch). Reprinted from Ref. 9 with permission.

Laboratory studies

The following studies may be indicated in jaundiced neonates:

Bilirubin measurement

Transcutaneous bilirubinometry using handheld devices performs better than visual assessment. In the presence of apparently mild jaundice, this may be sufficient to assure that total bilirubin levels are safely below intervention levels. In infants with moderate jaundice, transcutaneous measurement may be used to select patients who require phlebotomy or capillary blood sampling for serum bilirubin measurement. In the

Table 2. Risk factors for development of severe hyperbilirubinemia in infants of 35 or more weeks' gestation (in approximate order of importance)*.

Major risk factors:

Predischarge TSB or TcB level in the high-risk zone (Fig. 1)

Jaundice observed in the first 24 hours

Blood group incompatibility with positive direct antiglobulin test, other known hemolytic disease (e.g. G6PD deficiency), elevated ETCO$_c$

Gestational age 35–36 week

Previous sibling received phototherapy

Cephalohematoma or significant bruising

Exclusive breastfeeding, particularly if nursing is not going well and weight loss is excessive

East Asian race[†]

Minor risk factors:

Predischarge TSB or TcB level in the high intermediate-risk zone

Gestational age 37–38 week

Jaundice observed before discharge

Previous sibling with jaundice

Macrosomic infant of a diabetic mother

Maternal age 25 years

Male gender

Decreased risk (these factors are associated with decreased risk of significant jaundice, listed in order of decreasing importance):

TSB or TcB level in the low-risk zone (Fig. 1)

Gestational age 41 week

Exclusive bottle feeding

Black race

Discharge from hospital after 72 hours

---

* Reprinted from Ref. 1 with permission.

[†] Race as defined by mother's description.

presence of extreme jaundice, transcutaneous measurement may be used to fast-track infants to rapid and aggressive therapy. Please note that such devices cannot be used to monitor the progress of phototherapy.

In most jaundiced infants, a total serum bilirubin level (TSB) is the only necessary test. This is assuming that jaundice is only moderate, presents on the second or third day of life, and in the absence of a history and/or physical findings suggestive of a pathologic process. The possible cause of jaundice must be sought in any infant with TSB levels needing treatment and/or rising rapidly towards such levels. Measurement of bilirubin fractions (conjugated vs unconjugated) in serum is not required in most infants. However, in the presence of an enlarged liver or spleen, petechiae, thrombocytopenia, or other findings suggesting liver or biliary disease, metabolic disease, or congenital infection, bilirubin fractions should be measured. In infants who remain jaundiced beyond the first 1–2 weeks of life and infants whose total serum bilirubin levels repeatedly rebound following treatment, measurement of the conjugated bilirubin fraction is indicated. Situations in which additional studies may be indicated are listed in Table 3.

Suggested additional studies

- Complete blood count
- Blood type and Rh determination in mother and infant
  Should be done in any infant needing treatment.
- Direct antibody test (DAT/Coombs) in the infant
  Should be done in any infant needing treatment.
- Peripheral blood film for erythrocyte morphology
- Reticulocyte count
- G-6-PD test
  Recommended for any infant receiving treatment and whose family history/ethnic origin suggest G6PD.

Table 3. Situations in which laboratory studies in addition to TSB may be indicated.

- Jaundice presents on the first or after the third day of life
- Infant appears anemic at birth
- Infant appears ill
- TSB is above intervention levels
- Significant jaundice persists beyond the second week of life
- Family/maternal/pregnancy/case histories suggest a pathologic process
- Physical examination reveals findings not explained by simple physiologic hyperbilirubinemia

- Serum albumin levels
  Recommended when TSB levels approach or exceed exchange levels
  (albumin binds bilirubin in a ratio of 1:1 at the primary high-affinity
  binding site).
- Check results of metabolic screen
  In particular, thyroid and galactosemia screen.
- Conjugated bilirubin levels
  Direct bilirubin measurements are often inaccurate and are generally
  not a sensitive tool for diagnosing cholestasis.
- Liver function tests
  Aspartate aminotransferase (ASAT or SGOT) and alanine amino-
  transferase (ALAT or SGPT) levels are elevated in hepatocellular
  disease. Alkaline phosphatase and γ-glutamyltransferase (GGT) levels
  are often elevated in cholestatic disease.
- Tests for viral and/or parasitic infection may be indicated in infants
  with hepatosplenomegaly, petechiae, thrombocytopenia, or other
  evidence of hepatocellular disease.
- Measurement of end-tidal carbon monoxide in breath
  End-tidal carbon monoxide in exhaled breath (ET_{CO}) may be used as
  an index of bilirubin production. A commercial apparatus is available.
- Blood-gas measurements
  The risk of bilirubin CNS toxicity is increased in acidosis, particularly
  respiratory acidosis.
- Imaging Studies
  Ultrasonography of the liver and bile ducts is indicated in infants with
  laboratory and/or clinical signs of cholestatic disease.

  A radionuclide liver scan for uptake of hepatoiminodiacetic acid
  (HIDA) may assist in the diagnosis of extrahepatic biliary atresia. We
  pre-treat patients with phenobarbital 5 mg/kg/d for 3–4 days before
  performing the scan.

Assessment of infants readmitted for prolonged jaundice

When jaundice continues beyond the first two weeks of life, obtaining the
lactation/nutrition history is a first priority. Evaluate the infant's weight
curve. Delay to regain birth weight may be associated with prolongation

of jaundice through increased enterohepatic circulation. Elicit the mother's impressions as far as adequacy of breast feeding. Does the baby appear satisfied after the breast meal? Does the baby appear hungry again within 1–2 hours after the meal, or does the baby appear too weak or too sleepy to complete the meal?

Explore the family history. Prolonged and/or pronounced jaundiced in older siblings may be significant, as may a history suggesting Gilbert syndrome. Check the results of the newborn metabolic screen for galactosemia and congenital hypothyroidism. A grey/whitish stool may suggest intra- or extrahepatic biliary atresia. Your threshold should be low for ordering supplementary studies as outlined previously in this section.

The most common cause of prolonged jaundice in newborn infants is probably so-called breast-milk associated jaundice. This is largely an innocent condition, but note that kernicterus has been described in infants in whom no other cause for severe jaundice was found. In the absence of specific diagnostic tests, the diagnosis of breast-milk associated jaundice can only be presumptive and more serious conditions need to be ruled out. Follow-up must be close with careful instruction of the parents.

Pathophysiology

Jaundice is caused by the accumulation of bilirubin, a breakdown product of heme catabolism. Heme catabolism releases the iron bound to heme for renewed use by the body and carbon monoxide for release through the respiration. Measurement of CO in exhaled air has been used to estimate bilirubin production, as one molecule of CO is produced for every molecule of bilirubin (Fig. 2). The heme from which bilirubin is produced stems largely from hemoglobin, but some is also derived from other compounds such as myoglobin, cytochromes, and catalase.

Neonatal physiologic jaundice results from simultaneous occurrence of the following two phenomena:

- *Bilirubin production is elevated* due to breakdown of fetal erythrocytes. This results from a shorter lifespan of fetal erythrocytes and a higher erythrocyte mass in neonates.
- *Hepatic excretory capacity is low* because of (i) low concentrations of the binding protein ligandin in the hepatocytes and (ii) low activity

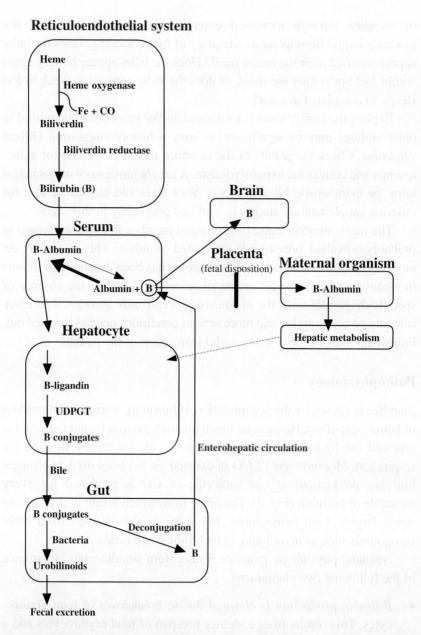

Figure 2. Schematic representation of the pathways of bilirubin metabolism and disposition. Modified from Ref. 10 with permission.

of glucuronyl transferase, the enzyme which binds bilirubin to glucuronic acid and makes it water-soluble (conjugation).

Bilirubin production

Catabolism of heme to bilirubin occurs in the reticuloendothelial system. Heme oxygenase catalyzes the production of biliverdin, releasing CO and iron. Biliverdin has a blue-green color and is water soluble. Biliverdin reductase then catalyzes the formation of bilirubin, a compound with strong yellow-to-orange color. The predominant form of bilirubin in humans is IXα, which, in the absence of light exposure, occurs almost exclusively as the 4Z,15Z isomer. The denotation "Z" refers to the intramolecular hydrogen bonds between the side chains. Bilirubin IXα (Z,Z) has very limited solubility in water and in many ways behaves like a lipid-soluble molecule. It is this solubility characteristic which permits transfer of bilirubin across tissue membranes, explaining its ability to enter the brain.

Bilirubin transport and binding

Bilirubin is transported in serum almost completely bound to albumin. There appears to be two bilirubin binding sites on albumin, with high and lower affinity respectively. Nanomolar concentrations of unbound ("free") bilirubin are present in serum during neonatal jaundice and this unbound fraction can transfer across membranes and equilibrate with bilirubin in tissues. Any substance (endogenous or exogenous) which competes for the same binding site on albumin may cause displacement of bilirubin into tissues, including the brain. Therefore all drugs used in neonatal medicine must be tested for their ability to displace bilirubin. Binding of bilirubin to albumin increases with postnatal age, but is reduced in sick infants. Bilirubin can also bind to erythrocytes and to other proteins such as α-fetoprotein and lipoprotein.

Processing of bilirubin in the liver

In the liver, bilirubin is transported into hepatocytes, where it binds to ligandin. Hepatocyte uptake of bilirubin increases with ligandin concentrations which are low at birth, but increase to reach adult values at 1–2 weeks of life. Ligandin concentrations may be increased by pharmacologic agents such as phenobarbital.

Bilirubin is bound to glucuronic acid (conjugated) in a reaction catalyzed by uridine diphospho-glucuronyltransferase (UDPGT). Bilirubin conjugation is critical because it makes bilirubin water-soluble, permitting transfer of conjugated bilirubin into bile. UDPGT activity is low at birth, but increases to adult values by 1–2 months. As for ligandin, certain drugs (phenobarbital, dexamethasone, clofibrate) increase UDPGT activity.

Intestinal handling of bilirubin

In the intestines, bilirubin is reduced to colorless tetrapyrroles by microbes in the colon. Some deconjugation may occur in the proximal small intestine, through β-glucuronidases located in the brush border. Unconjugated bilirubin can be reabsorbed into the circulation, increasing the total plasma bilirubin pool. This cycle of uptake, conjugation, excretion, deconjugation and reabsorption is called *enterohepatic circulation*. Enterohepatic circulation may be significant in the newborn infant, in part due to limited nutrient intake in the first days of life, which delays intestinal transit.

When establishment of breast feeding is difficult, significant postnatal weight loss may occur, accompanied by risk of jaundice through increased enterohepatic circulation. This *breast feeding jaundice* is probably different from *breast milk jaundice*.

Factors which may be present in the breast milk of some mothers may also increase the enterohepatic circulation of bilirubin (*breast milk jaundice*). β-glucuronidase may uncouple bilirubin from its binding to glucuronic acid. The risk of breast milk jaundice appears to be increased in infants who have genetic polymorphisms in the coding sequences of the UDPGT1A1 or OATP2 genes.[11] The mechanism that causes this phenomenon is still uncertain. However, it appears that supplementation with breast milk substitutes may reduce the degree of breast milk jaundice (see further in the section on management).[12]

Non-physiologic jaundice

Blood group incompatibilities (e.g. Rh, ABO) may increase bilirubin production. Rh isoimmunization has been an important cause of severe jaundice, but is now less common in industrialized countries because of immune prophylaxis in Rh-negative women. ABO incompatibility is now the most common cause of blood group incompatibility mediated neonatal jaundice in these countries. However, in developing countries, Rh isoimmunization is still common and an important cause of kernicterus.

Nonimmune hemolytic disorders (spherocytosis, G-6-PD deficiency) may also cause increased jaundice. Interaction between such conditions and genetic variants in bilirubin conjugation (e.g. Gilbert sydrome), as well as genetic variants of other proteins and enzymes involved in bilirubin metabolism, may be important in individual cases. Thus, infants who have Gilbert syndrome or who are compound heterozygotes for the Gilbert promoter and structural mutations of the UDPGT1A1 coding region appear to be at increased risk of significant hyperbilirubinemia.[13]

The increased risk of jaundice in infants with hypertrophic pyloric stenosis may also be due to a Gilbert-type variant. Genetic polymorphism for OATP-2 increases the risk of developing significant neonatal jaundice threefold. When OATP-2 polymorphism is combined with a variant UDPGT1A1 gene, the risk is augmented 22-fold.[11] Ligandin polymorphism may also cause higher TSB levels.

Extravasation of blood, such as in bruising or fractures, is accompanied by increased red cell lysis and higher bilirubin production. For a list of other possible causes of non-physiologic jaundice, see Table 1.

Management of the Jaundiced Neonate

Decisions on the management of jaundice in neonates involve assessment of individual as well as cohort risk, questions of discharge and follow-up, need for therapy and choice among therapeutic options. Examples of individual risk factors are significant bruising or family history of Gilbert syndrome. Examples of cohort risk are gestational age <37 weeks or exclusive breast feeding.

We treat neonatal jaundice to prevent kernicterus. A secondary target is to avoid exchange transfusion, a procedure associated with risk. Unfortunately, there is no evidence from sufficiently powered randomized controlled trials to guide decisions for management of neonatal jaundice. Kernicterus is a rare event, so that any trial with kernicterus as an end point would have to enroll a very large number of patients. However, as kernicterus should also be an avoidable event, any trial with that event as an outcome measure is ethically unthinkable.

Most guidelines for management of neonatal jaundice are based on small case series from the 1950s.[14,15] These data showed that the risk of kernicterus was limited when TSB was less than 20 mg/dL (342 μmol/L), and increased dramatically when TSB was greater than 30 mg/dL (513 μmol/L). Based on these data, the intervention limit for exchange transfusion was for many years 20 mg/dL, although in recent guidelines, this limit has been raised. Case reports show that some otherwise healthy infants may tolerate TSB levels of up to 40 mg/dL (684 μmol/L) without suffering harm. However, other infants may apparently develop kernicterus at maximum TSB levels <20 mg/dL (342 μmol/L). These data must be interpreted with caution because a clear distinction was not always made between a pale yellow brain (present in all individuals with significant hyperbilirubinemia) and the deeper staining of the basal ganglia accompanied by cell destruction, as would be required for a pathoanatomical diagnosis of kernicterus.

Vulnerability to the neurotoxic effects of bilirubin varies between individuals and this must be taken into account when managing jaundiced infants. In addition, the risk of developing severe jaundice is also variable. Thus, an infant who has both a low risk of developing significant jaundice and low vulnerability to bilirubin neurotoxicity is probably at very low risk of kernicterus. On the opposite side of the spectrum, an infant at high risk of severe jaundice and with high vulnerability to bilirubin neurotoxicity must be assumed to be at high risk for kernicterus. Management of neonatal jaundice should therefore ideally consist of an individualized assessment with regard to risk status. Risk factors for development of severe jaundice are listed in Tables 1 and 2.

Assessment of vulnerability to bilirubin neurotoxicity relies, in part, on data from clinical experience and in part from experimental studies. In addition, there may be risk factors that we are currently not aware of, the

Table 4.   Factors/conditions which may increase the risk of bilirubin neurotoxicity.

Prematurity
Hemolytic disorders
Sick infant:

  Sepsis
  Acidosis
  Respiratory failure

Reduced bilirubin binding to albumin:

  Immature albumin (as in prematurity)
  Binding competitors (drugs, i.v. lipids, free fatty acids)

Increased permeability of the blood-brain barrier:

  Hyperosmolality
  Hypercapnia
  Increased brain blood flow

recognition of which must await further research. All conditions which increase bilirubin entry into the brain must reasonably be assumed to increase the risk of neurotoxicity. A list of risk factors which may be associated with increased neurotoxicity is found in Table 4.

The AAP guidelines[1] recommend that all infants be examined for jaundice by qualified health personnel in the first few days of life. The timing of follow-up should be adjusted to the age at discharge and was suggested as follows:

Infant Discharged	Should Be Seen by Age
Before age 24 h	72 h
Between 24 and 47.9 h	96 h
Between 48 and 72 h	120 h

For some newborns discharged before 48 hours, two follow-up visits may be required, the first visit between 24 and 72 hours and the second between 72 and 120 hours. Clinical judgment should be used in determining followup. Earlier or more frequent follow-up should be provided for those who have risk factors for hyperbilirubinemia (Table 2), whereas those discharged with few or no risk factors can be seen after longer intervals.

Treating the jaundiced infant

Phototherapy, intravenous immune globulin and exchange transfusion are the most widely used therapeutic modalities in infants with neonatal jaundice. In some clinical circumstances, adjunct therapies may be considered.

In all infants who have risk factors for neurotoxicity (Table 4), treatment for these conditions should be applied along with the treatment directed towards hyperbilirubinemia. When increased risk for neurotoxicity is present, it is commonly recommended that treatment of hyperbilirubinemia be started at lower TSB levels than those which would apply to a healthy infant. A reduction of intervention levels by 3–6 mg/dL (50–100 μmol/L) is often suggested, although the evidence base for these numbers is virtually non-existent.

Prior to initiating treatment, the infant should be examined and assessed as discussed previously. If weight loss is greater than average, the infant should be offered the breast frequently, or a breast milk substitute if the supply of mother's milk appears inadequate. To reduce enterohepatic circulation of bilirubin, enteral nutrition should be prioritized. Oral supplementation with water or dextrose water is not recommended. There is also no evidence that parenteral hydration is helpful in the management of neonatal jaundice and it should only be used if it is indicated for other reasons than jaundice, of if enteral nutrition is contraindicated or impossible due to bowel or other abdominal disease.

Phototherapy

Phototherapy is the most frequently used treatment in neonates with unconjugated hyperbilirubinemia. Equipment for delivering phototherapy should be available in all units where babies are delivered or otherwise cared for. Maintenance and use of phototherapy equipment merits the same care and attention given to other technical equipment and their use. Unfortunately, there is evidence to suggest that this is not always the case, resulting in less effective and, therefore, more prolonged treatment.

Phototherapy works because three reactions occur when bilirubin is exposed to light[16]:

- *Photo-oxidation* was initially believed to be principal chemical reaction in phototherapy. Although bilirubin is bleached by light, this process is slow and probably contributes very little to the therapeutic effect of phototherapy. However, some photo-oxidation products can be found in urine during phototherapy.
- *Configurational isomerization* occurs very rapidly and changes some of the predominant 4Z,15Z bilirubin isomers to water-soluble isomers in which one or both of the intramolecular bonds are opened (*E,Z*; *Z,E*; or *E,E*). The side chains which are bound together in the Z configuration are now freed to attach to water molecules. In human infants receiving phototherapy, the 4Z,15E isomer is dominant and may constitute 20% or more of circulating bilirubin after a few hours of phototherapy. This proportion is not significantly influenced by the intensity of light.
- *Structural isomerization* happens when there is intramolecular cyclization, resulting in the formation of *lumirubin*. This process increases with the intensity of light. During phototherapy, lumirubin may constitute 2–6% of the total serum bilirubin concentration.

The photoisomers of bilirubin are excreted in bile and to some extent, in urine. The half-life of lumirubin in serum is much shorter than that of *E* isomers and lumirubin is the principal isomer recovered from bile during phototherapy. Thus, although the *E* isomers predominate in serum, the therapeutic effect of phototherapy as far as lowering the serum bilirubin level may owe more to lumirubin.

Phototherapy can be administered in several ways. To highlight the benefits and limitations of the different approaches, some basic principles regarding wavelength and types of light will be discussed, along with comments and suggestions regarding each system.

(i) *Wavelength*: Bilirubin absorbs light primarily around 450–460 nm. The ability of light to penetrate skin is also important, and longer wavelengths penetrate better. Lamps with output focused in the blue region of the spectrum (460–490 nm) appear to be most effective. In practice, white, blue and turqoise/green lights are used.

(ii)   A *dose-response relationship* appears to exist between the amount of irradiation and reduction in serum bilirubin up to an irradiance level of 30–40 μW/cm^2/nm.[17] Older phototherapy units often deliver much less energy, some near the minimally effective level (approximately 6 μW/cm^2/nm). Newer phototherapy units, when properly configured, may deliver irradiance above the 40 μW/cm^2/nm believed to be the saturation level.

(iii) *Distance between infant and light source* is an important determinant of the irradiance delivered to the infant's skin, as irradiance decreases with increasing distance. This distance should not be greater than 50 cm (20 in) and can be less (down to 10 cm), as long as the infant's temperature is monitored.

(iv)   *The amount of bilirubin that is irradiated* also contributes to the efficiency of phototherapy. Irradiating a large area of jaundiced skin increases the number of bilirubin molecules exposed to light. By the same mechanism, the effect of phototherapy increases with serum (and consequently skin) bilirubin concentration.

(v)   *The nature and character of the light source* may affect energy delivery. With quartz halide spotlights, irradiation levels are maximal at the center of the circle of light and decrease sharply towards the perimeter of the circle. Large infants and infants who can move away from the center of the circle may receive less efficient phototherapy.

(vi)   *Spectral power* is a key concept in phototherapy and keeping this concept in mind will help you to maximize the effect of phototherapy. Spectral power is irradiance times the size of the irradiated area. In other words, high irradiance and large exposed skin surface will increase the spectral power. This is why fiberoptic pads, although they deliver high irradiance, deliver low spectral power due to the limited area. Thus, although fiberoptic pads may be fine for routine phototherapy, they may be insufficient as the sole source of light in extreme jaundice. However, in the latter circumstance, the 2004 AAP guidelines suggest that a fiberoptic pad may be used as an adjunct light source from below, while exposing the infant to fluorescent or LED lights from above and sides.[1]

(vii) *Types of light source*: Blue fluorescent tubes are widely used for phototherapy. Narrow-spectrum blue lamps (*special blue*) appear to work best, while ordinary blue fluorescent lamps are probably equivalent to standard white daylight lamps. Narrow spectrum blue LED lamps are a recent addition and provide very high irradiance.

White (daylight) fluorescent tubes are less efficient than special blue lamps. However, reducing the distance between infant and lamps will improve efficiency. Use of reflecting materials may also help. Thus, in low income countries where the cost of special blue lamps may be prohibitive, efficient phototherapy can be accomplished with white lamps.[18]

White quartz lamps have a significant blue component in their light spectrum. The energy field is strongly focused towards the center, with significantly less energy delivered at the perimeter. Because the lamps are fixed to the overhead heater unit, energy delivery cannot be increased by moving lights closer to the infants.

Fiberoptic light is also used for phototherapy. These units deliver high energy levels, but to a limited surface area. Efficiency in infants of average size may be comparable to that of conventional low-output overhead phototherapy units, but not to that of overhead units used with maximal output. For small/preterm infants with a small body surface, the proportion of their total body surface irradiated by a fiberoptic pad will be much larger than for an infant of average size. Consequently, fiberoptic phototherapy is likely to work better for small/preterm infants.

"Double" and "triple" phototherapy, i.e. the concurrent use of two or three phototherapy units, is sometimes used to treat infants with very high TSB levels. The studies that showed benefits with this approach were performed with low-yield phototherapy units. Newer phototherapy units provide much higher levels of irradiance. Whether double or triple phototherapy also confers a benefit with high energy units has not been adequately tested.

(viii) *Indications for phototherapy* are often presented in tabular form or as graphs, which relate intervention levels to the infant's postnatal age. The graph recommended by the AAP[1] is shown in Fig. 3.

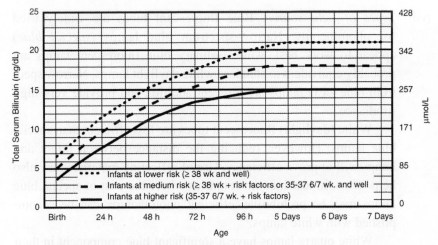

* Use total bilirubin. Do not subtract direct reacting or conjugated bilirubin.
* Risk factors = isoimmune hemolytic disease, G6PD deficiency, asphyxia, significant lethargy, temperature instability, sepsis, acidosis, or albumin < 3.0g/dL (if measured)
* For well infants 35-37 6/7 wk can adjust TSB levels for intervention around the medium risk line. It is an option to intervene at lower TSB levels for infants closer to 35 wks and at higher TSB levels for those closer to 37 6/7 wk.
* It is an option to provide conventional phototherapy in hospital or at home at TSB levels 2-3 mg/dL (35-50mmol/L) below those shown but home phototherapy should not be used in any infant with risk factors.

Figure 3. Guidelines for phototherapy in hospitalized infants of 35 or more weeks' gestation.

Note: These guidelines are based on limited evidence and the levels shown are approximations. The guidelines refer to the use of intensive phototherapy which should be used when the TSB exceeds the line indicated for each category. Infants are designated as "higher risk" because of the potential negative effects of the conditions listed on albumin binding of bilirubin, the blood-brain barrier, and the susceptibility of the brain cells to damage by bilirubin. "Intensive phototherapy" implies irradiance in the blue-green spectrum (wavelengths of approximately 430–490 nm) of at least 30 W/cm^2 per nm (measured at the infant's skin directly below the center of the phototherapy unit) and delivered to as much of the infant's surface area as possible. Note that irradiance measured below the center of the light source is much greater than that measured at the periphery. Measurements should be made with a radiometer specified by the manufacturer of the phototherapy system. If total serum bilirubin levels approach or exceed the exchange transfusion line (Fig. 4), the sides of the bassinet, incubator, or warmer should be lined with aluminum foil or white material. This will increase the surface area of the infant exposed and increase the efficacy of phototherapy. If the total serum bilirubin does not decrease or continues to rise in an infant who is receiving intensive phototherapy, this strongly suggests the presence of hemolysis. Infants who receive phototherapy and have an elevated direct-reacting or conjugated bilirubin level (cholestatic jaundice) may develop the bronze-baby syndrome.

Reprinted from Ref. 1 with permission.

The AAP graph uses TSB values as basis for intervention recommendations. Some practitioners add a test for serum albumin at higher TSB levels because bilirubin entry into the brain increases when the bilirubin-albumin ratio exceeds unity. Tests for bilirubin-albumin binding or unbound bilirubin levels are used by some, but have thus far not gained widespread acceptance.

Recommendations for the use of phototherapy vary widely. Practitioners in North America are advised to follow the 2004 AAP guidelines,[1] with attention to the 2009 update.[6] The AAP guidelines are well researched and are presented with appropriate detail. They can undoubtedly be used as a starting point for creation of national and/or local guidelines. Clinicians in different ethnic or geographic regions should apply guidelines as pertinent to their own populations and must consider factors that are unique to their medical practice settings. Such factors may include racial characteristics, prevalence of congenital hemolytic disorders, as well as the implications of how health care is organized for management of neonatal jaundice.

(ix) *Practical points in administration of phototherapy*: The infant should be naked and the eyes should be covered to reduce risk of retinal damage. Diapers should be used only if necessary and cut to minimum workable size. The distance between the infant's skin and the light source should be no greater than 50 cm (20 in) when using fluorescent lamps. This distance may be reduced down to 10–20 cm if temperature homeostasis is monitored to reduce the risk of overheating. Note that quartz lamps must *not* be brought close to the infant due to the risk of burns.

Cover the inside of the bassinet with reflecting material; white linen works well, but tin foil may also be used.[1,19] With the addition of a white curtain around the phototherapy unit and bassinet, energy delivery can be multiplied several fold. The AAP defines intensive phototherapy 30 μW/cm^2/nm or higher in the 430–490 nm band delivered to as much of the infant's surface area as possible,[1] and the use of reflecting surfaces can help to achieve that goal.

If temperature homeostasis is maintained, fluid loss is not significantly increased by phototherapy. Routine fluid supplementation is not necessary. The infant should be monitored for weight loss, urine output, and urine specific gravity; fluid intake should be adjusted accordingly. In infants who are orally fed, the preferred fluid is milk because it serves as a vehicle to transport bilirubin out of the gut.

Timing of TSB testing after start of therapy must be individualized. In infants admitted with extreme serum bilirubin values (>500 μmol/L or 30 mg/dL), a follow-up TSB should probably be obtained after no more than 1–2 hours of therapy. In infants with more moderate elevations of serum bilirubin, monitoring every 6–12 hours is probably adequate.

Expectations regarding efficacy of phototherapy depend on the circumstances. In the first 1–3 days of life, TSB will still be rising and a significant reduction of the rate of increase may be a satisfactory result. When TSB is close to its expected peak, phototherapy should result in a measurable reduction of TSB levels within a few hours. In general, the higher the starting TSB, the more dramatic the initial rate of decline. A TSB reduction of 30–40% during the first 24 hours may be expected with intensive phototherapy.[20]

In most circumstances, brief interruptions of phototherapy for feeding and nursing procedures can be permitted. In infants being treated for extreme jaundice (approaching or above exchange transfusion limits), interruption of phototherapy should not be permitted until TSB has been reduced adequately, neurological symptoms (if present) have abated, or exchange transfusion can begin.

Discontinuation of phototherapy is a matter of judgment and individual circumstances should be considered. In practice, phototherapy is discontinued when serum bilirubin levels fall 25–50 μmol/L (1.5–3 mg/dL) below the level that triggered the initiation of phototherapy. Serum bilirubin levels may rebound after treatment has been discontinued and follow-up tests should be obtained within 6–12 hours after discontinuation. If phototherapy is used for infants with hemolytic diseases or is initiated early and discontinued before the infant is 3–4 days old, a follow-up bilirubin measurement within 24 hours after discharge is recommended.[21]

Indications for prophylactic phototherapy are debatable as phototherapy does not do much good in an infant who is not clinically jaundiced. Although generally quite innocuous, phototherapy is not without potential risks and should be dosed appropriately like any other drug or therapy. It seems most rational to apply truly effective phototherapy once serum (and skin) bilirubin has reached levels at which light may do some good.

A device for measuring the irradiance delivered by the phototherapy equipment should be available wherever phototherapy is used. This will help to configure the set-up to deliver optimal irradiance and spectral power and to intermittently check that the set-up works as intended. However, it is not necessary to measure irradiance routinely for every baby under phototherapy lights.[1]

Side effects of phototherapy

Phototherapy is very safe and, in the vast majority of those treated, has no serious side effects. However, some adverse effects and complications have been noted (see Table 5).

Intravenous immune globulin (IVIG)

IVIG has been used in the treatment of several immunologically mediated conditions. In Rh, ABO, or other blood group incompatibilities that cause significant neonatal jaundice, IVIG may reduce the need for exchange transfusions.[21] The 2004 AAP guidelines suggest a dose range for IVIG of 500–1000 mg/kg (AAP 2004). The dose can be repeated 2–3 times. When combined with intensive phototherapy, exchange transfusion can be avoided in the majority of cases.[22] We do not use IVIG in the presence of hydrops because there is no documentation that this is safe or likely to be successful.

Exchange transfusion

Exchange transfusion is indicated to prevent bilirubin neurotoxicity when other therapeutic modalities have proven insufficient to curtail the rise of

Table 5.   Side effects of phototherapy.

Insensible water loss

— data suggest that this is not very important

— fluid balance should be monitored

Loose stools

— increased fecal water loss may create a need for fluid supplementation.

Retinal damage

— covering the eyes of infants in phototherapy with eye patches is routine

DNA-strand breakage

— *In vitro* and animal data have not shown any implication for treatment of human neonates

Increased skin blood flow

— redistribution of blood flow may occur in small premature infants

— increased incidence of patent ductus arteriosus has been reported

Hypocalcemia

— appears to be more common in premature infants under phototherapy lights

Deterioration of amino acids in total parenteral nutrition solutions

Burns

— resulting from failure to replace UV filters

the TSB level. The procedure may be also be indicated in infants with ery-throblastosis who present with severe anemia, hydrops, or both, even in the absence of high serum bilirubin levels. The AAP guidelines for exchange transfusion are shown in Fig. 4.[1] These guidelines distinguish between three risk categories: low, intermediate and high, which corre-spond to three levels of suggested intervention. The intervention limits increase from birth and plateau at four days of age. Intervention levels associated with exchange transfusion are higher than those of phototherapy, as seen in a comparison of Figs. 3 and 4.

In addition to controlling extreme hyperbilirubinemia, an exchange transfusion can achieve four goals[23]:

(i) Removing erythrocytes which are antibody coated
(ii) Correcting anemia

(iii) Removing maternal antibody

(iv) Removing other potentially toxic byproducts of hemolysis

In the early days, the principal indications for exchange transfusion were anemia (cord hemoglobin <11 g/dL), elevated cord bilirubin level (>70 μmol/L or 4.5 mg/dL), or both. A rapid rate of increase in the serum bilirubin level (>15–20 μmol/L/h or 1 mg/dL/h) was also an indication for the procedure, as was a more moderate rate of increase (>8–10 μmol/L/h or 0.5 mg/dL/h) in the presence of moderate anemia (11–13 g/dL).

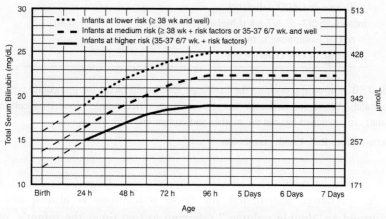

- The dashed lines for the first 24 hours indicate uncertainty due to a wide range of clinical circumstances and a range of responses to phototherapy.
- Immediate exchange transfusion is recommended if infant shows signs of acute bilirubin encephalopathy (hypertonia, arching, retrocollis, opisthotonos, fever, high pitched cry) or if TSB is ≥5 mg/dL (85 μmol/L) above these lines.
- Risk factors - isoimmune hemolytic disease, G6PD deficiency, asphyxia, significant lethargy, temperature instability, sepsis, acidosis.
- Measure serum albumin and calculate B/A ratio (See legend)
- Use total bilirubin. Do not subtract direct reacting or conjugated bilirubin
- If infant is well and 35-37 6/7 wk (median risk) can individualize TSB levels for exchange based on actual gestational age.

Figure 4. Guidelines for exchange transfusion in infants at 35 or more weeks' gestation.

Note that these suggested levels represent a consensus of most of the committee but are based on limited evidence, and the levels shown are approximations. See Table 6 for risks and complications of exchange transfusion. During birth hospitalization, exchange transfusion is recommended if the TSB rises to these levels despite intensive phototherapy. For re-admitted infants, if the TSB level is above the exchange level, repeat TSB measurement every two to three hours and consider exchange if the TSB remains above the levels indicated after intensive phototherapy for six hours. The following B/A ratios can be used together with but not in lieu of the TSB level as an additional factor in determining the need for exchange transfusion:

Figure 4.   (*Continued*)

Risk Category	B/A Ratio at Which Exchange Transfusion Should be Considered:	
	TSB mg/dL/Alb, g/dL	TSB μmol/L/Alb, μmol/L
Infants 38 0/7 wk	8.0	0.94
Infants 35 0/7–36 6/7 wk and well or 38 0/7 wk if higher risk or isoimmune hemolytic disease or G6PD deficiency	7.2	0.84
Infants 35 0/7–37 6/7 wk if higher risk or isoimmune hemolytic disease or G6PD deficiency	6.8	0.80

If the TSB is at or approaching the exchange level, send blood for immediate type and crossmatch. Blood for exchange transfusion is modified whole blood (red cells and plasma) crossmatched against the mother and compatible with the infant.

Reprinted from Ref. 1 with permission.

An exchange transfusion for these indications is almost always performed as "double volume," referring to two times the infant's, estimated blood volume of 80–85 mL/kg, i.a.w. 160–170 mL/kg. About 85% of the infant's red cells will be removed by a double volume exchange transfusion, while an estimated 110% of the circulating bilirubin will be removed.[24] The reason why >100% of estimated circulating bilirubin can be removed is that tissue bilirubin equilibrates with bilirubin in the blood during the exchange. In fact, only about 25% of total body bilirubin stores will be removed. For this reason, although the post-exchange TSB level can be expected to be about 60% of the starting level, a rebound to about 70–80% of pre-exchange levels can be expected after completion of the exchange. In the days when exchange transfusions were common, it was not unusual to have to perform multiple exchange transfusions in infants with severe hemolysis.

Intensive phototherapy is recommended during preparation for an exchange transfusion. In infants who show signs of neurotoxicity, phototherapy can also be continued during the exchange transfusion, e.g. by putting a fiberoptic pad or blanket underneath the infant, or by performing the procedure under overhead phototherapy lights.

Side effects and complications associated with exchange transfusions

Exchange transfusion was once a common procedure. The number of infants requiring exchange transfusion is now much smaller and even large NICUs may perform only a few procedures per year. This means that new generations of pediatricians and neonatologists in training do not have the opportunity to become thoroughly familiar with the procedure. Lack of experience must necessarily translate into increased risk when performing the procedure.[25] Reported mortality has ranged from 0.3–2% overall, with up to 8% in sick infants.[23] Other complications have been reported in 6–12% of infants, with the higher number applying to infants who were sick when the procedure as performed. An abbreviated list of possible complications is presented in Table 6. These data strongly suggest that exchange transfusions are increasingly becoming procedures that should be centralized to NICUs, and further that intensive phototherapy and IVIG are therapeutic options that should be pursued vigorously before embarking on an exchange transfusion.

Table 6. Complications associated with exchange transfusions.

(a) Vascular — embolization, thrombosis, vasospasm, infarct, perforation
(b) Cardiac — arrythmia, arrest, excessive volume load
(c) Fluids/electrolytes — hyperkalemia, hypoglycemia, hypernatremia, hypocalcemia, hypercalcemia (too rapid injection of calcium), acidosis
(d) Hemorrhage — thrombocytopenia, insufficient coagulation factors, too much anticoagulant in donor blood
(e) Infection — bacteriemia, hepatitis, CMV-infection, AIDS, malaria.
(f) Assorted — hemoglobinemia/-uria, hyperkalemia due to hemolysis resulting from too much warming of donor blood, hypo-/hyperthermia, GVH, NEC, hypothermia

---

Management of jaundice in very low birth weight infants

Premature, very low birth weight infants are believed to be more vulnerable to bilirubin toxicity than infants born at term. A study from the NICHD Neonatal Network found an association between peak total serum bilirubin levels in the first two weeks of life in ELBW infants, and death, hearing impairment and neurodevelopmental impairment in survivors.[26] A number of reasons for this apparent vulnerability have been proposed, such as reduced bilirubin binding by immature albumin in low concentration, increased risk of bilirubin displacement from drugs, parenteral nutrition solutions and stabilizers (e.g. benzyl alcohol), increased permeability of the blood-brain barrier (e.g. through hyperosmolality and respiratory acidosis) and decreased ability of the brain to detoxify bilirubin.

Guidelines for management of jaundice in VLBW and ELBW infants have not been validated by randomized, controlled studies. In the hierarchy of evidence-based medicine, these guidelines belong in the "expert opinion" category. Some general principles should be kept in mind:

(i) Phototherapy is more likely to increase insensible water loss in VLBW and ELBW infants,[27] so close surveillance of fluid balance is warranted. For the same reason, prophylactic phototherapy should not be given.

(ii) Exchange transfusion is a high-risk procedure in VLBW and ELBW infants, particularly if they are unstable and should be reserved for neurotoxic emergencies. Aggressive phototherapy and IVIG (when indicated) should be the principal tools.

(iii) Early TSB measurement (within first 24 hours) and close follow-up until stabilized (q12–24 h).[28]

Several different tables of intervention limits have been published.[28,29] Some describe limits according to birthweight, others according to gestational age. One example of a treatment graph is shown in Fig. 5. As no claims can be made for the scientific "correctness" of this or any other graph or table, you should view this as a suggestions only. Treatment at lower TSB levels is likely to be indicated whenever risk factors beyond prematurity are present.

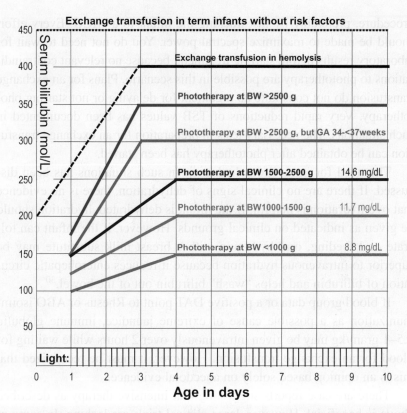

Figure 5. Partial view of chart with suggested intervention limits for phototherapy and exchange transfusion by consensus in the Norwegian Pediatric Association. Note that a choice was made to represent birth weights rather than gestational ages. Exchange transfusion *may* be indicated if TSB rises 50–100 μmol/L (3–6 mg/dL) above the suggested phototherapy limits for VLBW and ELBW infants. However, exchange transfusion is a high risk procedure for ELBW infants and should be avoided except in neurotoxic emergencies. Reproduced by permission.

Management of infants with extreme jaundice

In any infant who returns to the hospital with significant jaundice within the first 1–2 weeks of birth, transcutaneous bilirubin should be measured immediately. High values should result in start-up of treatment without delay. If a TcB device is not available, or if the infant presents with any neurological symptom, the infant should be put in intensive phototherapy as an emergency procedure, preferably by fast-tracking the infant to a NICU. Every effort should be made to maximize spectral power. You do not need to wait for laboratory results before starting treatment, because no relevant contraindications to phototherapy are possible in this scenario. Plans for an exchange transfusion do not constitute an argument for delaying or not starting phototherapy. Very rapid reductions of TSB values has been documented in such situations. The necessary tests in preparation for an exchange transfusion can be obtained after phototherapy has been started.

The need for intravenous hydration in such situations has been discussed. If there are no clinical signs of dehydration, there is no evidence that overhydration is helpful. If the infant is dehydrated, hydration should be given as indicated on clinical grounds. However, if the infant can tolerate oral feeding, oral hydration with a breast milk substitute may be superior to intravenous hydration because it reduces enterohepatic circulation of bilirubin and helps "wash" bilirubin out of the bowel.[30]

If blood group data or a positive DAT point to Rhesus or ABO isoimmunization as a possible cause of extreme jaundice, immune globulin 0.5–1 gram/kg may be given intravenously over 2 hours while waiting for blood for an exchange transfusion. However, it must be recognized that this is an opinion based solely on anecdotal evidence.

There are case reports suggesting that intensive therapy as described above is beneficial. However, large clinical trials are lacking. In some of the published cases, exchange transfusions were not carried out, even if the infants had presented with neurological symptoms,[4] and the patients survived without neurological sequela. However, given the limited number of such cases published, it is prudent to carry out an exchange transfusion.

Other therapies

In infants with breast milk jaundice, interruption of breastfeeding for 24–48 hours and feeding with breast milk substitutes may help to reduce the bilirubin level. Supplementing feeds of breast milk with 5 mL of a breast milk substitute reduces the level and duration of jaundice in breast milk–fed infants.[12] Because this latter intervention causes less interference with the establishment of the breastfeeding dyad, this approach tends to be our first step.

A new therapy currently under development consists of blockage of heme oxygenase through the use of metal mesoporphyrins and protoporphyrins. Heme can be excreted directly through the bile; therefore inhibition of heme oxygenase does not cause accumulation of unmetabolized heme. Before this treatment can be applied on a wide scale, important questions regarding the long-term safety of the drugs must be answered. Also, in light of data suggesting that bilirubin may play an important role as a free radical quencher, a more complete understanding of this putative role for bilirubin is desirable before general inhibition of its production can be recommended.

References

1. AAP Subcommittee on Hyperbilirubinemia. (2004) Management of hyperbilirubinemia in the newborn infant 35 or more weeks of gestation. *Pediatrics* **114**: 297–316.

2. Volpe JJ. (2008) Neurology of the Newborn. 5th ed. Elsevier, Philadelphia.

3. Harris MC, Bernbaum JC, Polin JR, Zimmerman R, Polin RA. (2001) Developmental follow-up of breastfed term and near-term infants with marked hyperbilirubinemia. *Pediatrics* **107**: 1075–1080.

4. Hansen TWR, Nietsch L, Norman E, Bjerre JV, Hascoet JM, Mreihil K, Ebbesen F. (2009) Apparent reversibility of acute intermediate phase bilirubin encephalopathy. *Acta Paediatrica* **98**: 1689–1694.

5. Johnson L, Bhutani VK, Karp K, Sivieri EM, Shapiro SM. (2009) Clinical report from the pilot USA Kernicterus Registry (1992 to 2004). *J Perinatol* **29**(Suppl. 1): S25–S45.

6. Maisels MJ, Bhutani VK, Bogen D, Newman TB, Stark AR, Watchko JF. (2009) Hyperbilirubinemia in the newborn infant > or = 35 weeks' gestation: An update with clarifications. *Pediatrics* **124**: 1193–1198.

7. Kramer LI. (1969) Advancement of dermal icterus in the jaundiced newborn. *Am J Dis Child* **118**: 454–458.

8. Maisels MJ, Deridder JM, Kring EA, Balasubramaniam M. (2009) Routine transcutaneous bilirubin measurements combined with clinical risk factors improve the prediction of subsequent hyperbilirubinemia. *J Perinatol* **29**: 612–617.

9. Bhutani VK, Johnson L, Sivieri EM. (1999) Predictive ability of a predischarge hour-specific serum bilirubin for subsequent significant hyperbilirubinemia in healthy term and near-term newborns. *Pediatrics* **103**: 6–14.

10. Hansen TWR. (2000) In Fetal and neonatal bilirubin metabolism. Maisels MJ, Watchko JF (eds.), *Neonatal jaundice.* Harwood Academic Publishers, London, pp. 3–20.

11. Huang MJ, Kua KE, Teng HC, Tang KS, Weng HW, Huangs CS. (2004) Risk factors for severe hyperbilirubinemia in neonates. *Pediatr Res* **56**: 682–689.

12. Gourley GR, Li Z, Kreamer BL, Kosorok MR. (2005) A controlled, randomized, double-blind trial of prophylaxis against jaundice among breastfed newborns. *Pediatrics* **116**: 385-391.

13. Watchko JF, Daood MJ, Biniwale M. (2002) Understanding neonatal hyperbilirubinemia in the era of genomics. *Semin Neonatol* **7**: 143–152.

14. Hsia DY, Allen FH Jr, Gellis SS, Diamond LK. (1952) Erythroblastosis fetalis. VIII. Studies of serum bilirubin in relation to Kernicterus. *New Engl J Med* **247**: 668–671.

15. Mollison PL, Cutbush M. (1954) Haemolytic disease of the newborn. In Gardner D (ed.), *Recent advances in pediatrics.* Churchill Ltd, London, pp. 110–132.

16. Maisel MJ, McDonagh AF. (2008) Phototherapy for Neonatal Jaundice. *New Engl J Med* **358**: 920–928.

17. Tan KL. (1977) The nature of the dose-response relationship of phototherapy for neonatal hyperbilirubinemia. *J Pediatr* **90**: 448–452.

18. De Carvalho M, De Carvalho D, Trzmielina S, Lopes JMA, Hansen TWR. (1999) Intensified phototherapy using daylight fluorescent lamps. *Acta Paediatr* **88**: 768–771.

19. Djokomuljanto S, Quah BS, Surini Y, Noraida R, Ismail NZN, Hansen TWR, Van Rostenberghe HLA. (2006) Efficacy of phototherapy for neonatal jaundice is increased by the use of low-cost white reflecting curtains. *Arch Dis Child* **91**: F439–F442.

20. Maisels MJ, Kring E.(2002) Bilirubin rebound following intensive phototherapy. *Arch Pediatr Adolesc Med* **156**: 669–672.

21. Rübo J, Albrecht K, Lasch P *et al.* (1992) High-dose intravenous immune globulin therapy for hyperbilirubinemia caused by Rh hemolytic disease. *J Pediatr* **121**: 93–97.

22. Huizing KMN, Røislien J, Hansen TWR. (2008) Intravenous immune globulin significantly reduces the need for exchange transfusions in infants with Rhesus and ABO incompatibility. *Acta Paediatr* **97:** 1362–1365.

23. Watchko JF. (2000) Exchange transfusion in the management of neonatal hyperbilirubinemia. In: Maisels MJ, Watchko JF (eds.), *Neonatal jaundice*. Harwood Academic Publishers, London, pp. 169–175.

24. Brown AK, Zuelzer WW, Robinson AR. (1957) Studies in hyperbilirubinemia. II. Clearance of bilirubin from plasma and extra vascular space in newborn infants during exchange transfusion. *Am J Dis Child* **93**: 274–286.

25. Watchko JF, Oski FA. (1992) Kernicterus in preterm newborns: Past, present, and future. *Pediatrics* **90**: 707–715.

26. Oh W, Tyson JE, Fanaroff AA, Vohr BR, Perritt R, Stoll BJ, Ehrenkranz RA, Carlo WA, Shankaran S, Poole K, Wright LL. (2003) Association between peak serum bilirubin and neurodevelopmental outcomes in extremely low birthweight infants. *Pediatrics* **112**: 773–779.

27. Grünhagen DJ, De Boer MGJ, De Beaufort AJ, Walther FJ. (2002) Transepidermal water loss during halogen spotlight phototherapy in preterm infants. *Pediatr Res* **51**: 402–405.

28. Cashore WJ. (2000) Bilirubin and jaundice in the micropremie. *Clin Perinatol* **27**: 171–179.

29. Maisels MJ, Watchko JF. (2003) Treatment of jaundice in low birthweight infants. *Arch Dis Child Fetal Neonat Ed* **88**: F459–F463.

30. Hansen TW. (1997) Acute management of extreme neonatal jaundice — the potential benefits of intensified phototherapy and interruption of enterohepatic bilirubin circulation. *Acta Paediatr* **86**: 843–846.

Chapter

Neonatal Infectious Diseases

Ira Adams-Chapman and Barbara J. Stoll

Neonatal Infections

Infectious diseases remain an important cause of neonatal morbidity and mortality across all gestational age groups. However, low birth weight infants share a disproportionate burden of disease and are more likely to die secondary to infection. Although the clinical signs and symptoms of neonatal infections are often subtle, some infants develop overwhelming multisystem organ dysfunction. The spectrum of pathogens causing infections in the newborn continues to shift, in part related to changes in medical practice, including the widespread use of intrapartum antibiotics and the increasing survival of extremely low birth weight infants. Clinicians must have a clear understanding of the epidemiology and risk factors associated with neonatal infection to ensure prompt diagnostic evaluation and appropriate treatment. Exploring opportunities to prevent neonatal infections are imperative to decrease infection-related mortality during the neonatal period.

Epidemiology

Worldwide, neonatal infections cause approximately 1.6 million deaths annually, particularly in resource-poor countries.[1] Although the burden of disease in the United States is less, infections continue to cause significant morbidity and mortality in the neonatal population. Epidemiologic patterns of pathogen distribution and antibiotic resistance vary between hospital, regions and countries, which highlight the important of active real-time local surveillance data.

Epidemiologic monitoring and research have been plagued by the lack of uniform definitions for infection in the neonatal population. Unfortunately, the lack of concordance between clinical signs, symptoms of sepsis and positive blood cultures, often leaves the clinician unclear about the appropriate course of treatment. In recent years, clinical investigators have attempted to define specific criteria for the major categories of infection in this population including infection, sepsis, clinical sepsis and/or systemic inflammatory response.[2–5]

Risk factors for sepsis

Risk factors for infection during the neonatal period vary based on postnatal age and associated comorbidities. Most congenital and early-onset neonatal infections are secondary to maternal infection during the pregnancy with associated hematogenous seeding of the fetus or exposure to infected body fluids during the birth process. Pregnancy complications such as maternal chorioamnionitis, maternal fever, preterm delivery and prolonged rupture of membranes have been associated with an increased risk of early-onset infection in the neonate.[2,5–7] Late-onset infections are often nosocomially acquired, particularly in the hospitalized low birth weight infant.

The overall risk for early- and late-onset sepsis varies inversely with gestational age and birth weight.[8–12] Stoll *et al.* reported an increased risk for late onset sepsis with increasing duration of catheter days, mechanical ventilation and delay in reaching full enteral feeds and decreasing gestational age and birth weight.[10] Even though these variables are surrogate markers for severity of illness, the need for devices that disrupt the integrity of the natural barriers to infection clearly increases the risk for infection in neonates.

Other aspects of the daily supportive care of the premature infant are also associated with an increased risk for infection, including central venous catheters, ventilators, nasal continuous positive pressure devices, skin care and cord care. Central venous catheters have become a mainstay in the care of extremely low birth weight infants. In a review of very low birth weight infants in the NICHD Neonatal Research Network, 46% had a percutaneously inserted central catheter (PICC), 15% had a peripheral arterial line and 8% had a surgically placed central line.[10] Several investigators have reported that the risk for infection increases with increasing duration of catheter days.[10,13] There is a lack of consensus regarding the recommended duration for umbilical catheters; however, similar to other central lines, the risk for infection increases with increased catheter days. It is imperative that neonatal intensive care units (NICU) have established practice guidelines regarding the care and maintenance of central venous catheters. (See Prevention Section)

Congenital Infections

Congenital infections are acquired before delivery or during the intrapartum period. The majority of these infections are secondary to either a primary exposure during the pregnancy resulting in hematogenous spread across the placenta, ascending infection through the cervix or contact with infected secretions during vaginal delivery. The acronym *TORCH* is commonly used to identify several common congenital infections that have similar clinical manifestations — *Toxoplasma gondii, Other, Rubella, Cytomegalovirus and Herpes. Human Immunodeficiency Virus (HIV), Treponema pallidum, coxsackievirus* and *Parvovirus B19* are also important pathogens to consider in the evaluation of neonates with suspected congenital infection.

HIV

Human Immunodeficiency Virus (HIV) is an important perinatally acquired viral infection that affects children across the globe. HIV is a major cause of mortality within the first year of life. Prevalence rates are highly variable with the greatest density in resource poor countries, sub–Saharan Africa, India and Southeast Asia.[14,15] In the United States, perinatal transmission is responsible for the majority of new cases of HIV in pre-adolescent children. Some cases of perinatal transmission occur *in utero*; however, the vast majority are acquired at the time of delivery. The risk for maternal-infant transmission in an HIV-positive mother who did not receive intrapartum treatment ranges from 12–40%.[15] Maternal viral load, prolonged rupture of membranes, low maternal CD4+ T-lymphocyte counts, chorioamnionitis and preterm delivery are associated with an increased risk of perinatal transmission.

Unfortunately, most perinatal HIV transmission in the United States is related to failure to identify maternal HIV-infection prior to the delivery.[16] The dramatic decline in perinatal HIV transmission rates with antiretroviral treatment of infected mothers during the pregnancy and intrapartum postnatal antiretroviral prophylaxis for the infant have led many to support universal HIV testing as a routine part of prenatal care using an "opt-out" consent.[16–18] Rapid HIV testing with "opt-out" consent is recommended for any woman with unknown HIV status so that appropriate prophylaxis can be offered to the neonate within 12 hours of birth.[16] The importance of identifying HIV status prior to delivery is highlighted by data showing that even for women diagnosed during labor, the risk of perinatal HIV transmission decreases by 60% with intrapartum prophylaxis with zidovudine and infant prophylaxis for six weeks compared to those with no prophylaxis.[19] There is a 50% risk reduction in perinatal HIV transmission when the mother fails to receive intrapartum prophylaxis but the infant receives zidovudine for six weeks.[19]

Elective cesarean delivery prior to the onset of labor or rupture of membranes has been associated with at least a 50% decrease in the risk of perinatal HIV transmission among HIV infected women who are not receiving antiretroviral therapy or those receiving zidovudine alone.[14,20] Furthermore, the American College of Obstetricians and Gynecologists (ACOG) recommends elective cesarean delivery at 38 weeks gestation for all HIV infected women with RNA levels greater than 1000 copies per ml even if the mother is receiving antiretroviral therapy.[21]

HIV infected women living in countries with safe and available infant feeding alternatives should not breastfeed because of a 9% to 15% excess risk of HIV transmission to the infant.[16]

Early-Onset Sepsis (EOS)

Early-onset infections occur during the first three to seven days of life (definitions vary) and are typically acquired during labor and/or delivery.

EOS remains a significant cause of neonatal morbidity and mortality in both preterm and term neonates. The overall, rate of EOS is approximately 1 case per 1000 live births[12]; however, low birth weight infants are disproportionately affected.[2,8,9] Stoll *et al.* reported EOS rates of 15.4 per 1000 live births in a cohort of VLBW infants. The distribution of pathogens associated with EOS has changed over time.[8,12,22]

A recent study from the National Institute of Child Health and Developmental (NICHD) Neonatal Research Network reports that GBS remains the most common pathogen among term infants with EOS (72%) while *E. coli* is the most common pathogen among preterm infants with EOS (87%).[12] Interestingly, 24% of the term infants were asymptomatic; however, overall 15% patients died. Mortality was higher among preterm infants (25%) and those with *E. coli* (33%).[12] Obstetrical risk factors associated with early onset sepsis (EOS) include maternal fever, chorioamnionitis, prolonged rupture of membranes and preterm delivery.[2,7,12]

Group B Streptococcus

Streptococcus agalactiae (Group B Streptococcus, GBS) is an important cause of EOS. Asymptomatic colonization in the gastrointestinal and genital tract occurs in approximately 15% to 40% of pregnant women and is the most likely source of intrapartum transmission.[23] For reasons that are unclear, African American women have higher rates of colonization and disease prevalence is higher among African American newborns of all gestational ages. Clinical manifestations of early-onset GBS infection include apnea, respiratory distress, sepsis, pneumonia and meningitis.

The 2002 guidelines for the prevention of early-onset neonatal GBS recommend universal screening at 35–37 weeks to identify women with rectovaginal GBS colonization who should receive intrapartum chemoprophylaxis.[24,25] Guidelines for the management of newborns born to mothers with a history of GBS colonization are outlined in (Fig. 1).

This successful and coordinated public health campaign resulted in an 80% decrease in the incidence of early-onset GBS disease from approximately 1.7 cases per 1,000 live births to 0.35 cases per 1,000 live births.[23] (CDC website) Rates of early-onset GBS disease were relatively stable for

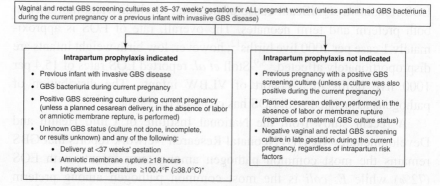

* If amnionitis is suspected, broad-spectrum antibiotic therapy that includes an agent known to be active against GBS should replace GBS prophylaxis.

Figure 1.   Indications for intrapartum antibiotic prophylaxis to prevent perinatal GBS disease under a universal prenatal screening strategy based on combined vaginal and rectal cultures collected at 35–37 weeks' gestation from all pregnant women. From Schrag S, Gorwitz R *et al.* (2002) Prevention of perinatal group B streptococcal disease. Revised guidelines from CDC. *MMWR Recomm Rep* **51**(RR-11): 1–22.

several years; however, recent data indicate a concerning upward trend, particularly among black term infants[24,26] (Fig. 2). Intrapartum antibiotic prophylaxis does not affect late-onset GBS disease, therefore, as expected, rates of late-onset GBS disease have remained relatively stable at approximately 0.36 cases per 1,000 live births.[24,26] Overall, black infants of all gestational ages are more likely to develop both early-onset and late-onset GBS disease. The reasons for racial differences are unclear, but are likely affected by the increased GBS colonization rates among black women. Ongoing surveillance and revision of the guidelines for GBS prophylaxis to minimize missed opportunities to prevent early-onset GBS are ongoing.

The successful efforts to decrease the burden of early-onset GBS disease were tempered by concerns that the widespread use of antibiotics would alter the distribution of pathogens and antibiotic susceptibility patterns. CDC surveillance data showed that 69% of *E. coli* strains were resistant to Ampicillin with a mortality rate of 41% among infected infants.[2] Indeed, the distribution of pathogens has dramatically shifted

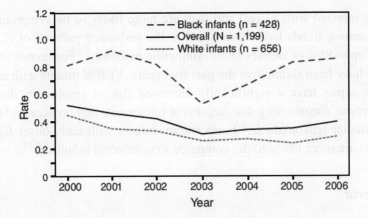

Figure 2. Rate* of early-onset[†] invasive group B streptococcal disease, by race and year — Active Bacterial Core surveillance system, United States,[‡] 2000–2006.[§]

* Per 1,000 live births.

[†] Occurring in infants aged <7 days.

[‡] Includes selected counties in California, Colorado, Connecticut, Georgia, Maryland, Minnesota, New Mexico, New York, Oregon, and Tennessee. Additional information available at http://www.cdc.gov/ncidod/dbmd/abcs.

[§] Rates for 2000–2006 include surveillance areas participating since 2000, with the addition of Colorado in 2001. New Mexico, where surveillance began in 2004, is not included in comparison of incidence over time. From Ref. 24.

over the past two decades for the VLBW population. Epidemiologic data from the NICHD Neonatal Research Network highlights this shift in pathogen distribution among very low birth weight infants. Gram negative agents have emerged as the most common pathogens causing EOS among preterm infants.[8] New technology for rapid detection of GBS in women with unknown GBS status and those who present in preterm labor is being investigated.[27] Furthermore, clinical trials are ongoing to evaluate the safety, efficacy and immunogenicity of vaccines targeting the most common serotypes of GBS.

E. coli

E. coli is the most common gram negative pathogen causing EOS among both term and preterm infants. In general, preterm infants are more likely to be infected with *E. coli* and they are more likely to be symptomatic. Concerning trends have been noted in the resistance patterns of *E. coli* with up to 85% of isolates being Ampicillin resistant.[8,9] Fortunately, these rates have been stable over the past five years. VLBW infants with early-onset sepsis have a significantly increased risk of respiratory distress syndrome, chronic lung disease, severe intracranial hemorrhage and periventricular leukomalacia.[8] Furthermore, infants with early-onset *E. coli* sepsis are more likely to die compared to uninfected infants.[8,9,12]

Listeria

Listeria monocytogenes is an aerobic, non-spore forming, gram-positive bacillus that rarely causes early-onset sepsis in the newborn. There is typically a history of a prodromal illness in the pregnant mother or one may elicit a history of potential exposure to contaminant food products, such as unpasteurized milk and cheese or uncooked poultry. Perinatal infection occurs secondary to transplacental transmission from the infected mother, or more rarely, after exposure during the birth process. Preterm delivery and chorioamnionitis are common and notable for the characteristic brown staining of the amniotic fluid. Affected infants develop pneumonia, sepsis or an erythematous rash. Late-onset disease is more likely to be associated with meningitis.[28]

Fungal

Although rare, cases of early-onset neonatal invasive candidiasis have been reported. Severe mucocutaneous candidiasis is the most common neonatal presentation; however, some infants develop disseminated disease.[29] In general, the mortality rate is very high in this clinical scenario.

Late-Onset Sepsis (LOS)

Globally, postnatal infections are a leading cause of death in the first year of life. Infections that occur after three days of age (7 days in some studies) are defined as late-onset infections and occur more frequently in the hospitalized premature infant. Many of these infections are nosocomially

Table 1. Distribution of pathogens associated with the first episode of late-onset sepsis: NICHD neonatal research network, from September 1, 1998 to August 31, 2000.[10]

Organism*	%
Gram-positive organisms	**70.2**
CONS	47.9
S aureus	7.8
Enterococcus spp.	3.3
Group B Streptococcus	2.3
Other	8.9
Gram-negative organisms	**17.6**
E coli	4.9
Klebsiella	4.0
Pseudomonas	2.7
Enterobacter	2.5
Serratia	2.2
Other	1.4
Fungi	**12.2**
C albicans	5.8
Candida parapsilosis	4.1
Other	2.3

acquired; however, infants may become colonized during the delivery process. Gram-positive organisms are the most common pathogens causing late-onset infections, of which 70% are caused by Coagulase-negative Staphylococci (CoNS)[10] (Table 1).

The rate of late-onset infection varies inversely with birth weight and gestational age. Stoll *et al.* reported rates of 43% among neonates with birth weight of 401–750 grams compared to 28% for those 750–1000 grams, 15% in those 1000–1250 grams and 7% in those >1200 grams.[10,11] VLBW infants with LOS had longer hospital lengths of stay (79 days vs 60 days), prolonged duration of mechanical ventilation, and took longer to reach full enteral feeds.[10] Infected infants also had an increased risk of death compared to uninfected infants (18% vs 7%) with the greatest risk being among those infected with gram-negative organisms or fungal infections.[10] Infants with gram-negative infections are more likely to have a more fulminant presentation with multisystem organ dysfunction and die within three days of the positive culture.[10] Stoll and colleagues reported a 3.5-fold increased risk of death in VLBW infants with gram-negative infection.[10] Compared to uninfected infants, those with gram-positive infection had a similar risk of death.[10]

Fungal

Fungal infections are an important cause of infection related morbidity and mortality among very low birth weight infants (VLBW). Colonization rates approach 60% in very low birth weight infants weighing <1500 grams, of whom, approximately 12% develop invasive fungal infection.[10,30] Similar to other nosocomial pathogens, the incidence of invasive fungal disease varies inversely with both gestational age and birth weight yielding infection rates of up to 20% among extremely low birth weight infants.[29,30] Other known risk factors include the use of broad spectrum antibiotics, the use of H-2 blockers, colonization at multiple sites and history of gastrointestinal surgery.[29,31–34]

Most infants have isolated bloodstream infection; however, disease can disseminate and cause meningitis, endopthalmitis, osteomyelitis or abscesses in the kidney, spleen or liver.[34] Even though meningitis is an infrequent complication, it is concerning that in a report by Benjamin *et al.* 48% of those with fungal meningitis had negative blood cultures.[31] These data highlight the importance of a thorough investigation for all possible sites of infection in neonates with fungal sepsis.

Persistent candidemia, despite initiating therapy, is common.[31] Delayed removal of central venous catheters in infants with invasive fungal disease prolongs the duration of candidemia and has also been associated with increased morbidity and mortality.[31,35,36] In a review of short-term outcomes in neonates with Candida infection who had early removal of central venous catheter compared to late removal of central venous catheter, Karlowicz and colleagues reported significantly shorter duration of candidemia and lower death rates in those with early removal of central venous catheters compared to those with late catheter removal.[36] Attributable mortality secondary to fungal sepsis is estimated to be at least a 25% among infected patients.[10,29,31] The mortality risk does not vary based on site of infection in ELBW infants.[37] Randomized controlled trials and systematic review suggest that prophylactic treatment with Fluconazole for the first six weeks of life decreases the rate of colonization and invasive fungal disease in VLBW infants.[29,30,38,39] Infants in the Fluconazole treatment group were less likely to die secondary to complications directly related to fungal infection; however, there were no differences in overall mortality rates compared to non-colonized infants.[30] However, current recommendations based on a recent meta-analysis of randomized controlled trials in this population do not recommend routine use of prophylactic Fluconazole in preterm infants secondary to the lack of apparent effect on decreasing mortality, fears about development of drug resistance and limited data regarding the long-term neurodevelopmental outcome of survivors.[39] Caution is advised in the interpretation of published reports secondary to the possibility of ascertainment bias in the treatment group because Fluconazole treatment may have reduced the sensitivity of cultures to detect the organism. Targeted use of Fluconazole prophylaxis may be considered in extremely premature infants and nurseries with high baseline prevalence rates of systemic candidiasis. Additional research is needed in this area.

Device-associated infections

Hospitalized newborns are at increased risk to develop device-associated infections secondary to the immaturity of their immune system and the disruption in natural barriers related to the need for invasive support devices, such as ventilators, central venous catheters and feeding tubes. These devices serve as potential reservoirs for various infections including bloodstream infections, pneumonia and urinary tract infections. In more recent reports, the national Healthcare Safety Network (NHSN) has recommended replacing the term "nosocomial infection" with "health care associated infections (HAI)."[40]

Catheter-associated blood stream infections (CABSI) are the most frequent device-associated, late-onset infection. The Centers for Disease Control and Prevention (CDC) define CABSI by the following

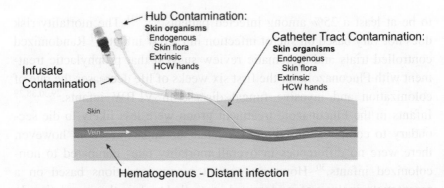

Figure 3. Pathogenesis of catheter-associated blood stream infections. From Garland JS, Uhing MR, (2009) Strategies to prevent bacterial and fungal infection in the neonatal intensive care unit. *Clinics in Perinatology* **36:** 1–13.

criteria: (1) a recognized pathogen isolated from one or more blood cultures or a known skin pathogen from two cultures; (2) one or more clinical signs of sepsis; (3) intravascular catheters in place at time of positive culture; (4) no other site of documented primary infection.[40] The three primary sources of contamination that result in CABSI are infusate, hub and catheter tract[41] (Fig. 3). Hub colonization is of particular concern in the low birth weight population, because typically these catheters are in place for a longer duration than in adult patients. Several investigators have documented hub colonization with the same bacterial prior to the development of a CABSI.[41–43] Maintaining a closed system by using extension tubing for medication administration is important to decrease the risk of line contamination. Mahieu and colleagues found correlation between risk of CABSI and the number of manipulations to the catheter; therefore, current recommendations are to perform dressing changes only when indicated and to use sterile technique when manipulating catheter position.[41]

Once infected, delayed catheter removal has been associated with increased duration of bacteremia and infection related complications. Benjamin *et al.* reported a 46% rate of complication in infants with fungal CABSI who had delayed catheter removal compared to 8% in those with prompt catheter removal (OR 9.8, 95% CI 2.2, 43.46).[35] Immediate removal of central venous catheters should be considered in infants infected with *Staphylococcus aureus* or nonenteric Gram-negative rods. CoNS infections are less likely to be associated with complications, but catheter removal should be considered after repeated positive cultures.[35]

Comprehensive yet targeted prevention strategies can effectively reduce the rate of CABSI in the NICU population. Several investigators have reported decreased rates of BSI after implementing BSI "bundles" which focus on minimizing the risk for catheter contamination from insertion until the catheter is removed.[44–47] Critical assessment regarding the relative need for all devices should be a part of daily care.

Diagnostic Evaluation

Sepsis is included in the differential diagnosis for many clinical scenarios in neonatology, particularly in the low birth weight infant. Often, the classic manifestations of sepsis are lacking, yet overshadowed by subtle clinical symptoms of unclear significance (Table 2). These nonspecific findings often prompt a full diagnostic evaluation for possible sepsis. Laboratory data are used to reassure the clinician that the likelihood of infection is low or provide additional evidence to support the clinical suspicion of infection. The sensitivity and specificity of any single diagnostic study is modest; however, combining multiple tests increases the negative predictive value and specificity. This inability to rely on currently available diagnostic tools highlights the importance of maintaining a high level of suspicion for neonatal sepsis and utilizing sound clinical judgment in the evaluation and treatment of suspected infection.

Table 2. Clinical signs and symptoms of sepsis.

Temperature instability — hypothermia/hyperthermia
Hyperglycemia
Respiratory distress
Apnea
Tachypnea
Poor feeding/feeding intolerance
Abdominal distension
Lethargy
Irritability

Inflammatory mediators

Researchers have sought for decades to identify the elusive "endogenous pyrogen" responsible for the systemic manifestations seen in patients with sepsis. Various inflammatory mediators are activated in response to sepsis. Researchers have attempted to identify appropriate threshold values of circulating cytokines that correlate with various infectious states. Understanding the phasic release of these mediators in response to infection provides an opportunity to facilitate early diagnosis of infants with sepsis.

The most commonly measured cytokine in clinical practice is C-reactive protein (CRP), which is an acute phase reactant synthesized by the liver within 6 hours after a stimulus. The sensitivity at the onset of disease manifestation is limited; however, both the sensitivity and predictive value increases with serial measurements or when combined with other proinflammatory mediators.[48,49] Researchers are actively working to identify other inflammatory mediators that might be used in a clinical setting to improve the early diagnosis of neonatal infection.

Blood cultures

Blood culture remains the gold standard for the diagnosis of neonatal sepsis; however, cultures are only positive in approximately 25% of patients with sepsis syndrome.[50–52] Sensitivity improves when volumes of at least 1 ml are collected from at least one peripheral site.[51,53,54] Research is ongoing to evaluate the utility of using molecular assays to detect bacterial DNA in the bloodstream.[50] Unfortunately, the sensitivity of this technology limits the ability to utilize it as the sole determinant of defined infection status. Pathogen-specific PCR testing is being developed to assist in the diagnosis of sepsis.[55]

White count

Complete Blood Count (CBC) is often used to help diagnose neonatal infection; however, this test is most useful at the extremes of normal ranges due to the wide variability in a normal neonate.[56] As an isolated measure, both sensitivity and negative predictive values are low, therefore, clinicians are cautioned against relying on CBC indices to guide treatment strategies in neonatal sepsis.[56,57] Several researchers have reported that neutropenia is more common of patients with culture proven sepsis.[56–58] In contrast, high neutrophil counts do not correlate well with infection.[57] The ratio between immature and total neutrophil count (I/T ratio) is frequently used in the diagnostic evaluation for neonatal sepias. It tends to be abnormal in symptomatic patients; however, it has a low negative predictive value in asymptomatic newborns.[48,56]

Lumbar puncture

The decision to perform a lumbar puncture is often deferred until a positive blood culture is obtained, which limits the predictive value of this test. Currently, there is no consensus regarding appropriate timing to perform a lumbar puncture in infants being evaluated for sepsis. However, there are several reports that suggest that we may be systematically under diagnosing meningitis in the VLBW population[58–60] including up to a 30% discordance rate between positive blood culture and positive CSF cultures among VLBW infants with culture-proven meningitis.[59,60] Furthermore, the biochemical findings in the CSF may not suggest infection despite the presence of positive CSF cultures.

Treatment

Due to the overwhelming concern for missing a case of neonatal sepsis, clinicians treat many infants for suspected sepsis who turn out to be uninfected. Withholding or delaying of treatment based on currently available diagnostic tools in unacceptable due to the low sensitivity of available diagnostic studies. Clinical judgment must be blended with diagnostic studies to identify those infants at highest risk for sepsis. The physical examination remains one of the most significant predictors of neonatal sepsis.

Bacterial sepsis

Ampicillin and Gentamicin remain the recommended empiric antibiotics for suspected early-onset neonatal infections. Because CoNS is the most common late-onset pathogen for VLBW infants, empiric antibiotics must provide coverage against this pathogen. While most *E.coli* isolates are sensitive to Gentamicin and other aminoglycosides, clinicians must be aware of the increasing Ampicillin resistance among *E. coli*. This is particularly important when choosing empiric antibiotic therapy in the ill or rapidly deteriorating neonate who is not responding to standard therapy. Empiric cephalosporin use should be limited, due to increased risk of antibiotic resistance. Once culture results are available, appropriate antibiotics should be chosen based on agent isolated and antibiotic sensitivity patterns. Vancomycin is often the drug of choice for infants at risk for device-associated infections. Liberal use of broad spectrum antibiotics is discouraged and should be used based on documented sensitivity profiles or unusual clinical circumstances when the patient is unresponsive to first line agents.

Fungal

Amphotericin B remains the preferred drug for treatment of systemic candidiasis due to concerns of Fluconazole-resistant Candida species. Lipid complex formulation of Amphotericin B are effective and less toxic; however, their use is restricted to patients with a history of renal dysfunction or intolerance to Amphotericin B secondary to the increased cost of this product.[29]

Viral

The benefits of treatment with antiviral agents vary based on the specific pathogen involved and the severity of associated clinical findings. Infants with suspected perinatal herpes infection should be treated as soon as possible with empiric acyclovir pending results of herpes cultures and clinical course. Consultation with an infectious disease specialist is often warranted to best establish risk-benefit for a specific patient with suspected viral infection. Mother-to-child perinatal transmission of HIV is decreased with antiretroviral treatment of the mother in the prenatal and intrapartum period and with prophylaxis of HIV-exposed neonates.

Prevention

Congenital and early-onset infections

Vaccine development is the focus for efforts to prevent congenital CMV infection. Immunization against rubella has markedly reduced congenital rubella in the US and other developed countries. Universal screening for GBS and HIV would help minimize missed opportunities to provide appropriate intrapartum prophylaxis and decrease rates of intrapartum transmission.

Late-onset infections

Nosocomial-acquired infections in the NICU are a common cause of late-onset infections which contribute to the late morbidity and mortality among newborns. Excess hospital costs secondary to increased length of hospital stay are also important considerations.[61]

Hand washing before and after each patient encounter is the cheapest and single most effective strategy to decrease rates of nosocomial infection. A variety of commercially available products are effective at decreasing the amount of resident and transient bacteria on the hands of health care workers. Hand antisepsis is required even if the provider wears gloves.

The most common nosocomial infections in the neonatal population are central line-associated blood stream infections (CLABSI); however, it is important to understand other aspects of supportive intensive care that increases the risk for infection. The premature infant is often dependent on extrinsic thermal support to maintain appropriate body temperature; for endotracheal intubation and ventilator support for respiratory insufficiency/distress and for intravenous access for fluid and nutritional support. Natural defense barriers are often immature or bypassed due to the need for artificial support. Effective and comprehensive strategies are needed to decrease the risk for nosocomial infections among preterm infants.

Prevention of catheter-related bloodstream infections (CRBSI) is critically important in the NICU due to the frequency of use in the vulnerable preterm population. Research has shown that CRBSI rates are lower in units that have a dedicated team of providers to perform insertion and daily maintenance care of intravenous lines. Many neonatal intensive care units have implemented "care bundles" outlining interventions designed to decrease CRBSIs. The key components of these bundles include: appropriate hand hygiene, skin antisepsis, adherence to sterile technique and barrier protection during insertion, dedicated central line care teams, prompt removal of catheters once they are no longer clinically indicated, and active surveillance. The 2010 Joint Commission Hospital Accreditation Program National Patient Safety Goals require the use of a catheter checklist and a standardized protocol for the insertion and maintenance care of central venous catheters.[62]

Peripheral intravenous catheters are the most commonly used device for vascular access in the neonate; however, unlike adult patients, there are limited data to base recommendations for duration of time they can remain *in situ*.[45,63] Non-tunneled, peripherally inserted central venous catheters, commonly referred to as PICC lines, are frequently used in the NICU. Surveillance data from the National Healthcare Safety Network (NHSN) Report shows that the relative risk for CLABSI is inversely related to birth weight. Infants <750 grams birth weight had approximately 3.7 infections per 1000 catheter days, compared to 2.0 infections per 1000 catheter days among those >2500 grams.[13] Similarly, rates of ventilator-associated pneumonia also varied inversely with birth weight.[13] The increased length of stay associated with extremely premature birth is reflected in an increase in absolute number of device days; however, overall utilization rates were stable. Despite these trends, it is encouraging that overall device-associated infections rates are lower in the current report compared to previous studies.[13] Ongoing surveillance is critically important.

Antibiotic lock

Data are limited regarding the use of antibiotic lock therapy in neonates.[64] Garland and colleagues reported a significantly lower rate of CABSI in patient randomized to antibiotic lock compared to control infants (2.3 vs 17.8 infections per 1000 catheter days).[64] Currently, routine use of antibiotic lock therapy is not recommended in neonates due to concerns that resistant strains of bacteria will develop, even though a single center trial and a meta-analysis of neonatal and pediatric patients suggest potential benefit.[65] Additional research is needed in this area.

Neurodevelopmental Outcome and Sepsis

Neurologic sequelae are common with many congenital infections, as one would expect based on the frequency of CNS involvement with the primary infection. Limited epidemiologic data are available regarding the neurodevelopmental outcome of infants with bacterial early-onset sepsis and late-onset sepsis, particularly in the term and late preterm populations. Preterm infants appear to be uniquely vulnerable to cytokine-induced neurologic injury. Various pathophysiologic mechanisms have been proposed including the stimulation of proinflammatory mediators which are directly cytotoxic to the developing neuronal tissues or influence on cerebral blood flow. Among preterm infants, several investigators have reported adverse neurodevelopmental outcomes in early infancy among infants with late-onset infection compared to uninfected groups.[11,66]

References

1. Vergnano S *et al.* (2005) Neonatal sepsis: An international perspective. *Arch Dis Child Fetal Neonatal Ed* **90**(3): F220–F224.
2. Schuchat A *et al.* (2000) Risk factors and opportunities for prevention of early-onset neonatal sepsis: A multicenter case-control study. *Pediatrics* **105**(1 Pt 1): 21–26.
3. Adams-Chapman. I, Stoll BJ. (2001) Systemic Inflammatory Response Syndrome, in Seminars in Pediatric Infectious Diseases, pp. 5–16.
4. American College of Chest Physicians/Society of Critical Care Medicine Consensus Conference: Definitions for sepsis and organ failure and guidelines for the use of innovative therapies in sepsis (1992). *Crit Care Med.* **20**(6): 864–874.
5. Goldenberg RL, Hauth JC, Andrews WW. (2000) Intrauterine infection and preterm delivery. *N Engl J Med* **342**(20): 1500–1507.

6. Gomez R *et al.* (1995) Premature labor and intra-amniotic infection. Clinical aspects and role of the cytokines in diagnosis and pathophysiology. *Clin Perinatol* **22**(2): 281–342.

7. Klinger G *et al.* (2009) Epidemiology and risk factors for early onset sepsis among very low birthweight infants. *American Journal of Obstetrics and Gynecology* **201**(1): 38.e1–38.e6.

8. Stoll BJ *et al.* (2002) Changes in pathogens causing early-onset sepsis in very low birth weight infants. *N Engl J Med* **347**(4): 240–247.

9. Stoll BJ *et al.* (2005) very low birth weight preterm infants with early onset neonatal sepsis: The predominance of gram-negative infections continues in the national institute of child health and human development neonatal research network, 2002–2003. *Pediatric Infectious Disease Journal* **24**(7): 635–639.

10. Stoll BJ *et al.* (2002) Late-Onset Sepsis in Very Low Birth Weight Neonates: The Experience of the NICHD Neonatal Research Network. *Pediatrics* **110**(2): 285–291.

11. Stoll, BJ *et al.* (2004) Neurodevelopmental and growth impairment among extremely low birth weight infants with neonatal infection. *JAMA* **292**(19): 2357–2365.

12. Stoll B. (2008) GBS and E. coli continue to put newborns at risk for early-onset sepsis (EOS): A surveillance study of 200,000 live births. *Pediatric Research* Abstract No. 750346.

13. Edwards JR *et al.* (2008) National Healthcare Safety Network (NHSN) Report, data summary for 2006 through 2007, issued November 2008. *American Journal of Infection Control* **36**(9): 609–626.

14. The mode of delivery and the risk of vertical transmission of human immuno-deficiency virus type 1 — a meta-analysis of 15 prospective cohort studies. The International Perinatal HIV Group (1999). *N Engl J Med* **340**(13): 977–987.

15. Human Immunodeficiency Virus Infection (2009). *Red Book* **2009**(1): 380a–400.

16. Committee on Pediatric, A. (2008) HIV testing and prophylaxis to prevent mother-to-child transmission in the United States. *Pediatrics* **122**(5): 1127–1134.

17. American Academy of, P., O. American College of, and Gynecologists (1999). Human Immunodeficiency Virus Screening. *Pediatrics* **104**(1): 128.

18. Branson BM *et al.* (2006) Revised recommendations for HIV testing of adults, adolescents and pregnant women in health-care settings. *MMWR Recomm Rep* **55**(RR-14): p. 1–17; quiz CE1-4.

19. Wade NA *et al.* (2004) Decline in perinatal HIV transmission in New York State (1997–2000). *J Acquir Immune Defic Syndr* **36**(5): 1075–1082.

20. The European Mode of Delivery Collaboration (1999). Elective caesarean-section versus vaginal delivery in prevention of vertical HIV-1 transmission: A randomised clinical trial, *Lancet* **353**(9158): 1035–1039.

21. ACOG committee opinion number 304, November 2004. Prenatal and perinatal human immunodeficiency virus testing: Expanded recommendations 2004. *Obstet Gynecol* **104**(5 Pt 1): 1119–1124.

22. Bizzarro MJ *et al.* (2005) Seventy-Five Years of Neonatal Sepsis at Yale: 1928–2003. *Pediatrics* **116**(3): 595–602.

23. Group B Streptococcal Infections (2009). *Red Book*, **2009**(1): 628–634.

24. MMWR C. (2009) Trends in Perinatal Group B Streptococcal Disease — United States, 2000–2006. [cited 2009; February 13, 2009/58:(05);109–112: [Available from: http://www.cdc.gov/mmwr/preview/mmwrhtml/mm5805a2. htm?s_cid=mm5805a2_e.

25. Phares CR *et al.* (2008) Epidemiology of invasive group B streptococcal disease in the United States, 1999–2005. *JAMA.* **299**(17): 2056–2065.

26. Trends in Perinatal Group B Streptococcal Disease — United States, 2000–2006. *JAMA*, 2009. **301**(12): 1218–1220.

27. Honest H, Sharma S, Khan KS. (2006) Rapid tests for group B streptococcus colonization in laboring women: A systematic review. *Pediatrics* **117**(4): 1055–1066.

28. Listeria monocytogenes Infections (Listeriosis) (2009). *Red Book* **2009**(1): 428–430.

29. Brecht MCL, McGuire W. (2008) Prevention and treatment of invasive fungal infection in very low birthweight infants. *British Medical Journal.*

30. Manzoni P *et al.* (2007) A multicenter, randomized trial of prophylactic fluconazole in preterm neonates. *N Engl J Med* **356**(24): 2483–2495.

31. Benjamin D, Stoll BJ, Fanaroff AA *et al.* (2006) Neonatal candidiasis among extremely low birth weight infants: Risk factors, mortality rates and neurodevelopmental outcomes at 18 to 22 Months. *Pediatrics* **117**: 84–92.

32. Cotten CM *et al.* (2006) The association of third-generation cephalosporin use and invasive candidiasis in extremely low birth weight infants. *Pediatrics* **118**(2): 717–722.

33. Benjamin Jr, DK *et al.* (2000) When to suspect fungal infection in neonates: A clinical comparison of candida albicans and candida parapsilosis fungemia with coagulase-negative staphylococcal bacteremia. *Pediatrics* **106**(4): 712–718.

34. Saiman LMM *et al.* (2000) Risk factors for candidemia in Neonatal Intensive Care Unit patients. *Pediatric Infectious Disease Journal* **19**(4): 319–324.

35. Benjamin Jr, DK *et al.* (2001) Bacteremia, central catheters, and neonates: When to pull the line. *Pediatrics* **107**(6): 1272–1276.

36. Karlowicz MG *et al.* (2000) Should central venous catheters be removed as soon as candidemia is detected in neonates? *Pediatrics* **106**(5): E63.

37. Benjamin DK Jr., Stoll BJ, Gantz MJ, Walsh MC, Sanchez PJ, Das A *et al.* (2010) Neonatal candidasis: Epidemiology, risk factors and clinical judgement. *Pediatrics* **126**(4): e865–e873.

38. Kaufman D *et al.* (2001) Fluconazole prophylaxis against fungal colonization and infection in preterm infants. *N Engl J Med* **345**(23): 1660–1666.

39. Clerihew LAN, McGuire W. (2007) Prophylactic systemic antifungal agents to prevent mortality and morbidity in very low birth weight infants. *Cochrane Database of Systematic Reviews* (4).

40. Horan TC, Andrus M, Dudeck MA. (2008) CDC/NHSN surveillance definition of health care-associated infection and criteria for specific types of infections in the acute care setting. *Am J Infect Control* **36**(5): 309–332.

41. Garland JS *et al.* (2008) Cohort study of the pathogenesis and molecular epidemiology of catheter-related bloodstream infection in neonates with peripherally inserted central venous catheters. *Infect Control Hosp Epidemiol* **29**(3): 243–249.

42. Mahieu LM *et al.* (2001) Catheter manipulations and the risk of catheter-associated bloodstream infection in neonatal intensive care unit patients. *J Hosp Infect* **48**(1): 20–26.

43. Salzman MB *et al.* (1993) A prospective study of the catheter hub as the portal of entry for microorganisms causing catheter-related sepsis in neonates. *J Infect Dis* **167**(2): 487–490.

44. Kilbride HW *et al.* (2003) Implementation of evidence-based potentially better practices to decrease nosocomial infections. *Pediatrics* **111**(4 Pt 2): e519–e533.

45. O'Grady NP *et al.* (2002) Guidelines for the prevention of intravascular catheter-related infections. *Infect Control Hosp Epidemiol.* **23**(12): 759–769.

46. Andersen C *et al.* (2005) Prospective evaluation of a multi-factorial prevention strategy on the impact of nosocomial infection in very-low-birthweight infants. *J Hosp Infect* **61**(2): 162–167.

47. Horbar JD *et al.* (2001) Collaborative quality improvement for neonatal intensive care. NIC/Q Project Investigators of the Vermont Oxford Network. *Pediatrics* **107**(1): 14–22.

48. Døllner H, Vatten L, Austgulen R. (2001) Early diagnostic markers for neonatal sepsis: Comparing C-reactive protein, interleukin-6, soluble tumour necrosis factor receptors and soluble adhesion molecules. *Journal of Clinical Epidemiology* **54**(12): 1251–1257.

49. Ng PC CS, Chui KM, Fok TF, Wong MY, Wong W, Wong RPO, Cheung KL. (1997) Diagnosis of late onset neonatal sepsis with cytokines, adhesion molecule and C-reactive protein in preterm very low birthweight infants. *Arch. Dis. Child. Fetal Neonatal Ed* **77**: F221–F227.

50. Reier-Nilsen T, Farstad T, Nakstad B, Lauvrak V, Steinbakk M. (2009) Comparison of broad range 16S rDNA PCR and conventional blood culture for diagnosis of sepsis in the newborn: A case control study. *BMC Pediatrics* **9**(5).

51. Schelonka RLCUMC *et al.* (1996) Volume of blood required to detect common neonatal pathogens. *Journal of Pediatrics* **129**(2): 275–278.

52. Saez-Llorens X, Chai MK, Yoder BA *et al.* (1995) Applications of new sepsis definitions to evaluate outcome of pediatric patients with severe systemic infections. *Pediatr Infect Dis J* **14**: 557–561.

53. Kellogg JA, Manzella JP, Bankert DA. (2000) Frequency of low-level bacteremia in children from birth to fifteen years of age. *J Clin Microbiol* **38**(6): 2181–2185.

54. Sarkar S *et al.* (2005) A study of the role of multiple site blood cultures in the evaluation of neonatal sepsis. *J Perinatol* **26**(1): 18–22.

55. Makhoul IR, YA, Smolkin T, Sujov P, Kassis I, sprecher H. (2006) V values of C-reactive protein, procalcitonin and Staphylococcus-specific PCR in neonatal late-onset sepsis. *Acta Paediatrica* **95**: 1218–1223.

56. Jackson GL *et al.* (2004) Are complete blood cell counts useful in the evaluation of asymptomatic neonates exposed to suspected chorioamnionitis? *Pediatrics* **113**(5): 1173–1180.

57. Escobar GJ *et al.* (2000) Neonatal sepsis workups in infants ≥ 2000 Grams at birth: A population-based study. *Pediatrics* **106**(2): 256–263.

58. Johnson CE *et al.* (1997) Term newborns who are at risk for sepsis: Are lumbar punctures necessary? *Pediatrics* **99**(4): e10-.

59. Stoll BJ *et al.* (2004) To tap or not to tap: High likelihood of meningitis without sepsis among very low birth weight infants. *Pediatrics* **113**(5): 1181–1186.

60. Smith PB, Garges H, Cotten CM *et al.* (2008) Meningitis in preterm neonates: Importance of cerebrospinal fluid parameters. *Am J Perinatol* **25**(7): 421–426.

61. Mahieu LM *et al.* (2001) Additional hospital stay and charges due to hospital-acquired infections in a neonatal intensive care unit. *J Hosp Infect* **47**(3): 223–229.

62. Accreditation Program. Hospital: National Patient Safety Goals. The Joint Commission Website. [cited 2009 September 25]; Available from: http://www.jointcommission.org/patientsafety/nationalpatientsafetygoals/.

63. Adams-Chapman IMD, Stoll BJMD (2002) Prevention of nosocomial infections in the neonatal intensive care unit. *Current Opinion in Pediatrics*. **14**(2): 157–164.

64. Garland JS *et al.* (2005) A vancomycin-heparin lock solution for prevention of nosocomial bloodstream infection in critically-ill neonates with peripherally inserted central venous catheters: A prospective, randomized trial. *Pediatrics* **116**(2): e198–e205.

65. Safdar N, Maki DG (2006) Use of Vancomycin-containing lock or flush solutions for prevention of bloodstream infection associated with central venous access devices: A meta-analysis of prospective, randomized trials. *Clinical Infectious Diseases* **43**(4): 474–484.

66. Hintz SR *et al.* (2005) Neurodevelopmental and growth outcomes of extremely low birth weight infants after necrotizing enterocolitis. *Pediatrics* **115**(3): 696–703.

Chapter

17

Brain Injury in Preterm and Term Infants

Seetha Shankaran

Introduction

The goal of this chapter is to discuss neonatal intracranial hemorrhage (ICH) and periventricular leukomalacia (PVL) in preterm infants and hypoxic-ischemic encephalopathy (HIE) in term infants. The chapter will cover clinical findings and pathophysiology associated with ICH, PVL and HIE. Treatment strategies, outcome and prevention of ICH, PVL and HIE based on evidence will be presented.

Neonatal Intracranial Hemorrhage (ICH) in Preterm Infants

Site of ICH in preterm infants

Intracranial hemorrhage (ICH) in preterm infants occurs in the following sites:

(a) germinal matrix (the subependymal area around the ventricles),
(b) intraventricular region (IVH, hemorrhage within the ventricular system),

(c) parenchyma of the cerebral hemispheres (periventricular hemorrhagic infarction, PVHI), and

(d) hemorrhage in the cerebellar regions.

Pathogenesis of ICH in preterm infants

The pathogenesis of ICH is due to the fragility of the germinal matrix, alterations in cerebral blood flow, injury to the endothelium of the vasculature, presence of inflammatory mediators and genetic factors. The germinal matrix is persistent in preterm infants until the infant reaches 34 weeks postmenstrual age. Many factors contribute to the fragility of the germinal matrix: the rich vascularization of this area, the paucity of selective proteins (such as glial fibrillary acidic protein), a lower level of fibronectin in this area and a reduced density of pericytes in the matrix.[1] All these factors increase the propensity for hemorrhage. Disturbances in cerebral blood flow are common because the circulation is pressure passive and there is an impaired auto regulation of cerebral blood flow. Any increase in the central venous pressure or increase in arterial blood pressure is reflected in the cerebral circulation, demonstrating lack of auto regulation. Lastly, the high metabolic demand of the precursor cells in the germinal matrix makes them exquisitely sensitive to free radical injury compounded by a decrease in antioxidants in preterm infants. There is also an increase in inflammatory mediators noted among neonates with severe grades of ICH. Lastly, genetic markers are now being shown to be associated with increase risk for hemorrhage. Neonates who have a mutation in Factor V Gene (Gln506-FV) are at higher risk for ICH.

Timing and frequency of neonatal ICH

Most intracranial hemorrhages (50%) occur within the first 24 hours of life and the majority of which (90%) are detected within 72 hours of age. Infants with early hemorrhages have a three-fold risk of progression of hemorrhage. Recent studies have documented that early hemorrhage may be associated with mode of delivery (vaginal) and low Apgar Scores at birth and later hemorrhages with low superior vena cava flow.[2] Based on data from the NICHD Neonatal Research Network, the frequency of germinal matrix ICH is approximately 10%, while that of IVH is 6%. The frequency of persistent ventricular dilation following IVH is 7% and that of parenchymal PVHI is approximately 9%.[3] Cerebellar hemorrhages are rare; the true incidence is unknown, but these hemorrhages are being noted with increasing frequency in autopsy findings; 15–25% of preterm infants who had an autopsy performed had cerebellar hemorrhages.

Risk and protective factors for ICH

The *prenatal protective factors* that have been demonstrated in large data bases include the presence of hypertension or preeclampsia in the mother, black race, female gender and antenatal corticosteroid use.[4] Even a partial course of antenatal corticosteroids is protective. The *prenatal risk factors* for neonatal ICH in preterm infants include breech presentation of the fetus, a lower birth weight and a lower gestational age. Vaginal (versus cesarean) delivery has not been clearly shown to increase the risk of hemorrhage. The *postnatal factors that are associated with risk* of ICH include: out-born birth, resuscitation in the delivery room, need for mechanical ventilation, occurrence of pneumothorax, and the presence of hypercarbia, acidosis, respiratory distress syndrome and use of rapid volume expansion. $Paco_2$ is the main regulator of cerebral blood and elevation of $Paco_2$ results in an increase of cerebral blood flow. Fluctuations in cerebral blood flow also increase the risk of severe intracranial hemorrhage. In a retrospective evaluation of 849 infants with a birth weight <1250 g, the maximum $Paco_2$, minimum $Paco_2$ and time/weighted average $Paco_2$ were all associated independently with severe ICH, in addition to the clinical variables of lower gestational age, lower five-minute Apgar score and need for mechanical ventilation. Antenatal steroid use and pregnancy-induced hypertension were protective against ICH in this study.[5]

Intraparenchymal periventricular hemorrhagic infarction (PHVI) usually involves the white matter, tends to be unilateral, is either localized or extensive and is due to a venous infarction.

Cerebellar hemorrhages are clinically silent; therefore these hemorrhages were diagnosed only in post mortem studies. In a study where 35 cases of cerebellar hemorrhage were matched with 70 preterm infants with normal cranial sonography, it was noted that 71% of the cerebellar hemorrhage were unilateral, 20% occurred in the vermian area while 9% had combined bihemispheric and vermian locations. In 23% of the cases, the cerebellar hemorrhage was isolated while in the remaining cases there was an association with supratentorial lesions. A multiple regression analysis revealed that risk factors associated with cerebellar hemorrhage were emergency cesarean section, the presence of a PDA and acidosis. The neonatal mortality and morbidity was significantly higher in the infants with cerebellar hemorrhage compared to the control infants in the study.[6]

Diagnosis of ICH in preterm infants

ICH in preterm infants may not be associated with symptoms of an acute deterioration or apnea since the majority of these infants may be receiving respiratory support. A large ICH may be preceded by a drop in hematocrit. The optimum way of diagnosing ICH is by cranial sonography. Ideally, the first sonographic study should be performed between day 5 and day 7 unless clinically indicated prior to this time. If any ICH is noted, infants should have serial weekly sonograms to evaluate progression of the ICH. If the initial ICH is completely normal a repeat cranial sonogram should be done around 32 weeks post menstrual age or between 3 to 5 weeks of age to capture any ischemic lesions that were not detected on the initial study. It should be noted that echo densities in early cranial ultrasounds may progress onto hemorrhagic or to ischemic brain injury.

Complications following neonatal ICH in preterm infants

The complications of neonatal ICH are related to the location and the severity of ICH. The majority of infants with ICH limited to the germinal matrix area have normal neurodevelopmental outcome. A recent study evaluating 20 month follow-up of infants with mild grades of ICH: hemorrhage in the germinal matrix or IVH without associated ventricular enlargement ($n = 104$) noted that developmental outcome was not as optimum as those neonates with normal cranial sonography ($n = 258$). Compared to infants with no ICH, infants with germinal matrix or IVH without ventriculomegaly had lower Bayley II Mental Developmental Index (MDI) scores (74 ± 16 vs 79 ± 14, $P < 0.01$), a higher frequency of infants with MDI scores < 70 (45% vs 25%, $P < 0.01$) and a higher rate of major neurologic abnormalities (13% vs 5%, $P < 0.05$) and neurodevelopmental impairment (47% vs 28%, $P < 0.05$).[7]

The most common complication of IVH is the occurrence of post hemorrhagic ventriculomegaly (PHVM), seen in 60 to 70% of preterm neonates with blood within the ventricular system. The majority of PHVM (65%) spontaneously arrest while the remaining infants with persistent increase in ventricular size require intervention. PHVM is due to obstruction of the ventricular system due to blood clots, basal arachnoiditis, and destruction of the white matter. The diagnosis of ventriculomegaly can best be evaluated by serial (weekly) sonograms. If serial ultrasounds demonstrate progressive increase in ventricular size, intervention is needed.

Pharmacological management of progressive ventriculomegaly has not been successful. Medications that have been evaluated include those administered to decrease CSF production (acetozolamide or furosemide) or medications to promote fibrinolysis (intraventricular streptokinase or tissue plasminogen activator). A RCT to evaluate the role of acetozolamide and furosemide in PHVM was published in 1998 where 177 infants with PHVM received either standard care or acetozolamide and furosemide. The trial was stopped early because mortality rate and disability were increased in the group receiving the treatment intervention.[8] A recent study evaluating the treatment of PHVM using drainage, irrigation and fibrinolytic therapy demonstrated that there was no benefit to ventricular drainage with streptokinase when compared to ventricular taps by reservoir catheter. The number of infants who had secondary intraventricular hemorrhage following irrigations with the fibrinolytic agent was higher than the reservoir therapy group.[9] Currently the majority of neonatal intensive care units remove CSF periodically following a reservoir placed in the ventricles when progressive PHVM occurs. Daily taps of the reservoir are preformed and when the infant is clinically stable and around 1.8 kg in weight placement of a ventriculoperitoneal shunt (VPS) occurs. It should be noted that blood clots within the ventricular system may be noted for up to six weeks following an IVH. The complications of VPS include infection, obstruction and injury to the optic tracts. Neuro-developmental outcome following PHVM is very discouraging. The NICHD Neonatal Research Network has presented the largest cohort study of outcome following PHVM where infants with no ICH ($n = 5167$) were compared with infants with IVH with no VPS ($n = 459$), infants with IVH with VPS ($n = 103$), cerebral parenchymal hemorrhage with no shunt ($n = 311$) and parenchymal ICH with VPS ($n = 125$). It was noted that the rate of cerebral palsy was 10% in the no ICH/no VPS group, 23% in the IVH/no VPS group, 37% in the parenchymal hemorrhage/no VPS, 57% IVH/VPS and 80% in the parenchymal hemorrhage/VPS group. The median MDI value for each of these groups was 82, 75, 72, 61 and 50 respectively.[10]

Unilateral PHVI results in a better outcome than bilateral PHVI. In a study of 69 infants <1500 g birth weight (52 unilateral, 17 bilateral PVHI), at 18–36 months the median MDI was higher among those with unilateral PHVI compared to those with bilateral PHVI (82 vs 49). The infants with unilateral PHVI had higher Psychomotor Developmental Index scores (median PDI, 53 vs 49) and were less likely to have moderate/severe CP than those with bilateral PHVI (37% vs 88%). By comparing the laterality of PHVI and presence of periventricular leucomalacia (PVL), and retinopathy of prematurity a better estimate of severe cognitive delay (MDI < 70) could be obtained.[11] A severity of PVHI scoring evaluating location PHVI ($\geq$ two territories of cerebral hemispheres), whether unilateral or bilateral and whether midline shift occurs is predictive of short-term outcome. Among 30 infants (12–66 months at follow-up), infants with higher PVHI scores had a much higher rate of cerebral palsy, visual field defects, gross motor and find motor abnormalities, as well as delays in language development.[12] In another study ($n = 25$) of infants with PHVI evaluated between 4 and 12 years of age, the rate of unilateral CP was 62% and bilateral CP was 14%. However, these infants had better functional outcome than previously thought as IQ was within 1 SD of the norm of preterm infants without PHVI in 60–80% of the children. Behavioral and executive function were very minimally impaired compared to preterm infants with no hemorrhage.[13]

Prevention of neonatal ICH in preterm infants

Antenatal prevention of ICH is a combination of prevention of preterm delivery, treatment of maternal complications and intrapartum fetal surveillance with obstetric intervention when needed. The use of pharmacological agents for the antenatal prevention of neonatal ICH such as phenobarbital and vitamin K has not been proven to be of benefit. Postnatal prevention of ICH includes supportive measures such as resuscitation with minimal distending pressure, adequate oxygenation and stabilization of blood pressure, minimal ventilation and avoidance of hypocarbia, minimal handling and surfactant therapy. Post natal pharmacological prevention of neonatal ICH has not been proven to be successful with phenobarbital, tranexamic acid, or pancuronium. Vitamin E does appear to be beneficial, although it has not been evaluated in a large RCT. The large multicenter trial of indomethacin for prophylaxis against hemorrhage in preterm infants (TIPP) study did demonstrate a decrease in neonatal ICH but no difference in neurodevelopmental outcome in infancy (the primary outcome of the study).[14] Indomethacin administered shortly after birth decreased severity of ICH in preterm infants, however at 12 years of age, follows up of participants demonstrated that preterm infants with severe brain injury had serious deficits in their neuropsychological profile while indomethacin did not affect intellectual function.[15]

Periventricular Leucomalacia (PVL)

The incidence of PVL is approximately 3% with a wide range (1–6%) in the NICHD Neonatal Research Network centers. The location of PVL is in the periventricular watershed region. PVL is an ischemic injury due to a decrease in cerebral blood flow and can be diffuse or localized. The clinical presentation is associated with any condition known to decrease systemic blood pressure including chorioamnionitis, severe respiratory distress, myocardial failure, sepsis, repeated apneic episodes and hypocarbia.[16–18] The cerebral blood flow velocity among infants with PVL has been noted to be decreased in all major cerebral arteries shortly after birth.[18] PVL is best diagnosed by sonography where the lesions initially appear echo dense and later appear as cavitations or Swiss cheese appearance.

Outcome following PVL is associated with both cognitive and motor deficits. The classification of PVL is based on location and extent of injury. It is important to examine whether PVL has developed into single or multiple cysts as a correlation has been noted with extent of PVL: grades II (small cystic areas) or III (extensive cystic areas) and outcome. In the study by Pierrat et al. over a 9-year period with 96 of 3451 infants (2.8%) with PVL, 50% of these infants had grade II cPVL. Grade II cPVL was noted to occur usually beyond a month of age and was often unilateral compared to Grade III cPVL. In many infants with grade II cPVL when the infant was 40 weeks post menstrual age the cyst were no longer visible on sonography. The rate and severity of CP was less common in Grade II PVL as compared to Grade III PVL.[19] Motor and cognitive developmental outcome after PVL has been shown to be correlated with the laterality, size and number of cystic lesions. Unilateral PVL was associated with lower rate of CP compared to bilateral PVL (66 vs 79%), and mental retardation (defined as IQ or developmental quotient <70) was noted in 35% with unilateral lesions compared to 43% with bilateral lesions. Small lesions are associated with 35% rate of CP compared to 94% with large lesions and the corresponding percentage of infants with MR is 11% versus 60%.[20]

Neonatal Hypoxic-Ischemic Encephalopathy in Term Infants

Neonatal encephalopathy

Neonatal encephalopathy due to hypoxia-ischemia occurs in 1 to 6 per 1000 live full term births in developed countries. Fifteen to 20% of affected newborns will die in the postnatal period and an additional 25% will sustain childhood disabilities. The presence of an abnormal neurologic examination in first few days of life is the single most useful predictor in childhood that a brain insult has occurred in the perinatal period. Neonates with mild encephalopathy do not have an increased risk of motor or cognitive deficits. Neonates with severe encephalopathy have an increased risk of death and an increased risk of cerebral palsy (CP) and mental retardation amongst survivors. Neonates with moderate encephalopathy have significant motor deficits, memory impairment, visual motor or visual perceptive dysfunction, increased hyper activity and delayed school readiness.[21,22]

The essential criteria suggested as prerequisites to a diagnosis of a hypoxic-ischemic insult resulting in moderate or severe encephalopathy in term newborn infants include: Metabolic acidosis with a cord pH <7 or a base deficit ≥12 mmol/L, early onset of encephalopathy, multi-system organ dysfunction and exclusion of other etiology such as trauma, coagulation disorders, metabolic disorders and genetic causes.[23]

Pathophysiology of neonatal hypoxic-ischemic brain injury

The pathophysiology of brain injury secondary to hypoxia-ischemia has been well studied. Hypoxia-ischemia is associated with two phases of pathologic events that culminate in brain injury (Table 1). These phases are primary and secondary energy failure based on characteristics of the cerebral energy state used to describe the temporal sequence in newborn animals.[24] Primary energy failure is characterized by reductions in cerebral blood flow and O_2 substrates. High-energy phosphorylated compounds such as ATP and phosphocreatine are reduced and tissue acidosis is prominent. This phase is an essential prerequisite for all deleterious events that follow. Primary energy failure is associated with acute intracellular

Table 1.   Mechanisms of damage in fetal/neonatal model of hypoxia ischemia.

Primary energy failure

- Increased release and decreased uptake of excitatory amino acids
- Loss of ionic homeostasis across membranes
- Decreased ATP production
- Generation of reactive oxygen species
- Activation of lipases and proteases

Secondary energy failure

- Activation of microglia — inflammatory response
- Activation of caspase proteins — trigger apoptosis
- Reduction in growth factors, protein synthesis
- Further accumulation of excitotoxic neurotransmitters

derangements such as loss of membrane ionic homeostasis, release/ blocked reuptake of excitatory neurotransmitters, defective osmoregulation and inhibition of protein synthesis.[25] Excessive stimulation of neurotransmitter receptors and loss of ionic homeostasis mediate an increase in intracellular calcium and osmotic dysregulation. Elevation in intracellular calcium triggers a number of destructive pathways by activating lipases, proteases and endonucleases.[26] Resolution of hypoxia-ischemia within a specific time interval reverses the fall in high-energy phosphorylated metabolites and intracellular pH and promotes recycling of neurotransmitters. The duration of time for hypoxia-ischemia to be successfully reversed and promote recovery will be affected by maturation, preconditioning events, substrate availability, body temperature and simultaneous disease processes. Although recovery of the cerebral energy state may occur following primary energy failure, a second interval of energy failure may occur at a time remote from the initiating event. Secondary energy failure differs from primary energy failure in that declines in phosphocreatine and ATP are not accompanied by brain acidosis.[24] The presence and severity of secondary energy failure depends on the extent of primary energy failure. The pathogenesis of secondary energy failure is not as well understood as primary energy failure, but likely involves multiple processes including accumulation of excitatory neurotransmitters, oxidative injury, apoptosis, inflammation, and altered growth factors and protein synthesis.[27–31]

The interval between primary and secondary energy failure represents a latent phase that corresponds to a therapeutic window. Initiation of therapies during the latent phase in perinatal animals has been successful in reducing brain damage and substantiates the presence of a therapeutic window. The duration of the therapeutic window is approximately 6 hours in near-term fetal sheep based on the neuroprotection associated with brain cooling initiated at varying intervals following brain ischemia.[32,33]

Current therapies for neonatal hypoxic-ischemic encephalopathy

The management of neonates with hypoxic-ischemic encephalopathy (HIE) has been limited to supportive intensive care. The latter includes correction of hemodynamic and pulmonary disturbances (hypotension, metabolic acidosis, and hypoventilation), correction of metabolic disturbances (glucose, calcium, magnesium and electrolytes), treatment of seizures and monitoring for other organ system dysfunction. This management approach does not target any component of the patho-physiological sequence leading to hypoxic-ischemic brain injury and is directed at avoiding injury from secondary events associated with hypoxia-ischemia.

Diagnosis of encephalopathy in term infants

A detailed history should be obtained regarding the pregnancy and intrapartum period as the first step in diagnosing encephalopathy. Any event likely to compromise blood or oxygen supply to the fetus should be examined. These events include a history of placental abruption, uterine rupture, amniotic fluid embolism, tight nuchal cord, cord prolapse/avulsion, maternal hemorrhage, trauma or cardio respiratory arrest, severe and sustained fetal bradycardia and prolonged labor. The majority of infants with encephalopathy do not have an obvious cause for the encephalopathy. There is currently no clear diagnostic test for encephalopathy due to hypoxia-ischemia. A history of maternal elevation of temperature is crucial as moderate elevation of temperature in the mother increases the risk of neonatal encephalopathy. A history of fetal tachycardia and maternal tachycardia may also raise suspicions of chorioamnionitis. Laboratory evaluations that should be performed include placenta pathology to evaluate the presence of placental infection. Elevated biomarkers (elevated cytokines) may improve the ability to predict outcome. All neonates should have a detailed neurologic examination to evaluate the presence of mild, moderate or severe encephalopathy.[34]

Hypothermia as neuroprotection: preclinical studies

There is established evidence in fetal and neonatal animal models, and across species, that cooling by a depth of 4–6°C vs controls has been neuroprotective while being well tolerated.[32,33,35–42] The duration of cooling in these studies varied from 3 to 72 hours, and each study compared a specific depth of cooling to controls. None of these studies comparing a specific depth of hypothermia to controls report any adverse effects except one report of a piglet shivering during the cooling. The mechanism of neuroprotection has been documented by many modalities, including a decrease in brain energy utilization measured by magnetic resonance spectroscopy, reduction of infarct size, decrease in neuronal cell loss, retention of sensory motor function, preservation of hippocampal structures and recovery of electroencephalographic activity[32,35,37,38,43,44] (Table 2). Neuroprotection with hypothermia is temperature specific, with progressively increased protection with increasing depth of temperature (up to a depth of 28°C). None of these studies comparing different depths of temperature to controls in the same models document adverse effects of hypothermia. In addition, adjusting brain temperatures from 28°C and 41°C did not alter any systemic variable in the piglet model except for heart rate, which directly correlated with brain temperature.

Hypothermia as neuroprotection: clinical studies

To date, four randomized controlled trials and one large pilot study have been published evaluating hypothermia as neuroprotection for term and near term infants with HIE. The multicenter Cool Cap Study involved 243 infants with moderate or severe encephalopathy and abnormal aEEG amplitude, who were either cooled to a temperature of 34 to 35°C for 72 hours or treated with temperature maintenance in the normothermia range with conventional care.[45] The primary outcome of the study was death or disability at 18 months. Cooling was provided by selective head

Table 2.   Mechanism of action of hypothermia.

* Reduces cerebral metabolism, prevents edema
* Decreases energy utilization
* Reduces/suppresses cytotoxic AA accumulation and NO
* Inhibits PAF inflammatory cascade
* Suppresses free radical activity
* Attenuates secondary energy failure
* Inhibits apoptosis (cell death)
* Reduces extent of brain injury

cooling with mild systemic cooling. Death or severe disability occurred in 66% of infants randomized to conventional care and 55% randomized to the cooled group, odds ratio (OR, 95% CI) 0.61 (0.34–1.09), $P = 0.10$. The effect of head cooling for infants with the most severe aEEG changes was not protective; on the other hand, the effect of head cooling for infants with less severe aEEG changes ($n = 172$) was protective with OR 0.42 (0.22–0.80; $P = 0.009$).

The large, randomized controlled pilot study performed at seven centers with 65 infants involved moderate systemic whole body hypothermia to 33°C for 48 hours compared to normothermia maintained at 37°C.[46] The safety report of this pilot study documented that infants in the hypothermia group had more significant bradycardia, longer dependence on pressor medications, higher prothrombin times, more seizures and need for more plasma and platelet transfusions. At 12 months of age, death or severe motor scores occurred in 52% of hypothermia group compared to 84% of normothermia group ($P = 0.02$). In a sub-group analysis, out-born infants were more likely to die than inborn infants, OR 10.7 (1.3–90.0).

The NICHD Neonatal Research Network trial of whole body hypothermia for infants with moderate and severe encephalopathy randomized 102 infants to hypothermia to 33.5°C for 72 hours and 106 control infants to conventional care.[47] The primary outcome was death or moderate/severe disability at 18 months of age. The infants in the hypothermia group had significantly lower heart rates than the infants in the control group throughout the 72 hour intervention period. There was no significant difference in systolic or diastolic blood pressure between groups. The frequency of adverse events during study intervention was low: one infant in each group had arrhythmia, two infants in the hypothermia group had acidosis, three infants in the hypothermia group and two control group infants had bleeding, and four cooled infants had altered skin integrity. The primary outcome was noted in 44% of infants in the hypothermia group compared to 62% of infants in the control group with a risk ratio of 0.72 (0.54–0.95). There was a trend for cooling to benefit infants in both moderate and severe encephalopathy groups.

The most recent RCT evaluating moderate hypothermia as neuroprotection is the Total Body Hypothermia for Neonatal Encephalopathy

(TOBY) trial.[48] Infants were eligible if moderate or severe encephalopathy was present and an abnormal background or seizures on the aEEG. The primary outcome was death or severe disability at 18 months. Of 325 infants enrolled, 163 underwent whole body cooling and 162 served as controls. In the cooled group, 42 infants died and 32 survived with severe neurodevelopmental disability, compared to 44 infants who died and 42 survived with severe disability (RR, 95% CI for either outcome 0.86 (0.68–1.07, $P = 0.17$). Infants in the cooled group had an increased rate of survival without neurological abnormality, RR 1.57(1.16–2.12). Among survivors, cooling resulted in reduced risks of CP and improved scores in the Mental and Motor Developmental Indices.

Elevated temperatures in infants with hypoxic-ischemic encephalopathy

The NICHD trial of whole body hypothermia demonstrated the occurrence of elevated core body temperature in the control group infants when temperatures were measured in a consistent manner in the 76 hours of study intervention and re-warming phases.[47] Of the 102 infants randomized to the usual care group, 28 infants had a median esophageal temperature $\geq$ 38°C. Higher core temperatures were associated with significant increases in risk of death or impairment in the control group.[49] In a secondary analysis of the Cool Cap trial, investigators also noted an association between elevated temperatures in the control group and increased risk of death or disability.[50] Hyperthermia after brain injury adds to the risk of more severe neurologic damage, and studies in adults consistently support association between higher core temperatures and worse outcome.[51] In the animal model, seizures associated with a hypoxic ischemic insult result in neuronal cell death, specifically within the hippocampus. The damage to the hippocampus occurs in the setting of spontaneously occurring hyperthermia of 1.5°C above normothermia; rat pups in whom hyperthermia was prevented during seizures displayed significant reduction in brain damage compared to controls. Neonatal rats subjected to hypoxic ischemic injury were noted to have selective and long lasting learning and memory impairments during behavioral tasks and hypothermia to 27°C significantly reduced the deficit in behavioral tasks, whereas hyperthermia aggravated the behavioral deficit and the brain injury.[52]

Four secondary analyses have been published from the NICHD RCT. In one study examining the relationship of elevated temperature after HIE, 22% of esophageal core temperatures measured among the control group infants were higher than 37.5°C. The odds of death or disability were increased 3.6 to 4-fold for each centigrade increase in the highest quartile of temperature in the control group.[49] Another study evaluating predictors of outcome has revealed that the classification and regression tree model, rather than the scoring system developed from identified variables and odds ratios, was superior to the early neurologic examination in predicting death/disability in this study.[53] A secondary study involving spot urine samples collected in 58 study participants revealed that a high urinary lactate to creatinine ratio was associated with death/disability.[54] Lastly, detailed analysis of the randomized controlled trial data revealed safety of hypothermia during the study intervention period, the entire hospital course and during follow-up to 18–22 months.[55]

Meta-analyses of trials

Three independent systematic reviews recently published have concluded that therapeutic hypothermia significantly (a) reduces both death and disability after perinatal encephalopathy (b) is safe and (c) outcomes are homogeneous both within and between trials.[56–58]

Gaps in knowledge regarding therapeutic hypothermia as neuroprotection

All the current published trials have evaluated hypothermia as a neuroprotective strategy with the primary outcome of death or disability at 18 months of age. To assess efficacy in childhood, assessments of school-age outcome are being evaluated in the Cool Cap and NICHD Network Trial. The role of cranial imaging in predicting outcome among infants undergoing hypothermia is currently being evaluated from MRI studies obtained in the NICHD trial. The role of initiating hypothermia beyond 6 hours of age in term infants is being examined as there is now evidence that effects of brain injury following hypoxia-ischemia in the preclinical model continues beyond the 6 hour therapeutic window. Hypothermia as neuroprotection for the 34–36 week gestation neonate with encephalopathy is also being investigated. The impact of hypothermia initiated during transport at <6 hours of age has not been demonstrated. The results of current whole body cooling trials, the ICE and European trials are pending. The optimum depth and duration of cooling for demonstrating better neuroprotection is unknown. The role of pharmacologic agents used along with hypothermia as neuroprotection for hypoxic ischemic brain injury is being actively investigated in preclinical studies. It should be noted that disability is high with severe HIE in spite of therapeutic hypothermia.

References

1. Ballabh P. (2010) Intraventricular hemorrhage in premature infants: Mechanism of disease. *Pediatric Research* **67**: 1–8.
2. Osborn DA, Evans N, Kluckow M. (2003) Hemodynamic and antecedent risk factors of early and late periventricular/intraventricular hemorrhage in premature infants. *Pediatrics* **112**: 33–39.
3. Stoll B, Hansen NL, Bell EF *et al.* (2010). Neonatal outcomes of extremely preterm infants from the NICHD Neonatal Research Network. *Pediatrics* **126**: 443–456.
4. Shankaran S, Bauer CR, Bain R *et al.* (1996) Prenatal and perinatal risk and protective factors for neonatal intracranial hemorrhage. *Arch Pediatr Adolesc Med* **150**: 491–497.
5. Fabres J, Carlo WA, Phillips V *et al.* (2007) Both extremes of arterial carbon dioxide pressure and the magnitude of fluctuations in arterial carbon dioxide pressure are associated with severe intraventricular hemorrhage in preterm infants. *Pediatrics* **119**: 299–305.
6. Limperopoulos C, Benson CB, Bassan H *et al.* (2005) Cerebellar hemorrhage in the preterm infant: Ultrasonographic findings and risk factors. *Pediatrics* **116**: 717–724.
7. Patra K, Wilson-Costello D, Taylor HG *et al.* (2006) Grades I-II intraventricular hemorrahge in extremely low birth weight infants: Effects on neurodevelopment. *J Pediatrics* **149**: 169–173.

8. International PHVD Drug Trial Group. (1998) International randomised controlled trial of acetazolamide and furosemide in posthaemorrhagic ventricular dilatation in infancy. *The Lancet* **352**: 433–440.

9. Whitelaw A, Evans D, Carter M *et al.* (2007) Randomized clinical trial of prevention of hydrocephalus after intraventricular hemorrhage in preterm infants: Brain-washing versus tapping fluid. *Pediatrics* **119**: e1071–e1078.

10. Adams-Chapman I, Hansen NI, Stoll BJ *et al.* For the NICHD Research Network (2008) Neurodevelopmental outcome of extremely low birth weight infants with posthemorrhagic hydrocephalus requiring shunt insertion. *Pediatrics* **121**: e1167–e1177.

11. Maitre NL, Marshall DD, Price WA *et al.* (2009) Neurodevelopmental outcome of infants with unilateral or bilateral periventricular hemorrhagic infarction. *Pediatrics* **124**: e1153–e1160.

12. Bassan H, Limperopoulos C, Visconti K *et al.* (2007) Neurodevelopmental outcome in survivors of periventricular hemorrhagic infarction. *Pediatrics* **120**: 785–792.

13. Roze E, Van Braeckel K, van der Veere CN *et al.* (2009) Functional outcome at school age of preterm infants with periventricular hemorrhagic infarction. *Pediatrics* **123**: 1493–1500.

14. Schmidt B, Davis P, Moddemann D *et al.* For the Trial of Indomethacin Prophylaxis in Preterms Investigators. (2001) Long-term effects of indomethacin prophylaxis in extremely-low-birth-weight infants. *N. Engl J Med* **344**: 1966–1972.

15. Luu TM, Ment LR, Schneider KC *et al.* (2009) Lasting effects of preterm birth and neonatal brain hemorrhage at 12 years of age. *Pediatrics* **123**: 1037–1044.

16. Shankaran S, Langer JC, Kazzi SN *et al.* For the National Institute of Child Health and Human Development Neonatal Research Network. (2006) Cumulative index of exposure to hypocarbia and hyperoxia as risk factors for periventricular leukomalacia in low birth weight infants. *Pediatrics* **118**: 1654–1659.

17. Okumura A, Hayakawa F, Kato T *et al.* (2001). Hypocarbia in preterm infants with periventricular leukomalacia: The relation between hypocarbia and mechanical ventilation. *Pediatrics* **107**: 469–475.

18. Fukuda S, Kato T, Kakita H *et al.* (2006) Hemodynamics of the cerebral arteries of infants with periventricular leukomalacia. *Pediatrics* **117**: 1–8.

19. Pierrat V, Duquénnoy C, van Haastert IC *et al.* (2001) Ultrasound diagnosis and neurodevelopmental outcome of localised and extensive cystic periventricular leukomalacia. *Arch Dis Child Fetal Neonatal Ed* **84**: F151–F156.

20. Holling EE, Leviton A. (1999). Characteristics of cranial ultrasound whitematter echolucencies that predict disability: A review. *Developmental Medicine and Child Neurology* **41**: 136–139.

21. Roberston CMT, Finer NN, Grace MGA. (1989) School performance of survivors of neonatal encephalopathy associated with birth asphyxia at term. *J Pediatr* **114**: 753–760.

22. Shankaran S, Woldt E, Koepke T *et al.* (1991) Acute neonatal morbidity and long-term central nervous system sequelae of perinatal asphyxia in term infants. *Early Hum Dev* **25**: 135–148.

23. American College of Obstetricians and Gynecologist and American Academy of Pediatrics. (2003) Neonatal encephalopathy and cerebral palsy. Defining the pathogenesis and pathophysiology. *Library of Congress* 1–93.

24. Lorek A, Takei Y, Cady EB *et al.* (1994) Delayed ("secondary") cerebral energy failure after acute hypoxia-ischemia in the newborn piglet: Continuous 48-hour studies by phosphorus magnetic resonance spectroscopy. *Pediatr Res* **36**: 699–706.

25. Johnston MV, Trescher WH, Ishida A *et al.* (2001) Neurobiology of hypoxic-ischemic injury in the developing brain. *Pediatr Res* **49**: 735–741.

26. Siesjo BK and Bengtsson F. (1989) Calcium fluxes, calcium antagonists, and calcium-related pathology in brain ischemia, hypoglycemia, and spreading depression: A unifying hypothesis. *J Cereb Blood Flow Metab* **9**: 127–140.

27. Fellman V, Raivio KO. (1997) Reperfusion injury as the mechanism of brain damage after perinatal asphyxia. *Pediatr Res* **41**: 599–606.

28. Liu XH, Kwon D, Schielke GP *et al.* (1999) Mice deficient in interleukin-1 converting enzyme are resistant to neonatal hypoxic-ischemic brain damage. *J Cereb Blood Flow Metab* **19**: 1099–1108.

29. Mehmet H, Yue X, Squier MV *et al.* (1994) Increased apoptosis in the cingulate sulcus of newborn piglets following transient hypoxia-ischaemia is related to the degree of high energy phosphate depletion during the insult. *Neurosci Lett* **181**: 121–125.

30. Tan WK, Williams CE, During MJ *et al.* (1996) Accumulation of cytotoxins during the development of seizures and edema after hypoxic-ischemic injury in late gestation fetal sheep. *Pediatr Res* **39**: 791–797.

31. Gluckman PD, Guan J, Williams C *et al.* (1998) Asphyxial brain injury — the role of the IGF system. *Mol Cell Endocrinol* **140**: 95–99.

32. Gunn AJ, Gunn TR, Gunning MI *et al.* (1998) Neuroprotection with prolonged head cooling started before postischemic seizures in fetal sheep. *Pediatrics* **102**: 1098–1106.

33. Gunn AJ, Bennet L, Gunning MI *et al.* (1999) Cerebral hypothermia is not neuroprotective when started after postischemic seizures in fetal sheep. *Pediatr Res* **46**: 274–280.

34. Sarnat HB, Sarnat MS. (1976) Neonatal encephalopathy following fetal distress: A clinical and electroencephalographic study. *Arch Neurol* **33**: 696–705.

35. Bona E, Hagberg H, Løberg EM *et al.* (1998) Protective effect of moderate hypothermia after neonatal hypoxia-ischemia: Short and long term outcome. *Pediatr Res* **43**: 738–745.

36. Busto R, Dietrich WD, Globus MYT *et al.* (1987) Small differences in intraischemic brain temperature critically determine the extent of ischemic neuronal injury. *J Cereb Blood Flow Metab* **7**: 729–738.

37. Carroll M, Beek O. (1992) Protection against hippocampal CA cell loss by post-ischemic hypothermia is dependent of delay of initiation and duration. *Metab Brain Dis* **7**: 45–50.

38. Colbourne F, Corbett D. (1994) Delayed and prolonged post-ischemic hypothermia is Neuroprotective in the gerbil. *Brain Research* **656**: 265–272.

39. O'Brien FE, Iwata O, Thornton JS *et al.* (2006) Delayed whole body cooling to 33 to 35C and the development of impaired energy generation consequential to transient cerebral hypoxia-ischemia in the newborn piglet. *Pediatrics* **117**: 1549–1558.

40. Sirimanne ES, Blumberg RM, Bossano D *et al.* (1996) The effect of prolonged modification of cerebral temperature on outcome after hypoxia-ischemic brain injury in the infant rat. *Pediatr Res* **39**: 591–597.

41. Thoresen M, Penrice J, Lorek A *et al.* (1995) Mild hypothermia following severe transient hypoxia-ischemic ameliorates delayed cerebral energy failure in the newborn piglet. *Pediatr Res* **5**: 667–670.

42. Thoresen M, Simmonds M, Satas S *et al.* (2001) Effective selective head cooling during posthypoxic hypothermia in newborn piglets. *Pediatr Res* **49**: 594–599.

43. Laptook AR, Corbett RJ, Sterett R *et al.* (1995) Quantitative relationship between brain temperature and energy utilization rate measured *in vivo* using P and H magnetic resonance spectroscopy. *Pediatr Res* **38**: 919.

44. Taylor DL, Mehmet H, Cady EB *et al.* (2002) Improved neuroprotection with hypothermia delayed by 6 hours following cerebral hypoxia-ischemia in the 14-day-old rat. *Pediatr Res* **51**: 13–19.

45. Gluckman PD, Wyatt J, Azzopardi DV *et al.* on the behalf of the Cool Cap Study Group. (2005) Selective head cooling with mild systemic hypothermia after neonatal encephalopathy: Multicenter randomized trial. *Lancet* **365**: 663–670.

46. Eicher DJ, Wagner CL, Katikaneni LP *et al.* (2005) Moderate Hypothermia in Neonatal Encephalopathy: Efficacy outcomes. *J Pediatr Neurol* **32**: 11–17.

47. Shankaran S, Laptook AR, Ehrenkranz RA *et al.* and the NICHD and Human Development Neonatal Research Network. (2005) Whole-body hypothermia for neonates with hypoxic-ischemic encephalopathy. *N Engl J Med* **353**: 1574–1584.

48. Azzopardi DV, Strohm B, Edwards AD *et al.* For the TOBY Study Group. (2009) Moderate Hypothermia to Treat Perinatal Asphyxial Encephalopathy. *N Engl J Med* **362**: 1051.

49. Laptook A, Tyson J, Shankaran S *et al.* (2008) Elevated temperature after hypoxic-ischemic encephalopathy: Risk factor for adverse outcomes. *Pediatrics* **122**: 491–499.

50. Wyatt JS, Gluckman PD, Liu PY *et al.* For the Cool Cap Study Group. (2007) Determinants of outcomes after head cooling for neonatal encephalopathy. *Pediatrics* **119**: 912–921.

51. Bramlett HM, Dietrich WD. (2007) Progressive damage after brain and spinal cord injury; pathomechanisms and treatment strategies. *Prog Brain Res* **161**: 125–141.

52. Mishima K, Ikeda T, Yoshikawa T *et al.* (2004) Effects of hypothermia and hyperthermia on attention and spatial learning deficits following neonatal hypoxia-ischemic insult in rats. *Behav Brain Res* **151**: 209–217.

53. Ambalavanan N, Carlo WA, Shankaran S *et al.* National Institute of Child Health and Human Development Neonatal Research Network. (2006) Predicting outcomes of neonates diagnosed with hypoxemic-ischemic encephalopathy. *Pediatrics* **118**: 2084–2093.

54. Oh W, Perritt R, Shankaran S *et al.* (2008) Association between urinary lactate to creatinine ratio and neurodevelopmental outcome in term infants with hypoxic-ischemic encephalopathy. *J Pediatr* **153**: 375–378.

55. Shankaran S, Pappas A, Laptook AR *et al.* Das A for the NICHD Neonatal Research Network. (2008) Outcomes of safety and effectiveness in a multi-center randomized controlled trial of whole body hypothermia for neonatal hypoxic ischemic encephalopathy. *Pediatrics* 122: e791–e798.

56. Shah PS, Ohlsson A, Perlman A. (2007) Hypothermia to treat neonatal hypoxic ischemic encephalopathy. *Arch Pediatr Adolesc Med* 161: 951–958.

57. Schulzke SM, Rao S, Patole SK. (2007) A systematic review of cooling for neuroprotection with hypoxic ischemic encephalopathy — are we there yet? *BMC Pediatrics* 7: 1–30.

58. Jacob S, Hunt R, Tarnow-Mordi W *et al.* (2007) Cooling for newborns with hypoxic ischemic encephalopathy. *Cochrane Database of Systemic Reviews* 4: 1–46.

Chapter 18

Retinopathy of Prematurity: Current Concepts in Pathogenesis and Treatment

Joseph M. Bliss

Introduction

Retinopathy of prematurity (ROP) is a vasoproliferative disorder of the developing retina. Since the original description of "retrolental fibroplasia" by Terry in 1942,[1] this disorder has been the focus of extensive study. As the survival of the smallest and most vulnerable infants has increased in recent decades, so has the prevalence of ROP and its potentially severe sequelae. Yet, recent advances in our understanding of its pathogenesis have led to promising new therapies that specifically target the mechanisms that lead to disease. This chapter will focus on these advances and review the current status of such targeted therapies.

ROP remains a serious and common problem among extremely low birth weight (ELBW) infants. In a recent, population-based study of all infants less than 27 weeks gestation born during a three year period from 2004–2007 in Sweden, ROP greater than Stage 2 was diagnosed in 34%. The rate was inversely proportional to gestational age, with the most immature babies at highest risk (80%, 62% and 48% at 22, 23 and 24 weeks, respectively).[2] Although blindness is the most severe adverse

419

outcome associated with this disorder, other visual disturbances including myopia, strabismus, glaucoma and amblyopia are frequent childhood complications.[3]

Historically, ROP has been wrought with confusion and controversy. The first suggestion that this disease of premature infants was associated with the liberal use of supplemental oxygen was raised in 1951 in both the United Kingdom and Australia.[4,5] Conflicting reports over the subsequent several years cast some doubt on these initial concerns, until more definitive trials were complete in 1954.[6] Subsequent strict limitation of supplemental oxygen for premature infants greatly reduced the incidence of end-stage ROP, but at the cost of increased mortality and spastic diplegia among survivors that unfortunately took many years to fully appreciate.[7] Thus, two "epidemics" of ROP have been described in industrialized countries; the first occurring in the 1940s and 1950s with the liberal use of supplemental oxygen and the second in the 1970s with the improved survival of infants at the extremes of prematurity who continue to be at greatest risk.[8] Current worldwide estimates indicate that over 50,000 children are blind from ROP, and suggest a "third epidemic" is underway. These data suggest that the risk of ROP-related blindness is associated with infant mortality rate (IMR), with low ROP rates in countries with high (>60/1000 live births) and low (<9/1000 live births) IMR. The ROP rate is highest in countries with IMR that is between these two extremes.[8] This interesting association likely occurs because countries with high IMR generally lack formalized systems for neonatal intensive care such that survival of extremely premature infants is unlikely, while those with low IMR have resources that allow minimization of risk. The "in between group" of countries may have neonatal care, but limited resources may result in the lack of optimal care and preclude extensive ROP screening and treatment programs.[9]

The current descriptions of the manifestations of ROP are based on the international classification developed by a group of ophthalmologists from six countries that was first described in 1984[10] and expanded in 1987[11] and 2005.[12] The classification system allows careful description of the location, extent and stage of disease. To describe location, the retina was divided into zones with the optic disc at the center (Fig. 1). Extent of disease is described in terms of "clock hours" of involvement. The stages of ROP are

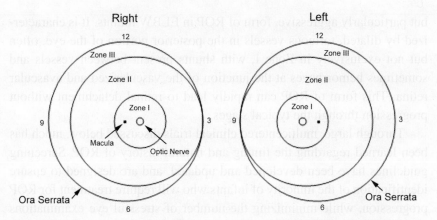

Figure 1. Schematic representation of the zone nomenclature used to describe location of ROP within the retina.[10] Numbers refer to "clock hours," used to describe extent of disease.

Table 1. Stages of ROP.

Stage	Description
1	Line of demarcation separating vascularized from avascular retina
2	Ridge with height and width that extends out of the retinal plane
3	Ridge with extraretinal fibrovascular proliferative tissue
4	Subtotal retinal detachment
4a	Extrafoveal subtotal detachment
4b	Retinal detachment that includes the fovea
5	Total retinal detachment

described in Table 1, with the higher stages indicative of more severe disease. The original classification scheme also introduced the concept of "plus" disease, an indication of progressive vascular incompetence. Features of plus disease include dilatation and tortuosity of the peripheral retinal vessels, vascular engorgement of the iris, papillary rigidity and vitreous haze. When ROP is present in zone I or posterior zone II and the retinal vessels are dilated and tortuous, progression can be rapid, requiring close follow-up and prompt treatment. More recently, the terms "pre-plus" and "aggressive posterior ROP (AP-ROP)" have been added to the classification system.[12] "Pre-plus" disease is used to describe vessels that are abnormally dilated and tortuous, but not to the extent that would be classified as plus disease. "AP-ROP" or "rush disease" describes an uncommon, but particularly aggressive, form of ROP in ELBW infants. It is characterized by dilated, tortuous vessels in the posterior portion of the eye, often but not exclusively in Zone I, with shunts present between vessels and sometimes hemorrhages at the junction of the vascularized and avascular retina. This form of ROP can rapidly lead to retinal detachment without progression through the typical stages.

Through large, multicentered clinical trials discussed below, much has been learned regarding the timing and natural history of ROP. Screening guidelines have been developed and updated, and are designed to ensure identification of the minority of infants who will require treatment for ROP progression, while minimizing the number of stressful eye examinations among these patients.[13] Screening is recommended for all infants with a birth weight of less than 1500 g or gestational age of 32 weeks or less. Screening should also be considered for select patients with gestational age greater than 32 weeks and between 1500–2000 g birth weight who have an unstable clinical course. The timing of initiation of screening varies because ROP is well known to correlate better with postmenstrual age than with chronologic age. Table 2 shows the current recommendations for

Table 2.   Timing of first eye examination.

Gestational Age at Birth (week)	Age at Initial Examination (week)	
	Postmenstrual	Chronologic
22	31	9
23	31	8
24	31	7
25	31	6
26	31	5
27	31	4
28	32	4
29	33	4
30	34	4
31	35	4
32	36	4

Adapted from Ref. 13.

timing of the first eye exam, based on gestational age at birth. Timing of subsequent exams and criteria for discontinuing screening exams are based on prior exam findings.

Pathogenesis

ROP is truly a developmental disease in the sense that the pathology observed is the direct result of normal developmental pathways disrupted by abrupt changes in the environment in which these pathways were to take place. Retinal vascular development begins in the first trimester and continues throughout gestation, reaching a mature state at approximately 36–40 weeks. Vascular development can be broadly classified into two distinct processes, vasculogenesis and angiogenesis. Vasculogenesis refers to *de novo* formation of primitive vessels through the differentiation of endothelial cell precursors. Angiogenesis is the formation of the complex network of blood vessels through budding or sprouting from existing vessels.[14] The vascular development of the retina has been studied in a number of species, including the rat, cat and dog, however the human situation is unique. In a term gestation, retinal vascular development reaches a mature state *in utero*, where arterial oxygen tension is generally less than 30 mmHg, whereas retinal development continues after birth in lower mammals at much higher oxygen tension. Careful histological assessment of human fetal retinas suggests that both vasculogenesis and angiogenesis occur.[14,15] At approximately 12 weeks gestation, mesenchymal cells migrate from the region of the optic nerve toward the periphery, and then aggregate to form vascular cords. The process of vasculogenesis is considered complete by 21 weeks and is restricted to the central two-thirds of the retina. Angiogenesis is responsible for the remainder of vascular development and is underway by 18 weeks, reaching maturity at or near term.

Angiogenesis in the retina is believed to be driven in response to "physiological hypoxia" resulting from increased metabolic demand of maturing neurons in the avascular retina.[16] When metabolic activity in the developing retina outpaces the ability of the existing circulation to supply oxygen, factors that stimulate angiogenesis are produced locally by neuroglia with vascular endothelial growth factor (VEGF) playing a prominent role. This VEGF-dependent vascularization is thought to be responsible for angiogenesis, but not vasculogenesis.[14] ROP primarily develops because of perturbations in this well-orchestrated developmental process that accompany extremely preterm birth. An overall summary of the pathogenesis and mediators involved is presented in Fig. 2 and described below in more detail. At least two mechanisms lead to disordered vascular development of the retina in these infants.[17] The first is hyperoxia. Retinal development that normally occurs in the setting of relatively low oxygen tension *in utero* ($PaO_2 \sim 30$ mmHg) now must occur in the higher oxygen tensions of the extrauterine environment ($PaO_2 \sim 55\text{--}80$ mmHg). More recently, the role of maternally derived factors that support retinal development has received increasing attention, and deficiency of these factors following preterm birth also contributes to ROP pathogenesis.[18]

Pathogenesis of ROP is best conceptualized to occur in two phases.[17,18] Phase I, or the vaso-obliterative phase, occurs secondary to the relative hyperoxia that occurs following preterm birth, even at ambient inspired oxygen concentrations, and is exacerbated by supplemental oxygen. Angiogenic factors like VEGF that are released in response to hypoxia are down-regulated, resulting in decreased angiogenesis and constriction/retraction of vessels already present. This phenomenon, coupled with the ongoing metabolic demand of the avascular retina leads to phase II, or the vaso-proliferative phase, in which the relative hypoxia leads to renewed induction of vasoactive growth factors through hypoxia-inducible factor (HIF) regulation. The damage incurred during phase I makes the existing blood vessels unable to adequately meet the increased demand, hypoxia persists, and expression of growth factors is further induced. Angiogenesis then becomes excessive in response, and abnormal growth ensues at the junction between the vascular and avascular retina. Subsequent fibrotic or cicatricial changes can lead to retinal folds or detachment with resulting visual impairment.

Several animal models of oxygen-induced retinopathy have been studied.[19] The mouse model is particularly useful because proliferative retinopathy can be induced in a reliable and reproducible fashion, it is quantifiable, and it allows genetic manipulation to facilitate hypothesis testing.[20] In this model, neonatal mice are exposed to 75% oxygen from postnatal day 7 to 12. Cessation of vessel growth with vessel regression is

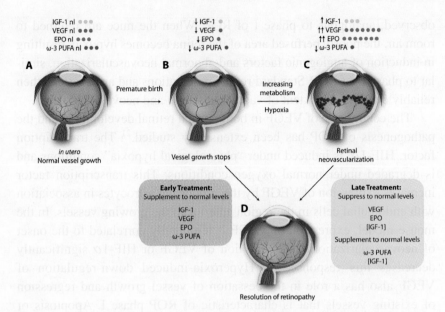

Figure 2. Schematic representation of IGF-I, VEGF, Epo and ω-3 PUFA control of blood vessel development in ROP. (**A**) *In utero*, VEGF is found at the growing front of vessels. IGF-I is sufficient to allow vessel growth, Epo is normal and ω-3 PUFAs are provided by the mother. (**B**) With premature birth and loss of the placenta, IGF-I and ω-3 PUFA levels fall and the relative hyperoxia of the extrauterine environment suppress VEGF and Epo. Vascular growth ceases. Both endothelial cell survival (Akt) and proliferation (mitogen-activated protein kinase) pathways are compromised. With low IGF-I and cessation of vessel growth, a demarcation line forms at the vascular front. Supplemental oxygen in some premature infants may further suppress VEGF and Epo, increasing inhibition of vessel growth. (**C**) As the premature infant matures, the developing, but nonvascularized retina, becomes hypoxic. VEGF and Epo increase in retina and vitreous. With maturation, the IGF-I level slowly increases. Without an external source, ω-3 PUFA levels will remain low. When the IGF-I level reaches a threshold at ~34 weeks gestation, with high VEGF and Epo levels in the vitreous, endothelial cell survival and proliferation driven by VEGF may proceed. Neovascularization ensues at the demarcation line, growing into the vitreous. (**D**) There are two ways to prevent the neovascular proliferation: (1) Inhibition of the neovascular phase. If elevated, VEGF and Epo vitreal levels are suppressed and IGF-1 is normalized and ω-3 PUFA is provided, normal retinal vessel growth can proceed. (2) Inhibition of the vessel loss phase. If IGF-1, Epo, and VEGF levels are increased to normal *in utero* levels in phase I, then vessel loss is suppressed and the neovascular phase II will not occur. With normal vascular growth and blood flow, oxygen suppresses VEGF expression so it will no longer be overproduced. Reproduced with permission from Ref. 18 via Copyright Clearance Center, Copyright © 2008 by Association for Research in Vision and Ophthalmology.

observed, analogous to phase I of ROP. When the mice are returned to room air, the poorly perfused area of the retina becomes hypoxic, resulting in induction of angiogenic factors and abnormal neovascularization, similar to phase II of ROP. Standard retinal preparations and analyses can then reliably quantify the extent of vaso-obliteration and neovascularization.

The central role of VEGF in both normal retinal development and the pathogenesis of ROP has been extensively studied.[21] The transcription factor, HIF-1α, is induced under "physiological hypoxia" conditions and is degraded under normal oxygen conditions. This transcription factor increases expression of VEGF by the supporting astrocytes in association with endothelial cells in the region anterior to the growing vessels. In the mouse model, expression of VEGF is temporally correlated to the onset of neovascularization, and inhibition of VEGF or HIF-1α significantly decreases this response.[18,22] Hyperoxia-induced down-regulation of VEGF also has a role in the cessation of vessel growth and regression of existing vessels that is characteristic of ROP phase I. Apoptosis of vascular endothelial cells that is induced by hyperoxia is reduced following administration of exogenous VEGF or the VEGF-receptor ligand, PIGF-1.[23]

The observation that inhibition of VEGF is insufficient to completely eliminate neovascularization in the mouse model of ROP fostered the search for additional factor(s) contributing to this pathology. Erythropoietin (Epo) is another HIF-regulated factor that likely has a role in the pathogenesis of ROP. This hormone is produced in the kidney in response to hypoxia and is well known to induce erythropoiesis in bone marrow and has been used clinically in the treatment of anemia of prematurity, as well as anemia associated with other chronic diseases. Epo and its receptors are expressed in the retina of the mouse with apparently similar patterns to that of VEGF. Epo is downregulated in the hyperoxic vessel loss phase and administration of exogenous Epo protects against vessel loss and the subsequent hypoxic phase hypervascularization,[24] suggesting that supplementation of Epo during phase I of ROP may be protective in terms of preventing vessel loss. In the proliferative phase II however, retinal Epo levels are highly induced and exogenous Epo enhances the pathological neovascularization. The effects of Epo and VEGF are independent and additive at this stage,[25] and inhibition of Epo with siRNA can prevent neovascularization.[26] These findings underscore the complexity of therapeutic intervention for ROP. Exogenous Epo may have a protective role in the early, hyperoxic phase I of ROP, while administration during the proliferative phase II may exacerbate the aberrant vessel growth and cause disease progression. Indeed, administration of recombinant Epo for anemia in preterm infants has been suggested as an independent risk factor for both the development of ROP as well as ROP requiring intervention.[27] These studies demonstrate the complexity of the pathogenesis of this disorder, the valuable information that can be gained from a viable animal model, and the need for cautious implementation of therapies involving biological molecules that have potentially multifaceted effects.

As described above, the association between oxygen and the pathogenesis of ROP is well established. However, this disorder, like most of the morbidities of prematurity, is clearly multifactorial in origin. To fully understand the risks associated with prematurity, one must consider not only the factors to which the preterm infant is exposed in the extrauterine environment, but also the conditions of the intrauterine environment that would otherwise have been of benefit in the term gestation. Two such elements that have received recent attention as they relate to ROP are insulin-like growth factor-1 (IGF-1) and ω-3 polyunsaturated fatty acids (PUFAs).

IGF-1 is present in the fetus and in the maternal serum at levels that increase throughout gestation and show a positive correlation with fetal size.[28] These levels fall after preterm birth due to loss of supply from the placenta and amniotic fluid.[29] A role for IGF-1 in ROP was suggested by the observation that IGF-1 knockout mice have abnormal development of retinal blood vessels and that IGF-1 allows maximal signaling by VEGF to increase survival of retinal endothelial cells.[30] Neovascularization characteristic of phase II of ROP is also dependent on IGF-1. IGF-1 expression is induced through growth hormone (GH), and transgenic mice expressing a GH-receptor antagonist or wild-type mice given a somatostatin analogue have decreased neovascularization in the mouse model of ROP. Systemic administration of IGF-1 restores neovascularization in these mice.[18] The association between low IGF-1 levels and ROP has also been substantiated in clinical studies. Mean serum levels of IGF-1 in premature infants are inversely associated with severity of ROP, and patients with genetic defects leading to low IGF-1 expression have diminished vascular density in the retina.[18,31] In fact, Lofqvist and colleagues devised an algorithm using birth weight, gestational age, IGF-1, IGFBP-3 and weight gain that predicted 100% of infants who will progress to Stage 3 ROP at least three weeks prior, as well as those who will reach threshold at least 5 weeks prior.[32] Together, these studies provide compelling evidence that IGF-1 has an important role in disease pathogenesis and that IGF-1 replacement may be a viable therapeutic option to prevent vessel loss during phase I. However, as in the case of Epo, timing of intervention is likely to be paramount. In the proliferative phase of ROP, an IGF-1 receptor antagonist decreases retinal neovascularization through suppression of VEGF signaling pathways, suggesting that IGF-1 plays a permissive role in VEGF-mediated angiogenesis.[18] Increased endogenous IGF-1 levels in the proliferative phase cause the effects of hypoxia-induced elevations in VEGF to be manifest and contribute to neovascularization, suggesting that inhibition of IGF-1 signaling may be beneficial in the later stage of disease.

Transplacental passage of PUFAs occurs from the mother to fetus in large amounts during the third trimester. Therefore, similar to IGF-1, preterm infants are relatively deplete in these nutrients. The major ω-3 PUFAs in the human retina are docosahexaenoic acid (DHA) and its precursor, eicosapentaenoic acid (EPA), while the major ω-6 PUFA is arachidonic acid (AA).[18,33] These fatty acids are primarily distributed in the membrane phospholipids of vascular and nerve cells. Their importance in the pathogenesis of ROP has been studied in the mouse model as well.[34] Mice were fed a defined, isocaloric diet enriched with 2% of the total fatty acids from either ω-3 PUFAs (DHA and EPA) or ω-6 PUFA (AA). This defined diet resulted in a two-fold shift in the retinal ω-3/ω-6 ratio and afforded a 50% protective effect against pathologic neovascularization in the mouse model. There was also a statistically significant decrease in vaso-obliteration during phase I in the mice fed the ω-3 enriched diet. Suppression of secretion of the inflammatory cytokine, TNF-α, from microglia and macrophages had a role in this protection.

Treatment

The CRYO-ROP study established the current standard of care for treatment of ROP.[35,36] This multicentered study evaluated 4099 babies with a birth weight under 1251 g by serial retinal examinations and identified 6% of them as progressing to "threshold" ROP, the stage at which the risk of blindness is 50% if untreated. Threshold was defined as stage 3 ROP with plus disease in zone I or II, involving at least five contiguous clock-hours or at least eight interrupted clock-hours. Unfavorable outcomes, defined as posterior retinal detachment, posterior retinal fold, or retrolental tissue that obscured the view of the posterior pole were reduced from 51% in control eyes to 31% in treated eyes, thereby establishing ablative therapy of the peripheral avascular retina as providing some benefit for this disease. Long-term follow-up of the CRYO-ROP study has demonstrated persistence of the beneficial effect of treatment. At 15 years, 30% of treated eyes had unfavorable structural outcomes, compared to 52% of control eyes.[37] A subsequent trial, the Early Treatment for ROP (ETROP) study, was conducted in an effort to improve visual outcomes by intervening sooner, at prethreshold, in those infants found to be at high risk based on the RM-ROP2 risk model.[38] In this study, prethreshold ROP was defined as any ROP in zone I (less than threshold); stage 2 with plus disease, stage 3 without plus disease or stage 3 with plus disease, but insufficient clock-hours to reach threshold in zone II. Infants at high-risk with prethreshold disease were randomized to ablative therapy vs control with treatment at threshold. Infants in the treatment arm had lower rates of unfavorable acuity outcomes at 9 months (14% vs 20%) and lower rates of unfavorable structural outcome at 6 months (5% vs 10%). In subgroup analysis, including high-risk, prethreshold eyes assigned to the control arm, characteristics of eyes that were less likely to progress to threshold were discerned. A clinical algorithm evolved from these analyses defined "Type I" and "Type II" ROP. Early ablation should be considered for prethreshold eyes with Type I ROP, defined as any stage of ROP with plus disease or stage 3 ROP (with or without plus disease) in zone I; or stage 2 or 3 with plus disease in zone II. Conservative management with continued serial exams was recommended for Type II ROP, defined as zone I, stage 1 or 2 with no plus disease; or zone II, stage 3 with no plus disease. Since the CRYO-ROP study, numerous reports have demonstrated that indirect laser photocoagulation for peripheral retinal ablation is at least as effective as cryotherapy in preventing unfavorable outcomes and is technically easier to administer and is better tolerated with fewer local and systemic adverse effects, so this modality has become standard.[39] The most recent guidelines issued by the relevant professional organizations recommend intervention for any stage of ROP with plus disease in zone I, stage 3 ROP in zone I (without plus disease), or stage 2 or 3 ROP in zone II with plus disease.[13]

Although peripheral retinal ablation is well accepted to improve outcomes for severe ROP, a significant number of infants are still left with serious sequelae despite therapy. Retinal detachments are generally managed with additional procedures such as vitrectomy or scleral buckling, but these procedures have not been subjected to randomized controlled trials. Improved structural outcomes have been reported with these procedures, but visual outcomes generally remain poor.[39] Efforts to identify strategies to prevent progression of disease or provide adjunctive therapies directed at key elements of disease pathogenesis are paramount to improving the visual outcomes in patients at risk, but so far, results have been disappointing or remain preliminary.

Because the vasoproliferative phase II of ROP pathogenesis is driven in response to hypoxic conditions in the avascular retina, considerable efforts have been undertaken to better define the optimal use of supplemental oxygen therapy as it relates to ROP. The Supplemental Therapeutic Oxygen for Prethreshold ROP (STOP-ROP) study was designed to determine if supplemental oxygen could reduce the progression from prethreshold to threshold disease.[40] Thirty centers enrolled 649 infants with prethreshold ROP in at least one eye and randomized them to receive supplemental oxygen to maintain oxygen saturations from 96%–99% or to the control arm with targeted saturations from 89%–94%. No statistically significant differences were found in the rate of progression to threshold or the number of infants requiring retinal ablation, while the supplemental oxygen group had increased pulmonary morbidity. Defining the optimal targets for oxygen therapy has proven to be an elusive goal. Avoidance of hyperoxia as well as large fluctuations in oxygenation saturation is likely beneficial and has been supported by case series.[41,42] A recent study at a single institution using historical controls demonstrated a decrease in prethreshold ROP from 17.5% to 5.6% following a decrease in saturation alarm limits from 87%–97% to 85%–93%, lending further support to the role of hyperoxia in progression of ROP.[43] The Eunice Kennedy Shriver National Institute of Child Health and Development (NICHD) sponsored Neonatal Research Network has recently published results of a multicentered, randomized controlled trial that included higher and lower targets for oxygen saturation with severe ROP as an endpoint.[44] This study randomized 1316 infants between 24 and 27 weeks of gestation to target oxygen saturation ranges of 85 to 89% or 91 to 95% in a blinded fashion. The primary outcome was a composite of severe ROP, death before hospital discharge, or both. The lower oxygen group was found to have a lower rate of severe ROP among survivors, 8.6% vs 17.9% in the higher oxygen group (RR = 0.52, 95% confidence interval 0.37–0.73). However, there was a statistically significant increase in death before discharge in the lower oxygen group, 19.9% vs 16.2% in the higher oxygen group (RR = 1.27, 95% confidence interval 1.01–1.60). The combined outcome of severe ROP or death did not differ significantly between groups. Longer-term neurodevelopmental assessments in these patients are planned but results are not yet available. Therefore, although data suggesting that limitation in oxygen supplementation has a favorable effect on ROP, continued vigilance for untoward effects is important. The optimal target for oxygen supplementation in these infants continues to be difficult to define.

The important role of VEGF in the pathogenesis of the vasoproliferative phase of ROP has prompted consideration of VEGF inhibition as a potential therapy. A monoclonal antibody against VEGF, bevacizumab (Avastin®, Genentech Inc.), is FDA-approved for the treatment of colorectal cancer, and has been used off-label for the treatment of age-related macular degeneration[45] and proliferative diabetic retinopathy[46] with encouraging results. Although currently limited to case reports and case series that lack randomization or control arms, this therapy has been applied in the setting of severe ROP and some potential benefit reported.[47] In addition to regression of ROP, anterior segment disease including tunica vasculosa lentis and persistent hyaloids arteries that can interfere with visualization of the fundus and preclude laser therapy seem to consistently benefit from this treatment and may be an additional indication for this therapy. Still, many questions remain including optimal dose and frequency, timing of therapy in disease progression and in relation to other therapies, effects on normal retinal growth and differentiation and potential systemic absorption and complications. Definitive answers to these questions await completion of randomized, controlled clinical trials investigating this novel therapy.

Several dietary supplements have also received attention as a means to prevent ROP and its sequelae. Early studies suggested that deficiencies of vitamin E are associated with ROP, but clinical trials of vitamin E supplementation yielded mixed results in terms of efficacy while finding increased rates of retinal hemorrhage, intraventricular hemorrhage (IVH), necrotizing enterocolitis and sepsis.[48] A meta-analysis found that in VLBW infants, decreases in severe ROP and blindness were associated with vitamin E supplementation, but sepsis rates were significantly increased.[49] These findings have limited its practical application. The antioxidant, D-penicillamine, has also been suggested to have efficacy in the prevention of ROP.[50] In a recent small open-label, non-randomized study, a 14-day course of enteral D-penicillamine decreased the incidence of ROP from 60% to 21% by eliminating stage I and II disease, but did not affect the need for surgery.[51] No short-term toxicities were noted. Further investigation of the potential benefit of this therapy is recommended. A systematic review of studies investigating the effect of supplementation of the essential nutrient, inositol, on respiratory distress syndrome and other morbidities of prematurity found a marked reduction in stage 4 ROP (RR = 0.09, 95% confidence interval 0.01–0.67), as well as other short-term morbidities including death and IVH.[52] Larger, randomized trials of inositol supplementation were also recommended. Based in part on the findings in the mouse model, evidence for benefit from PUFA supplementation has been sought in clinical trials as well. There has been some evidence that enhanced retinal sensitivity and visual acuity can be achieved with PUFA supplementation in preterm infants, and ROP was included as an outcome of interest in a recent systematic review.[53] Although no clear differences in rates of ROP were found between control and PUFA supplemented infants, the studies were generally limited by small numbers and low rates of disease. The role of PUFA supplementation in preterm infants will undoubtedly receive additional attention in the coming years and may become a part of the interventions available to attenuate ROP development.

Conclusions

Since it was first described in 1942, our understanding of the pathogenesis of ROP and methods to treat or prevent its complications has made tremendous strides. The role of oxygen and tissue hypoxia, the importance of mediators such as VEGF and IGF-1, and careful assessment of risk factors and epidemiology of this disorder have all contributed to important advances in management and the development of novel therapeutic strategies that are still being carefully evaluated. Until significant reductions in the rates of preterm birth are achieved, infants will continue to be at risk for this disease. Results of ongoing clinical trials, however, will better define the optimal combination of preventive strategies in the form of oxygen administration and dietary supplements, and therapeutic adjuncts to retinal ablation like VEGF inhibition that specifically target the pathophysiology. Through these combined efforts, the considerable progress gained in the prevention of the severe visual sequelae of ROP is likely to be significantly augmented.

References

1. Terry TL. (1944) Retrolental fibroplasia in the premature infant V: Further studies on fibroplastic overgrowth of the persistent tunica vasculosa lentis. *Trans Am Ophthalmol Soc* **42**: 383–396.

2. The EXPRESS Group. (2009) One-year survival of extremely preterm infants after active perinatal care in Sweden. *JAMA* **301**: 2225–2233.

3. Sylvester CL. (2008) Retinopathy of prematurity. *Semin Ophthalmol* **23**: 318–323.

4. Crosse VM. (1951) The problem of retrolental fibroplasia in the city of Birmingham. *Trans Ophthalmol Soc UK* **71**: 609–612.

5. Campbell K. (1951) Intensive oxygen therapy as a possible cause of retrolental fibroplasia: A clinical approach. *Med J Aust* **2**: 48–50.

6. Kinsey VE, Hemphill FM. (1955) Etiology of retrolental fibroplasia and preliminary report of cooperative study of retrolental fibroplasia. *Trans Am Acad Ophthalmol Otolaryngol* **59**: 15–24; discussion, 40–11.

7. Silverman WA. (2004) A cautionary tale about supplemental oxygen: The albatross of neonatal medicine. *Pediatrics* **113**: 394–396.

8. Gilbert C. (2008) Retinopathy of prematurity: A global perspective of the epidemics, population of babies at risk and implications for control. *Early Hum Dev* **84**: 77–82.

9. Gilbert C, Rahi J, Eckstein M, O'Sullivan J, Foster A. (1997) Retinopathy of prematurity in middle-income countries. *Lancet* **350**: 12–14.

10. The Committee for the Classification of Retinopathy of Prematurity. (1984) An international classification of retinopathy of prematurity. *Arch Ophthalmol* **102**: 1130–1134.

11. The International Committee for the Classification of the Late Stages of Retinopathy of Prematurity. (1987) An international classification of retinopathy of prematurity II: The classification of retinal detachment. *Arch Ophthalmol* **105**: 906–912.

12. The International Committee for the Classification of the Late Stages of Retinopathy of Prematurity. (2005) The international classification of retinopathy of prematurity revisited. *Arch Ophthalmol* **123**: 991–999.

13. American Academy of Pediatrics Section on Ophthalmology, American Academy of Ophthalmology, American Association for Pediatric Ophthalmology and Strabismus. (2006) Screening examination of premature infants for retinopathy of prematurity. *Pediatrics* **117**: 572–576.

14. Hughes S, Yang H, Chan-Ling T. (2000) Vascularization of the human fetal retina: Roles of vasculogenesis and angiogenesis. *Invest Ophthalmol Vis Sci* **41**: 1217–1228.

15. Chan-Ling T, McLeod DS, Hughes S *et al.* (2004) Astrocyte-endothelial cell relationships during human retinal vascular development. *Invest Ophthalmol Vis Sci* **45**: 2020–2032.

16. Chan-Ling T, Gock B, Stone J. (1995) The effect of oxygen on vasoformative cell division. Evidence that "physiological hypoxia" is the stimulus for normal retinal vasculogenesis. *Invest Ophthalmol Vis Sci* **36**: 1201–1214.

17. Heidary G, Vanderveen D, Smith LE. (2009) Retinopathy of prematurity: Current concepts in molecular pathogenesis. *Semin Ophthalmol* **24**: 77–81.

18. Smith LE. (2008) Through the eyes of a child: Understanding retinopathy through ROP the Friedenwald lecture. *Invest Ophthalmol Vis Sci* **49**: 5177–5182.

19. Madan A, Penn JS. (2003) Animal models of oxygen-induced retinopathy. *Front Biosci* **8**: d1030–d1043.

20. Smith LE, Wesolowski E, McLellan A *et al.* (1994) Oxygen-induced retinopathy in the mouse. *Invest Ophthalmol Vis Sci* **35**: 101–111.
21. Penn JS, Madan A, Caldwell RB *et al.* (2008) Vascular endothelial growth factor in eye disease. *Prog Retin Eye Res* **27**: 331–371.
22. Jiang J, Xia XB, Xu HZ *et al.* (2009) Inhibition of retinal neovascularization by gene transfer of small interfering RNA targeting HIF-1alpha and VEGF. *J Cell Physiol* **218**: 66–74.
23. Shih SC, Ju M, Liu N *et al.* (2003) Selective stimulation of VEGFR-1 prevents oxygen-induced retinal vascular degeneration in retinopathy of prematurity. *J Clin Invest* **112**: 50–57.
24. Chen J, Connor KM, Aderman CM *et al.* (2008) Erythropoietin deficiency decreases vascular stability in mice. *J Clin Invest* **118**: 526–533.
25. Watanabe D, Suzuma K, Matsui S *et al.* (2005) Erythropoietin as a retinal angiogenic factor in proliferative diabetic retinopathy. *N Engl J Med* **353**: 782–792.
26. Chen J, Connor KM, Aderman CM *et al.* (2009) Suppression of retinal neovascularization by erythropoietin siRNA in a mouse model of proliferative retinopathy. *Invest Ophthalmol Vis Sci* **50**: 1329–1335.
27. Suk KK, Dunbar JA, Liu A *et al.* (2008) Human recombinant erythropoietin and the incidence of retinopathy of prematurity: A multiple regression model. *J Aapos* **12**: 233–238.
28. Reece EA, Wiznitzer A, Le E *et al.* (1994) The relation between human fetal growth and fetal blood levels of insulin-like growth factors I and II, their binding proteins, and receptors. *Obstet Gynecol* **84**: 88–95.
29. Langford K, Nicolaides K, Miell JP. (1998) Maternal and fetal insulin-like growth factors and their binding proteins in the second and third trimesters of human pregnancy. *Hum Reprod* **13**: 1389–1393.
30. Hellstrom A, Perruzzi C, Ju M *et al.* (2001) Low IGF-I suppresses VEGF-survival signaling in retinal endothelial cells: Direct correlation with clinical retinopathy of prematurity. *Proc Natl Acad Sci USA* **98**: 5804–5808.
31. Hellstrom A, Carlsson B, Niklasson A *et al.* (2002) IGF-I is critical for normal vascularization of the human retina. *J Clin Endocrinol Metab* **87**: 3413–3416.
32. Lofqvist C, Andersson E, Sigurdsson J *et al.* (2006) Longitudinal postnatal weight and insulin-like growth factor I measurements in the prediction of retinopathy of prematurity. *Arch Ophthalmol* **124**: 1711–1718.

33. SanGiovanni JP, Chew EY. (2005) The role of omega-3 long-chain polyun-saturated fatty acids in health and disease of the retina. *Prog Retin Eye Res* **24**: 87–138.

34. Connor KM, SanGiovanni JP, Lofqvist C *et al.* (2007) Increased dietary intake of omega-3-polyunsaturated fatty acids reduces pathological retinal angiogenesis. *Nat Med* **13**: 868–873.

35. Cryotherapy for Retinopathy of Prematurity Cooperative Group. (1990) Multicenter trial of cryotherapy for retinopathy of prematurity. One-year outcome — Structure and function. *Arch Ophthalmol* **108**: 1408–1416.

36. Palmer EA, Flynn JT, Hardy RJ *et al.* (1991) The Cryotherapy for Retinopathy of Prematurity Cooperative Group. Incidence and early course of retinopathy of prematurity. *Ophthalmology* **98**: 1628–1640.

37. Palmer EA, Hardy RJ, Dobson V *et al.* (2005) 15-year outcomes following threshold retinopathy of prematurity: Final results from the multicenter trial of cryotherapy for retinopathy of prematurity. *Arch Ophthalmol* **123**: 311–318.

38. Good WV. (2004) Final results of the early treatment for retinopathy of prematurity (ETROP) randomized trial. *Trans Am Ophthalmol Soc* **102**: 233–248; discussion 248–250.

39. Clark D, Mandal K. (2008) Treatment of retinopathy of prematurity. *Early Hum Dev* **84**: 95–99.

40. The STOP-ROP Multicenter Study Group. (2000) Supplemental therapeutic oxygen for prethreshold retinopathy of prematurity (STOP-ROP), a random-ized, controlled trial I: Primary outcomes. *Pediatrics* **105**: 295–310.

41. Chow LC, Wright KW, Sola A. (2003) Can changes in clinical practice decrease the incidence of severe retinopathy of prematurity in very low birth weight infants? *Pediatrics* **111**: 339–345.

42. Cunningham S, Fleck BW, Elton RA *et al.* (1995) Transcutaneous oxygen levels in retinopathy of prematurity. *Lancet* **346**: 1464–1465.

43. Vanderveen DK, Mansfield TA, Eichenwald EC. (2006) Lower oxygen saturation alarm limits decrease the severity of retinopathy of prematurity. *J AAPOS* **10**: 445–448.

44. SUPPORT Study Group of the Eunice Kennedy Shriver NICHD Neonatal Research Network. (2010) Target ranges of oxygen saturation in extremely preterm infants. *N Engl J Med* **362**: 1959–1969.

45. Schouten JS, La Heij EC, Webers CA *et al.* (2009) A systematic review on the effect of bevacizumab in exudative age-related macular degeneration. *Graefes Arch Clin Exp Ophthalmol* **247**: 1–11.

46. Arevalo JF, Garcia-Amaris RA. (2009) Intravitreal bevacizumab for diabetic retinopathy. *Curr Diabetes Rev* **5**: 39–46.

47. Micieli JA, Surkont M, Smith AF. (2009) A systematic analysis of the off-label use of bevacizumab for severe retinopathy of prematurity. *Am J Ophthalmol* **148**: 536–543 e532.

48. Mantagos IS, Vanderveen DK, Smith LE. (2009) Emerging treatments for retinopathy of prematurity. *Semin Ophthalmol* **24**: 82–86.

49. Brion LP, Bell EF, Raghuveer TS. (2003) Vitamin E supplementation for prevention of morbidity and mortality in preterm infants. *Cochrane Database Syst Rev*: CD003665.

50. Phelps DL, Lakatos L, Watts JL. (2001) D-Penicillamine for preventing retinopathy of prematurity in preterm infants. *Cochrane Database Syst Rev*: CD001073.

51. Christensen RD, Alder SC, Richards SC *et al.* (2007) D-Penicillamine administration and the incidence of retinopathy of prematurity. *J Perinatol* **27**: 103–111.

52. Howlett A, Ohlsson A. (2003) Inositol for respiratory distress syndrome in preterm infants. *Cochrane Database Syst Rev*: CD000366.

53. Smithers LG, Gibson RA, McPhee A *et al.* (2008) Effect of long-chain polyunsaturated fatty acid supplementation of preterm infants on disease risk and neurodevelopment: A systematic review of randomized controlled trials. *Am J Clin Nutr* **87**: 912–920.

Chapter  19

Neonatal Surgery

François I. Luks

Prenatal Diagnosis of Surgical Conditions

Less than 1% of infants have a *congenital* surgical anomaly. Infants may also *acquire* a condition that requires surgical intervention. In the past, most congenital anomalies were diagnosed at birth or beyond. The availability of sophisticated prenatal imaging has significantly increased the rate of prenatal detection for many of these conditions. Advanced knowledge of a congenital anomaly can be a source of much anxiety for future parents and, in some cases, lead to a desire to terminate the pregnancy. On the other hand, prenatal diagnosis offers the possibility for families and health care professionals to be better prepared, and in many cases, minimize diagnostic and therapeutic delays.[1,2]

Obstructions of the foregut prevent absorption of swallowed amniotic fluid, and will tend to produce polyhydramnios. The combination of polyhydramnios and a "double bubble" in the upper abdomen suggests distension of the stomach and the first portion of the duodenum. This is highly suspicious of atresia or extrinsic duodenal compression. More distal obstructions are less commonly associated with polyhydramnios, as swallowed fluid is absorbed by the intestine proximal to the obstruction; ultrasound will show multiple dilated loops of intestines.

Oligo- or anhydramnios, in the absence of rupture of the membranes or clinical signs of amniotic leak, suggests decreased fetal urinary excretion.

439

Possible causes are absence of kidneys (Potter syndrome) or lower urinary tract obstruction, which in boys is most often due to posterior urethral valves.

Elevation of alpha-fetoprotein (AFP) in amniotic fluid or maternal serum suggests leakage of fetal proteins through a breach in the integumental integrity of the fetus. Maternal serum AFP (MSAFP) screening is most often used to detect open neural tune defects (myelomeningocele or spina bifida),[3] but elevation of MSAFP is also seen with gastroschisis.

Neonatal Surgery

Although many surgical conditions can now be diagnosed *in utero*, the vast majority of these can best be treated after birth. Advance knowledge may, however, help determine the ideal timing, mode and place of delivery. Surgical conditions of the newborn may require immediate intervention, within minutes or hours of life, or may benefit from a more detailed diagnostic work-up and delayed treatment. In some cases, elective intervention later in infancy or childhood may be preferable. The most acute surgical problem in the newborn typically involves the upper airways and the lungs, as the newborn transitions from placental support to independent breathing.

The EXIT Procedure

The *Ex-utero*-Intrapartum procedure (EXIT) refers to a modified Cesarean section that allows access to the newborn's airway before the umbilical cord is clamped. Also called Operation On Placental Support (which makes for an unfortunate acronym[4]), this approach requires particular planning and a multidisciplinary team of obstetrical specialists, obstetrical anesthetists, neonatologists, pediatric surgeons or otolaryngologists, respiratory therapists and neonatal and operating room nurses. It requires meticulous myometrial hemostasis and sufficient uterine relaxation to prevent full delivery and separation of the placenta, and preservation of umbilical blood flow. As the head and neck of the infant are delivered, access to the distal airways is obtained by intubation or tracheostomy. Only then can the cord be clamped and the delivery completed.[5] Indications for the EXIT procedure include large head- and neck tumors and masses (most commonly cervical teratomas or cystic hygromas) and, less commonly, severe micrognathism and large cystic lung lesions.

Neonatal Surgery for Congenital Anomalies

Congenital diaphragmatic hernia (CDH)

Congenital diaphragmatic hernia is a common surgical condition of the newborn, occurring in 1 in 2,000 live births. Previously thought to be almost universally fatal, CDH can now be treated successfully in a majority of cases. The CDH Registry is a world-wide consortium of treatment centers that regularly updates the overall survival and complication rates for CDH. The most recent report from the CDH Registry indicates that isolated CDH not associated with chromosomal or cardiac anomalies has an overall survival rate in excess of 70%.[6] The most severe forms of the disease and those associated with complex syndromes have a poorer outcome.

Attempts at stratifying the risk of CDH based on the degree of pulmonary hypoplasia or other perinatal parameters have been frustrating and to date, no single factor can predict survival or death with reasonable accuracy. Nevertheless, the combination of several parameters can be helpful. The most commonly used measure of pulmonary hypoplasia is the lung-to-head ratio (LHR), which normalizes the size of the contralateral lung by using head circumference as a surrogate for gestational age (Fig. 1). An LHR greater than 1.4 is generally considered to indicate good prognosis (normal LHR is greater than 2.5). An LHR between 1.0 and 1.4 is considered an intermediate risk, but the presence of part of the liver in the chest worsens the prognosis.[7] These infants, and those whose LHR is less than 1.0, will often need aggressive postnatal management, including extracorporeal membrane oxygenation (ECMO). Therefore, it would stand to reason to recommend delivery of these infants in tertiary centers with ECMO capabilities and experienced neonatal critical care teams. Surgical correction of the defect is never an emergency in these infants, and can typically be delayed by several days. This allows stabilization of

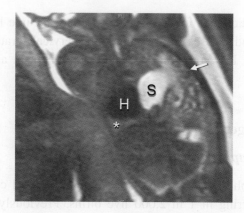

Figure 1.   Prenatal magnetic resonance imaging (MRI) in left-sided congenital diaphragmatic hernia. Coronal image showing stomach (S) and intestinal loops in the left
hemithorax (arrow), deviation of the heart (H) into the right hemithorax and a small
wedge-shaped right lung (asterisk).

the infant during the transitional phase from fetal to adult circulation, as
pulmonary hypertension (persistent fetal circulation) is more detrimental
than actual lung hypoplasia.

Surgical correction of the CDH is usually performed through an
abdominal incision, more rarely through the chest. After reduction of
the viscera into the abdomen, the diaphragm is closed; in all but the
largest defects, there is sufficient native diaphragmatic tissue to allow
primary closure. In some cases, including agenesis (or absence) of the
diaphragm, a synthetic patch may be needed. In these cases, the risk of
recurrent diaphragmatic hernia reaches 45%. Infants with diaphragmatic hernia face many complications, including gastroesophageal
reflux, feeding difficulties, pulmonary hypertension, reactive airway
disease and the many side effects of prolonged ventilation and ECMO.
Of note, the guarded prognosis and relatively high morbidity mainly
refers to the form of CDH that present immediately at birth.
Asymptomatic CDH may be diagnosed beyond the immediate neonatal
period (from several hours of life to sometimes years later), on a
routine chest radiograph. This form of the disease carries none of the
stigmas of symptomatic CDH.

Esophageal atresia and tracheoesophageal fistula (EA/TEF)

The trachea arises as a frontal diverticulum of the foregut around the fourth week of embryonic development, and undergoes growth and dichotomous branching into the left and right bronchial trees. Interruption of the esophagus, with or without fistulization with the trachea, is presumed to occur around that time. Although the exact mechanism for this anomaly is not know, several experimental models have been developed (most notably, the adriamycin mouse model[8]). Defective signaling of sonic hedgehog (Shh) and other homeobox genes is believed to play a central role in the maldevelopment of the esophagus and the trachea, as well as other anomalies commonly seen with EA/TEF.[9,10] The combination of several of these anomalies constitutes the VATER (or, more accurately, VACTERL) association, which refers to Vertebral, Anorectal, Cardiac, Tracheo-Esophageal, Renal and Limb anomalies.

Esophageal atresia and tracheoesophageal fistula can present in various ways. The most common type (type C), occurring in approximately 85% of all cases, consists of a proximal blind pouch and a distal tracheoesophageal fistula. Pure esophageal atresia without fistula (type A) is the second most common (5–10%) and is often the most difficult to manage. Because the distal esophageal pouch is not tethered to the trachea by a fistula, that segment is often short and the distance between the two esophageal halves is significant (so-called long gap EA).This form of esophageal atresia is most easily recognized because of the complete isolation of the distal intestinal tract: a plain radiograph of the abdomen shows a complete absence of intestinal gas (Fig. 2). Because the fetus cannot swallow, this condition may be recognized *in utero* (wide proximal esophageal pouch) and is often associated with polyhydramnios and premature delivery. Other forms of EA/TEF include, in decreasing order of frequency, type D (EA with proximal AND distal fistulas), type E ("H" or "N" type tracheoesophageal fistula without EA) and type B (EA with proximal fistula). All these forms, except the isolated TEF without EA, present shortly after birth and are characterized with choking, excessive salivation and inability to pass a nasogastric tube. The diagnosis may be confirmed by instilling a very small amount of barium (not water-soluble contrast, which is often

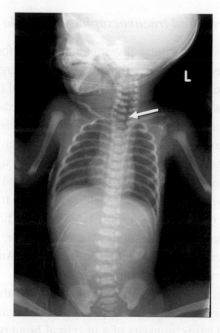

Figure 2. Chest and abdominal radiograph of a newborn with esophageal atresia without tracheo-esophageal fistula (type A). Note tip of catheter in an air-filled, distended upper esophageal pouch (arrow) and absence of gas in the abdomen.

hypertonic and may cause pulmonary edema if aspirated), showing the characteristic blind upper esophageal pouch. However, a contrast study is rarely necessary, given the typical clinical presentation and plain chest radiograph view of the nasogastric tube coiled in the proximal esophagus.

Waterston[11] initially described three situations, based on prematurity, degree of aspiration pneumonitis and overall clinical status, and recommended primary repair only in the strongest newborns (Waterston class A). All others underwent a temporizing gastrostomy and frequent aspiration of the upper pouch until definitive repair could be performed safely. This classification is now modified[12] and most newborns with straightforward TEF now undergo an attempt at definitive repair within the first few days of life. A preoperative echocardiography is useful to rule out associated cardiac anomalies (seen in 20% of patients and the most common of the VACTERL associations).

More recently, thoracoscopic repair of TEF and EA has been described, and an increasing number of surgeons are becoming facile with this approach. The advantages of a minimally invasive alternative are not yet clear, particularly compared with small muscle-sparing thoracotomy incisions. There may be increased incidence of postoperative anastomotic leaks after thoracoscopic repair[13] and long-term outcome is not yet known. Nevertheless, it is likely that minimally invasive surgery will gradually evolve beyond its learning curve and become an accepted approach.[14]

Long-gap esophageal atresias (with or without a concomitant tracheo-esophageal fistula) offer the greatest challenge. If known preoperatively (such as with type A, or pure EA), a gastrostomy is performed and the infant is allowed to grow. It is accepted that the esophagus will grow somewhat for the first few months of life, thereby reducing the gap. However, there is little to be gained from waiting more than 4–6 months and delaying repair much further increases the risk of complications, such as aspiration pneumonitis, pneumonia and sudden death. Esophageal replacements, using a segment of colon or small bowel, or fashioning a gastric tube, may be necessary to bridge the gap; however, these techniques have fallen out of favor with the recognition that the native esophagus, even if abnormal, provides better function.[15] Preoperative lengthening procedures have been advocated, including tethering the ends of each esophageal pouch to the chest wall, to stretch the segments as the child's chest cavity grows.[16] However, it is unclear whether this and other inventive techniques truly alter the success of delayed primary repair of the esophagus.

Postoperative complications are not uncommon, and include anastomotic leaks (typically requiring prolonged periods of esophageal rest) and the development of anastomotic strictures. These can be the result of a healing leak or relative ischemia at the anastomosis. A significant percentage of infants with EA/TEF (up to 30%) will require at least one postoperative esophageal dilation. The morbidity of EA/TEF also includes a high incidence of gastroesophageal reflux, tracheomalacia, reactive airway disease and asthma.

Cystic lung lesions

Congenital pulmonary airway malformations (CPAM) consist of a diverse number of anomalies of the lung. Large congenital cystic adenomatoid malformations of the lung (CCAM) may cause fetal hydrops and may require *in utero* intervention. If they are composed of a few large cysts, needle decompression or pleuroamniotic shunt insertion may be indicated. If they are more solid and cause compression of the mediastinal vessels, the only option may be open fetal surgery. The vast majority of CPAMs, however, tend to regress in the third trimester of gestation.[17] Most newborns are asymptomatic, but delayed intervention may still be advisable because of the long-term risks of these lesions. In some cases, the infant presents in respiratory distress, requiring urgent intervention at birth. Large, persistent lesions may have caused enough pulmonary compression to result in relative pulmonary hypoplasia. Some authors have advocated resection of these lesions in the delivery room through an EXIT procedure (see above).[5] However, this technique is more commonly reserved for airway obstruction, rather than pulmonary hypoplasia; conventional airway management is preferable, followed by surgical decompression or resection if necessary. Large cystic lesions typically communicate with the tracheobronchial tree via microscopic pores of Kohn — and may cause significant air-trapping (simulating a tension pneumothorax) or abscess formation within the lung. Urgent drainage of the "pneumatoceles" must be followed by thoracotomy and resection of the lesion and involved lobe. If chronic *in utero* compression of the lung has occurred, the degree of pulmonary hypoplasia may mandate aggressive respiratory management, which may include ECMO.

Abdominal Conditions

Abdominal wall defects

The two most common types of abdominal wall defects are gastroschisis and omphalocele. Gastroschisis refers to a paramedian defect, typically to the right of the umbilicus. Gastroschisis is more common than omphalocele (1 in 2,500–4,500 live births vs 1 in 4,000–7,000), and its incidence appears to be on the rise. It tends to occur in younger mothers. It is most commonly isolated, although it is associated with an intestinal atresia in 5–10% of the cases. Conversely, omphalocele is more often seen in complex chromosomal and other anomalies, some of which may have a dire prognosis.

These include Pentalogy of Cantrell (omphalocele, diaphragmatic defect, sternal cleft, pericardial defect and cardiac anomalies), cloacal exstrophy (also termed OEIS, for omphalocele-exstrophy-imperforate anus-spinal defects), and some chromosomal disorders, including trisomies 13 and 18. As a result, some obstetricians and perinatologists have offered a grim prognosis to parents of a fetus or infant with omphalocele. However, the prognosis of isolated omphalocele, without other major anomalies detected by prenatal ultrasonography, carries a prognosis similar to that of gastroschisis.[18,19]

Since most abdominal wall defects can be detected prenatally, some have advocated perinatal intervention (timing, place and mode of delivery) and even aggressive fetal treatment. The main concern is the thickened peel often seen on the intestinal loops in gastroschisis, believed by some to be a result of prolonged exposure to the supposedly caustic effect of amniotic fluid. Despite many speculations, there is currently no evidence to support this theory, or the practice of early delivery by Cesarean section.[20]

Management of abdominal wall defects depends on the size of the defect and the type of viscera that have herniated. Whereas primary closure was offered for most newborns with gastroschisis, a delayed approach is now used for all but the smallest defects. Bedside placement of a silicone rubber (Silastic®) "silo" to protect the exposed viscera can now be done with minimal sedation, as the elastic ring at the base of the silo is deployed intra-abdominally to form a watertight seal, thereby protecting intestinal loops from dehydration, infection and hypothermia. The infant does not typically require ventilatory support. Once adaptation of the abdominal cavity and gravity (as well as active squeezing of the silo) have resulted in near-reduction of the viscera, a delayed repair of the defect is performed under general anesthesia (typically between 5–8 days of life). Postoperative ileus is the rule and can persist for 10–15 days. Once intestinal transit returns, gradual feeding of the baby can be started. If nasogastric output remains copious for more than three weeks, an atresia must be suspected and a contrast radiograph may be required for diagnosis.

Omphaloceles are usually not associated with damaged intestinal wall, as they are most commonly covered by the umbilical membrane.

"Ruptured" omphaloceles are treated like gastroschisis. So-called "giant" omphaloceles represent a unique challenge, particularly when a large part of the liver is herniated. The chronic anterior displacement of the liver will have created a tortuous and angled inferior vena cava, and acute reduction of the herniation may result in kinking of the cava and acutely impaired venous return to the heart, leading to failure. A more gradual reduction must therefore be achieved, and several techniques have been described to bridge the period before definitive closure of the abdominal skin and fascia. The practice of covering a giant omphalocele with skin flaps without fascial repair is no longer popular, as it creates a significant, chronic and debilitating ventral hernia. Alternative techniques include progressive pressure bandages, muscle and fascial rotational flaps and the use of tissue expanders.[21]

Survival for infants born with isolated abdominal wall defects exceeds 90%, and long-term quality of life is excellent. However, malabsorption and slow weight gain may occur in the first year in children with gastroschisis; intestinal obstruction, midgut volvulus, and necrotizing enterocolitis are occasionally seen.

Hirschsprung disease

Hirschsprung disease occurs in approximately 1 in 4,000–7,000 live births. It is characterized by arrested caudad migration of the ganglion cells in the submucosal and subserosal autonomic neural plexus of the colorectal wall. This aganglionosis always involves the most distal segment of the rectum, down to the level of the dentate line (the internal sphincter, itself an area of physiologic hypoganglionosis). The length of aganglionosis and its cephalad transition with normal bowel is highly variable; however, the majority of children (70–75%) have rectosigmoid involvement, while 10–25% of cases involve the descending colon. Total colonic (or even ileo-colic) aganglionosis is rare, occurring in 5–12% of all cases of Hirschsprung disease. Hirschsprung disease is more common in boys (4:1 ratio), but the disease in girls is more often of the long-segment variety: 50–60% of patients with extensive (total colonic or small bowel) aganglionosis are girls. For reasons that remain unclear, Hirschsprung disease is rare in premature infants.

Absence of ganglion cells results in an inability for the rectum to relax, resulting in partial or total obstruction of the proximal large bowel. In long-segment cases, the obstruction is complete and immediate, and results in abdominal distension and bilious vomiting shortly after birth. Inability to pass meconium within the first 24 hours (which >95% of normal neonates should do) and explosive release of stools after digital examination of the rectum are highly suspicious of Hirschsprung disease. A contrast enema may show a transition zone, between a dilated proximal colon and a narrow rectum. However, colonic distension may not yet be fully established in the newborn period. Nevertheless, a rectal diameter that is inferior to the diameter of the sigmoid or the colon is highly suspicious for Hirschsprung disease (Fig. 3). Ultimately, the diagnosis must be confirmed by biopsy. This can be performed at the bedside, without anesthesia, using a suction biopsy device to obtain a partial thickness, mucosa and submucosa specimen of the rectum. If the suction rectal biopsy is inconclusive, an operative rectal biopsy under direct vision may be required. Hematoxylin-eosin staining (H&E) of the specimen is generally sufficient; absence of ganglion

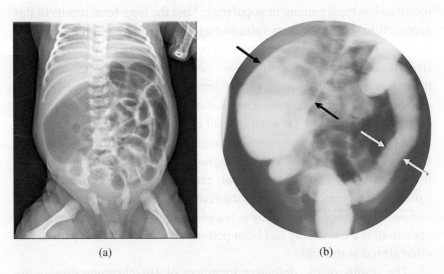

(a)   (b)

Figure 3. Hirschsprung disease. (a) Plain abdominal radiograph showing multiple dilated intestinal loops, suggesting a distal obstruction. (b) Barium enema of the same patient. Note caliber of the aganglionic distal colon and rectum (white arrows) is inferior to the caliber of the proximal, normal colon (black arrows).

cells in the submucosal plexus is accompanied by hypertrophy or proliferation of nerve endings. Immunohistochemical staining for acetyl-cholinesterase (AChE) has been well described, as there is an increased staining for AChE in the absence of acetylcholine-secreting ganglion cells. However, special stains are more time-consuming and are rarely used acutely, for frozen sections during a pull-through operation. As a result, most centers have learned to rely solely on H&E stains.[22]

The immediate treatment of Hirschsprung disease is intestinal decom-pression (nasogastric tube) and intravenous hydration. The definitive treatment of the disease involves removal of the aganglionic segment of intestine and anastomosis of normal bowel to the anorectal junction. Decades ago, a neonatal colostomy proximal to the aganglionic segment was deemed the safest approach, delaying definitive pull-through until at least four months. Following early success with neonatal pull-through, many surgeons now perform definitive resection and anastomosis within the first few days or weeks of life.[23] A laparoscopic approach to the oper-ation was introduced in the early 1990s, and is now an acceptable form of treatment. More recently, a fully transanal approach (without abdominal incision) has been gaining in popularity,[24] but the long-term results of this approach have not yet been validated against the more traditional opera-tions.[25] There are three main types of operations for Hirschsprung disease (regardless of the actual approach — open, laparoscopic or transanal). All three aim to avoid damage to the retrovesical neural plexus between bladder and anterior rectum. The Duhamel operation is a hybrid rectal reservoir consisting of the anterior wall of the native, aganglionic rectum and a posterolaterally anastomosed ganglionic bowel. The Swenson oper-ation is a straight pull-through of ganglionic colon to the dentate line, and in the Soave operation, the proximal, ganglionic bowel is pulled through a mucosa-free muscular cuff of distal rectum, and anastomosed to the den-tate line. Typically, a colostomy is not used at the time of the pull-through operation; if a colostomy had been performed in the newborn period, it is often closed at this time.

The results of the definitive treatment of Hirschsprung disease are overall good, but not perfect. Bouts of constipation and fecal impaction are common; however, incontinence is rare, except in children with associated anomalies, such as Down syndrome. Typically, symptoms improve by 5–15 years.[26] The most dangerous complication of the disease is enterocolitis, a fulminant systemic infection characterized by severe foul-smelling diarrhea, dehydration and sepsis. Treatment must be aggressive and includes bowel rest, intravenous antibiotic therapy, intravenous hydration and mechanical bowel cleansing. Although early recognition usually leads to good outcome, enterocolitis continues to be the major cause of mortality. The pathophysiology of enterocolitis involves stasis and bacterial overgrowth of the bowel, and its risk may be increased if there is a postoperative anorectal stricture or if the patient has concomitant neuronal intestinal dysplasia (an elusive condition that involves generalized colonic dysmotility).[27]

Intestinal atresia

Atresia of a segment of the intestinal tract is most often caused by a single vascular accident during fetal life. As the fetus heals without scar formation and the intestinal content of the fetus is sterile, tissue necrosis leads to resorption, resulting in a continuity gap. Occasionally, the condition is not an isolated *in utero* accident, but is the consequence of an underlying genetic or familial condition. The most common association is cystic fibrosis and *in utero* volvulus of a segment of small bowel (through sheer weight of the meconium-filled loop), resulting in vascular occlusion and necrosis (see meconium ileus). Most forms of intestinal atresia present as a lower intestinal obstruction with abdominal distension and vomiting. An abdominal radiograph shows multiple dilated loops of bowel; the presence of meconium on a rectal examination, and even bowel movements, do not rule out a complete obstruction, which may be very proximal or may have developed late *in utero*. As with all forms of obstruction, immediate treatment aims at hydration and gastrointestinal decompression (nasogastric tube). The presence of multiple loops of distended bowel and air-fluid levels (on a lateral decubitus film) suggest distal small bowel obstruction; the finding of one or only a few, severely distended loops suggests a high jejunal atresia. A contrast enema has been recommended in the past, to confirm the presence of an unused, "microcolon" and to rule out multiple atresias. In reality, colonic atresias are rare, and multiple, distal atresias must still be ruled out at the time of surgical exploration. Operative treatment consists of end-to-end anastomosis if there is only mild size discrepancy between proximal, dilated bowel and distal bowel. If the size difference is greater, tapering of the proximal, dilated segment can be performed, or a protective stoma may be created to allow decompression and normalization of the proximal bowel.

Atresias can present in various forms — with a simple intraluminal web or with actual interruption of the entire bowel wall; with or without a gap in the mesentery. While the classification is mostly academic, multiple atresias (so-called "string of sausages") and Christmas tree- or apple peel atresia stand out by their guarded prognosis. In multiple atresias, the main goal is to preserve as much intestinal length as possible and avoid short-bowel syndrome. A similar concern exists with apple peel atresia, particularly because of the tenuous blood supply in this condition: apple peel atresia usually results from *in utero* midgut volvulus (see below) and occlusion of the main jejuno-ileal branches of the superior mesenteric artery. The colon is spared, and some distal ileum may survive on retrograde flow through a branch of the ileocolic branch of the right colic artery. This results in a diminutive distal small bowel with very short mesentery wrapped around a single ileocolic vessel, and any attempt to straighten out the intestine or dissect the mesentery may result in bowel ischemia. Not uncommonly, these infants are plagued with absorptive difficulties in the first months of life. If adequate intestinal length is preserved, however, ultimate bowel adaptation is the norm.[28]

Duodenal atresia is probably not a result of an *in utero* vascular accident, as with jejunal and ileal atresia. It is believed to be a result of incomplete vacuolization or recanalization. Duodenal atresia is also more commonly associated with other anomalies. Thirty percent of duodenal atresias are associated with trisomy 21.

Duodenal atresia can present as an intraluminal web, without disruption of the duodenal continuity, or as a complete atresia. It typically occurs at the second portion of the duodenum, near the ampulla of Vater and the junction with the pancreatic head. Because most duodenal atresias occur just distal to the ampulla, vomiting is usually bilious. An annular pancreas may cause a partial or complete extrinsic duodenal obstruction, or it can be present together with a true duodenal atresia. Infants with duodenal atresia do not typically present with abdominal distension, since the small and large bowel are collapsed. Severe gastric distension may be present, but after nasogastric decompression, the abdomen will typically appear scaphoid. With complete duodenal obstruction, no distal intestinal air is seen, and the characteristic "double bubble" (stomach and proximal duodenum) provides the diagnosis. No further studies are usually necessary, and surgical exploration should be performed. Incomplete duodenal obstruction will result in a double bubble pattern and scattered distal intestinal gas. Partial obstruction may be intrinsic, from an incomplete or perforated duodenal web; or extrinsic, from an annular pancreas or compression by Ladd's bands (see malrotation, below) or a midgut volvulus. While duodenal atresia and annular pancreas are not surgical emergencies, midgut volvulus is — and any suspicion of complete or incomplete duodenal obstruction warrants a rapid work-up. An upper gastrointestinal contrast study is the most expeditious way to document the degree of obstruction and to rule out malrotation or midgut volvulus.

Meconium ileus and meconium peritonitis

Meconium ileus refers to intestinal obstruction caused by the inability of the newborn to pass thick, tenacious meconium. This condition is almost always associated with cystic fibrosis. As with other causes of intestinal obstruction, newborns with meconium ileus present with severe abdominal distension, bilious vomiting and inability to pass meconium. The diagnosis of meconium ileus may be suspected on a plain abdominal radiograph by the presence of numerous distended intestinal loops without air-fluid levels on a lateral decubitus film (as the thick meconium does not layer out). Other characteristic radiological findings are a soap-bubble appearance of the intestinal content (as gas is trapped within the viscous meconium) and the impression of a soft tissue mass, most often in the right lower quadrant — which represents inspissated meconium in the terminal ileum. A water-soluble iso-osmolar contrast enema will show a small-caliber, unused colon and diffuse reflux into the meconium-filled distal small bowel. In an otherwise stable infant, an attempt at non-operative treatment is reasonable. First described by Helen Noblett in 1969,[29] the technique uses the hygroscopic properties of a hyperosmolar water-soluble enema to loosen up the thick, viscous meconium and meconium pellets.

Because of the hygroscopic effect, dehydration is a real danger and these infants should be aggressively hydrated intravenously before and after the procedure.

If relief of the obstruction is unsuccessful, surgical intervention is indicated. At exploration, the radiological findings are confirmed, with distended, doughy appearing meconium-filled distal small bowel loops and an empty microcolon. The distal ileum is opened and the sticky, tarry appearing meconium is evacuated manually. This is followed by warm saline irrigations. A diagnosis of cystic fibrosis must be confirmed.

Complicated meconium ileus refers to meconium peritonitis, meconium ileus-associated volvulus and atresia, or perforation during the initial, non-operative management of the disease. Meconium peritonitis is a sterile peritonitis secondary to *in utero* perforation of an intestinal loop. The perforation usually seals once the loop of bowel is decompressed, and inflammation causes the leaked meconium to be walled off by a thick rind of serosa from adjacent intestinal loops (meconium pseudocyst). The specks of leaked meconium ultimately appear as echogenic foci on prenatal ultrasound and as calcifications on a postnatal radiograph. Often, these infants present with impressive abdominal distension and a red, inflamed abdominal wall. While the distension may cause significant respiratory compromise, these infants are usually less sick than they appear. Surgical exploration is necessary, but not before adequate stabilization and intravenous hydration has been initiated.

Meconium plug syndrome

Meconium plug syndrome is distinctly different from meconium ileus. It refers to a distal intestinal obstruction (most often at the level of the ascending or transverse colon) by a plug of inspissated stool, proximal to which there is accumulation of normal meconium. Dislodgment of the plug results in rapid decompression of the proximal bowel and passage of normal stools. Meconium plug syndrome is therefore not associated with cystic fibrosis. It is typically seen in full-term infants, and is more common in infants of diabetic mothers. It has also been associated with perinatal stress and hypoglycemia, leading some to suspect a transient disturbance in glucose metabolism, and a glucagon surge in particular.[30]

Meconium plug syndrome is synonymous with "small left colon syndrome," an older term that reflects the typical location of the obstruction (i.e. mid-transverse colon, with proximal dilation and an unused, small caliber descending colon).

Meconium plug syndrome presents like any other distal intestinal obstruction. An abdominal radiograph shows multiple dilated loops of bowel, but without the soap bubble appearance or lack of air-fluid levels seen in meconium ileus. Gestational diabetes or fetal/neonatal distress raises suspicion, and an iso-osmolar water-soluble contrast enema is typically diagnostic and therapeutic in dislodging the plug. Because the typical appearance of meconium plug syndrome is a distended proximal colon and a collapsed, constricted distal colon and sigmoid, it may be confused with Hirschsprung disease. Ten to fifteen percent of infants with meconium plug syndrome will, in fact, prove to have aganglionosis.[31]

Intestinal malrotation

At around the fourth week of embryonic development, and shortly after infolding of the future heart, the intestinal tract, too, lateralizes. A complex process that involves rapid elongation of the primitive gut and "rotation" of its various parts (a process that probably involves asymmetrical proliferation, cell migration and apoptosis/resorption, rather actual mechanical rotation) leads to the normal anatomic relationships of the midgut. The duodenum describes a 270° counterclockwise loop, and ends up lying posterior to the root of the superior mesenteric artery and vein. To the left of the mesenteric vessels, the bowel becomes intraperitoneal (duodeno-jejunal junction). Simultaneously, the colon develops into a frame that describes a 270° clockwise loop from cecum to sigmoid. The cecum itself does not have a mesentery, but sits against the posterior abdominal wall and the retroperitoneum. As a result, the small bowel mesentery is tethered posteriorly between the duodeno-jejunal junction (ligament of Treitz) in the left upper quadrant and the cecum (ileocecal valve) in the right lower quadrant. This wide two-point fixation normally prevents complete twisting of the mesentery on its axis.

If proper intestinal rotation does not occur or is halted, non- or incomplete rotation may lead to poor or dangerous fixation of the posterior

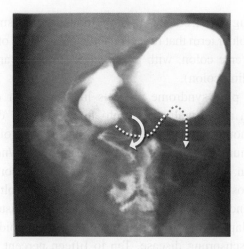

Figure 4. Intestinal malrotation. Upper gastrointestinal contrast study shows stomach (upper left) and duodenum, which remains to the right of the midline (curved arrow) instead of describing the typical "C"-loop to the left of the midline (dotted line).

mesentery. In complete nonrotation (the more correct term for malrotation), the duodenum does not describe the typical "C"-loop and remains to the right of the midline (Fig. 4). The small bowel lies mostly to the right, and the first portion of the large bowel (cecum and ascending colon) is fixed just to the left of the midline in the upper abdomen, adjacent to the duodenojejunal junction. Thus, posterior fixation of the small bowel mesentery consists of a very narrow pedicle, which can easily twist and cause complete obstruction of the superior mesenteric vessels. This results in ischemia and necrosis of the entire midgut, embryologically defined from the proximal jejunum to the transverse colon.

The surgical intervention for malrotation (Ladd's procedure) aims at reducing the risk of midgut volvulus. It is not possible to recreate the normal anatomic relationships of the intestinal tract, but the root of the mesentery (two-point fixation between duodenum and cecum) can be widened by dissecting the avascular adhesive bands that connect them. Ultimately, the duodenum will lie well into the right upper quadrant and the cecum and ascending colon well into the left. The root of the mesentery, while still narrower than with normal rotation, is now wide enough to significantly decrease the risk of subsequent volvulus. Typically, an appendectomy is performed as well, since its abnormal location on the left side of the abdomen would make appendicitis much more difficult to diagnose in the future.

Anorectal malformations

There is a wide spectrum of anomalies commonly termed anorectal malformations, from low imperforate anus and anteriorly displaced anus to high forms of imperforate anus and cloacal anomalies. The definitive treatment of these conditions is often complex, and the results are not uniformly gratifying. All present with some degree of low intestinal obstruction, which must be dealt with acutely in the neonatal period.

Inspection of the perineum at birth should alert one to the absence of an anal opening — but a normally formed natal cleft, perineal body, and a functional external sphincter complex may, on rare occasions, mask the actual absence of an opening. High forms of imperforate anus are more obvious and are often associated with hypoplasia of the perianal region and a flat ("rocker bottom") perineum without a well-defined sphincter complex. Low forms of imperforate anus are more common in girls — and are usually associated with a fistula between the rectal pouch and the perineum. Even if this rectoperineal conduit is not the anatomic anal canal and is not surrounded by an appropriate sphincter muscle complex, it is sufficient for stool evacuation. It is therefore appropriate to treat these infants conservatively, gradually dilating the fistula to allow normal bowel movements. Definitive surgery can then be postponed until the child is several months old and the anatomy can be better defined. In more complex anorectal anomalies, creation of a colostomy is the safe first step. Full work-up can then be undertaken to map out the precise anorectal and urogenital anatomy. These complex anomalies include cloacal malformations, where the rectourinary fistula drains into a common urogenital sinus, which represents the common channel of vagina and urethra. A combination of cysto-vaginoscopy, pelvic ultrasonography and various contrast imaging studies are required to map out the exact anatomic relationships, which vary from patient to patient. Consequently, reconstructive surgery will have to be indidualized, and its success will depend on the severity of the atresia and the presence of associated anomalies.

Boys more often have a high form of imperforate anus and almost never have a true perineal fistula (a rectourinary fistula is almost always present, but it terminates in the posterior urethra or, rarely, the bladder). Therefore, these infants require an intervention to relieve the distal obstruction. Within the first 24–48 hours of life, a colostomy is created, and the infant is allowed to feed and grow. As with girls, definitive surgery can safely be performed at a few months of age.

Infants with anorectal malformations have a high incidence of associated anomalies. In addition to the VACTERL association (see above), many have urinary tract anomalies, sacral deformation and lower extremity disorders, such as talipes. Up to 10% of children with anorectal malformations have tethered cord — spine ultrasonography may be useful, but not as diagnostic as magnetic resonance imaging (MRI).[32] It is important to remember that tethered cord may not become symptomatic until after the first year of life, and its effect on anorectal and urinary continence may worsen an already compromised prognosis.

Biliary anomalies

The two main surgically correctible causes of neonatal jaundice are choledochal cyst and biliary atresia. Choledocal cysts can be isolated (fusiform or diverticular) or part of a diffuse intra- and extrahepatic process such as Caroli's disease.

Ultrasonography usually provides the diagnosis. Additional studies, such as nuclear (HIDA) scanning, may be helpful, but endoscopic retrograde cholangiopancreatography (ERCP) is often not feasible in very young children. In recent years, magnetic resonance cholangiopancreatography (MRCP) has offered a minimally invasive alternative, and its usage is increasing rapidly.[33,34] Treatment of choledochal cyst is surgical resection and anastomosis of a Roux-en-Y limb of small bowel to the proximal bile ducts (hepatico-jejunostomy).

The most serious surgical cause of neonatal jaundice is biliary atresia. Multiple anatomic variations have been reported, but all but the strictly extrahepatic forms of the disease require the same intervention.

Previously called "inoperable" biliary atresia, the absence of intrahepatic bile ducts is associated with bile ductular proliferation that can be drained through the hilar region of the liver (the porta hepatis, at the confluence of the left and right branches of the portal vein). This operation, initially described by Morio Kasai,[35] leads to adequate bile drainage and complete resolution of the jaundice in a quarter of the patients. An additional 50% will experience some improvement, but will gradually develop bridging fibrosis and cirrhosis, ultimately requiring liver transplantation. Roughly one quarter of patients will not show improvement after a Kasai portoenterostomy.[36]

Work-up of infants with suspected biliary atresia must be expeditious, as the overall chances of success of the Kasai operation decrease if the patient is older than 8–10 weeks. This is further complicated by the fact that many infants do not present with severe jaundice until several weeks of life. Direct hyperbilirubinemia and a non-visualized gallbladder on ultrasonography raise the suspicion of biliary atresia. A HIDA scan, preferably after a 3–5 day course of phenobarbital to stimulate cytochrome P450 function and bile secretion by the liver, typically demonstrates rapid uptake of the tracer by the liver. Delayed images show persistence of a bright hepatic signal and absence of tracer in the intestinal tract. The definitive diagnosis of biliary atresia is established surgically. An intraoperative cholangiogram through an often diminutive gallbladder will fail to visualize intrahepatic bile ducts (even if the distal bile ducts are patent). A wedge biopsy of the liver confirms absence of normal bile ducts and bile ductular proliferation.

Acquired disorders

Necrotizing enterocolitis (NEC) and idiopathic spontaneous intestinal perforation (SIP)

The medical aspect of NEC is discussed elsewhere in this Handbook. Surgical intervention is reserved for complications of NEC. These include interstinal perforation with peritonitis, bowel necrosis and impending perforation, and failure of non-operative treatment. The aim of surgical intervention is to control the peritonitis and remove the irreversibly necrotic intestine. Preservation of intestinal length is important, but not always possible — short bowel syndrome is a serious long-term complication.

Because of the significant surgical risk of laparotomy and general anesthesia, percutaneous drainage of leaked intestinal content was proposed decades ago as a temporizing measure. The original concept was to allow fluid resuscitation, after which percutaneous drainage was followed by laparotomy. Because of the anecdotal survival of these infants without a subsequent laparotomy, peritoneal drainage became a popular definitive treatment of perforated NEC in extreme low birthweight infants (<1000 g). Following several retrospective studies showing acceptable survival, particularly in micropremies (<750 g),[37] a multicenter prospective randomized trial showed equivalent survival at 90 days, length of hospitalization and dependence on total parenteral nutrition between peritoneal drainage and laparotomy.[38] A follow-up study is currently under way to examine long-term morbidity of both approaches.

SIP can occur in the premature infant without underlying NEC. It is most commonly seen within the first days of life, and can present with acute and severe abdominal distension. An abdominal radiograph shows large amounts of peritoneal free air, which is often clearly visible over the liver even on a decubitus film. While the sudden distension may cause some respiratory impairment, these infants are surprisingly stable overall. Bedside peritoneal drainage is considered the treatment of choice by many, and results are typically good, often without the need for a subsequent laparotomy (the perforation seals itself). A more detailed description of this condition is presented elsewhere in this Handbook.

Midgut volvulus

The most dramatic acute surgical condition of the newborn is midgut volvulus, an acquired disorder that occurs in children with intestinal malrotation (see above).The typical presentation is sudden bilious vomiting and rapid, progressive deterioration of the child. The abdomen is not typically distended (and may be frankly scaphoid), as the obstruction occurs at the level of the duodeno-jejunal junction. However, acute gastric distension may mask this. In addition, advanced volvulus and generalized ischemic damage to the midgut (from jejunum to mid-colon) may cause edema of the intestinal wall and fluid accumulation within the lumen, resulting in generalized abdominal distension.

Any bilious vomiting in a newborn or infant raises the immediate suspicion of midgut volvulus, and the diagnosis must be promptly made (or ruled out). An abdominal radiograph may be non-specific, and because the colon of the newborn does not yet have well-developed haustrations, it can be difficult to differentiate it from small bowel. Therefore, diagnosis of malrotation or volvulus requires a contrast study. The most definitive study is an upper gastrointestinal series. The third portion of the duodenum does not cross the midline in malrotation; with midgut volvulus, the duodenum and proximal jejunum are twisted and show an apple peel or bird's beak sign, particularly on a lateral film.

Surgical exploration must be performed emergently. The small bowel is exteriorized, gently untwisted, and its viability assessed. If rapid return of perfusion is seen, a Ladd's procedure is completed (see above).

References

1. Luks FI, Carr SR, Feit LR *et al.* (2003) Experience with a multidisciplinary antenatal diagnosis and management model in fetal medicine. *J Matern Fetal Neonatal Med* **14**(5): 333–337.

2. Crombleholme TM, D'Alton M, Cendron M *et al.* (1996) Prenatal diagnosis and the pediatric surgeon: The impact of prenatal consultation on perinatal management. *J Pediatr Surg* **31**(1): 156–162; 162–163.

3. Canick JA, Kellner LH, Bombard AT. (2003) Prenatal screening for open neural tube defects. *Clin Lab Med* **23**(2): 385–394, ix.

4. Skarsgard ED, Chitkara U, Krane EJ *et al.* (1996) The OOPS procedure (operation on placental support): *In utero* airway management of the fetus with prenatally diagnosed tracheal obstruction. *J Pediatr Surg* **31**(6): 826–828.

5. Hedrick HL, Flake AW, Crombleholme TM *et al.* (2005) The *ex utero* intrapartum therapy procedure for high-risk fetal lung lesions. *J Pediatr Surg* **40**(6): 1038–1043; 1044.

6. Seetharamaiah R, Younger JG, Bartlett RH *et al.* (2009) Factors associated with survival in infants with congenital diaphragmatic hernia requiring

extracorporeal membrane oxygenation: A report from the Congenital Diaphragmatic Hernia Study Group. *J Pediatr Surg* **44**(7): 1315–1321.

7. Jani J, Keller RL, Benachi A *et al.* (2006) Prenatal prediction of survival in isolated left-sided diaphragmatic hernia. *Ultrasound Obstet Gynecol* **27**(1): 18–22.

8. Calonge WM, Martinez L, Lacadena J *et al.* (2007) Expression of homeotic genes Hoxa3, Hoxb3, Hoxd3 and Hoxc4 is decreased in the lungs but not in the hearts of adriamycin-exposed mice. *Pediatr Surg Int* **23**(5): 419–424.

9. Spilde TL, Bhatia AM, Mehta S *et al.* (2003) Defective sonic hedgehog signaling in esophageal atresia with tracheoesophageal fistula. *Surgery* **134**(2): 345–350.

10. Dawrant MJ, Giles S, Bannigan J, Puri P. (2007) Adriamycin mouse model: A variable but reproducible model of tracheo-oesophageal malformations. *Pediatr Surg Int* **23**(5): 469–472.

11. Teich S, Barton DP, Ginn-Pease ME *et al.* (1997) Prognostic classification for esophageal atresia and tracheoesophageal fistula: Waterston versus Montreal. *J Pediatr Surg* **32**(7): 1075–1079; 1079–1080.

12. Poenaru D, Laberge JM, Neilson IR *et al.* (1993) A new prognostic classification for esophageal atresia. *Surgery* **113**(4): 426–432.

13. Bax KM, van Der Zee DC. (2002) Feasibility of thoracoscopic repair of esophageal atresia with distal fistula. *J Pediatr Surg* **37**(2): 192–196.

14. Ron O, De Coppi P, Pierro A. (2009) The surgical approach to esophageal atresia repair and the management of long-gap atresia: Results of a survey. *Semin Pediatr Surg* **18**(1): 44–49.

15. Lessin MS, Wesselhoeft CW, Luks FI *et al.* (1999) Primary repair of long-gap esophageal atresia by mobilization of the distal esophagus. *Eur J Pediatr Surg* **9**(6): 369–372.

16. Till H, Rolle U, Siekmeyer W *et al.* (2008) Combination of spit fistula advancement and external traction for primary repair of long-gap esophageal atresia. *Ann Thorac Surg* **86**(6): 1969–1971.

17. Roggin KK, Breuer CK, Carr SR *et al.* (2000) The unpredictable character of congenital cystic lung lesions. *J Pediatr Surg* **35**(5): 801–805.

18. Porter A, Benson CB, Hawley P *et al.* (2009) Outcome of fetuses with a prenatal ultrasound diagnosis of isolated omphalocele. *Prenat Diagn* **29**(7): 668–673.

19. Blazer S, Zimmer EZ, Gover A *et al.* (2004) Fetal omphalocele detected early in pregnancy: Associated anomalies and outcomes. *Radiology* **232**(1): 191–195.

20. Huang J, Kurkchubasche A, Carr S *et al.* (2002) Benefits of term delivery in infants with antenatally diagnosed gastroschisis. *Obstet Gynecol* **100**(4): 695.

21. Martin AE, Khan A, Kim DS *et al.* (2009) The use of intra-abdominal tissue expanders as a primary strategy for closure of giant omphaloceles. *J Pediatr Surg* **44**(1): 178–182.

22. Martucciello G, Pini Prato A, Puri P *et al.* (2005) Controversies concerning diagnostic guidelines for anomalies of the enteric nervous system: A report from the fourth *International Symposium on Hirschsprung's disease* and related neurocristopathies. *J Pediatr Surg* **40**(10): 1527–1531.

23. Teitelbaum DH, Coran AG. (2003) Primary pull-through for Hirschsprung's disease. *Semin Neonatol* **8**(3): 233–241.

24. Podevin G, Lardy H, Azzis O *et al.* (2006) Technical problems and complications of a transanal pull-through for Hirschsprung's disease. *Eur J Pediatr Surg* **16**(2): 104–108.

25. Jester I, Holland-Cunz S, Loff S *et al.* (2009) Transanal pull-through procedure for Hirschsprung's disease: A 5-year experience. *Eur J Pediatr Surg* **19**(2): 68–71.

26. Fortuna RS, Weber TR, Tracy TF, Jr. *et al.* (1996) Critical analysis of the operative treatment of Hirschsprung's disease. *Arch Surg* **131**(5): 520–524; discussion 524–525.

27. Feichter S, Meier-Ruge WA, Bruder E. (2009) The histopathology of gastrointestinal motility disorders in children. *Semin Pediatr Surg* **18**(4): 206–211.

28. Festen S, Brevoord JC, Goldhoorn GA *et al.* (2002) Excellent long-term outcome for survivors of apple peel atresia. *J Pediatr Surg* **37**(1): 61–65.

29. Noblett HR. (1969) Treatment of uncomplicated meconium ileus by Gastrografin enema: A preliminary report. *J Pediatr Surg* **4**(2): 190–197.

30. Stewart DR, Nixon GW, Johnson DG *et al.* (1977) Neonatal small left colon syndrome. *Ann Surg* **186**(6): 741–745.

31. Ellis H, Kumar R, Kostyrka B. (2009) Neonatal small left colon syndrome in the offspring of diabetic mothers-an analysis of 105 children. *J Pediatr Surg* **44**(12): 2343–2346.

32. Kim SM, Chang HK, Lee MJ *et al.* (2010) Spinal dysraphism with anorectal malformation: Lumbosacral magnetic resonance imaging evaluation of 120 patients. *J Pediatr Surg* **45**(4): 769–776.

33. Fitoz S, Erden A, Boruban S. (2007) Magnetic resonance cholangiopancreatography of biliary system abnormalities in children. *Clin Imaging* **31**(2): 93–101.

34. Hamada Y, Tanano A, Takada K *et al.* (2004) Magnetic resonance cholangiopancreatography on postoperative work-up in children with choledochal cysts. *Pediatr Surg Int* **20**(1): 43–46.

35. Kasai M, Suzuki H, Ohashi E *et al.* (1978) Technique and results of operative management of biliary atresia. *World J Surg* **2**(5): 571–579.

36. Hartley JL, Davenport M, Kelly DA. (2009) Biliary atresia. *Lancet* **374**(9702): 1704–1713.

37. Lessin MS, Luks FI, Wesselhoeft CW, Jr. *et al.* (1998) Peritoneal drainage as definitive treatment for intestinal perforation in infants with extremely low birth weight (<750 g). *J Pediatr Surg* **33**(2): 370–372.

38. Moss RL, Dimmitt RA, Barnhart DC *et al.* (2006) Laparotomy versus peritoneal drainage for necrotizing enterocolitis and perforation. *N Engl J Med* **354**(21): 2225–2234.

PART

IV

Follow-Up Care
of High-Risk Infants

PART

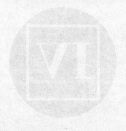

IV

Follow-Up Care
of High-Risk Infants

Chapter 20

Follow-Up Assessment of High-Risk Infants

Betty R. Vohr and Bonnie E. Stephens

Rationale for Follow-Up of Infants cared for in a Neonatal Intensive Care Unit

Advances in perinatal and neonatal management of very low birth weight (VLBW) infants (<1500 grams) have resulted in increased survival of fragile "high-risk" infants, including those with special health care needs. These high-risk preterm survivors have increased post-discharge morbidities including neurologic, sensory, cognitive, visual-motor/fine motor, speech and language, motor function, coordination, functional skills for daily living, and behavior and they may be technology dependent for prolonged periods of time. The changes in survival are associated with a constant emergence of new interventions and a changing environment of the intensive care unit (NICU). Therefore, it is critically important that as new technologies or concepts of care are introduced, that they be evidence based and evaluated for both safety and efficacy. As a consequence, most tertiary care programs in the United States and all neonatal training programs have a structured follow-up program to evaluate outcomes.

Objectives of a Follow-Up Program

To be successful, follow-up programs must identify the program objectives. A workshop on the follow-up care of high risk infants sponsored by the National Institute of Child Health and Human Development (NICHD), the National Institute of Neurologic Disorders and Stroke and the Centers for Disease Control and Prevention held in 2002, established guidelines for the provision of Follow-up Services which were published in 2004.[1] The workshop concluded that two primary areas of responsibility for Neonatal Follow-up Programs are surveillance and research. These areas of responsibility will be expanded to include clinical management and education goals.

Clinical

The Follow-up Program has opportunities to provide comprehensive evaluations of growth, neurologic status, development, pulmonary status, feeding, and behavior. Clinical objectives include improving the health and developmental outcomes of high risk infants, providing support to families and reducing family stress. The provision of feedback to both the family and the medical home after each visit supports the concept of an effective medical home for NICU graduates. A follow-up clinic may provide a mechanism for the provision of seamless comprehensive medical, psychosocial, and early intervention services to NICU graduates.[2]

Surveillance and quality assurance

A mechanism of data management greatly facilitated by electronic medical records should be in place to systematically monitor neonatal characteristics, morbidities and interventions during the stay in the NICU and the neurologic, developmental, medical and behavioral outcomes post-discharge. This data base provides the opportunity to monitor quality indicators for the individual NICU, summarize data about center outcomes for specific conditions such as periventricular leukomalacia or chronic lung disease and summarize annual outcome data that can be utilized in policy development. Data derived from surveillance of neonatal and post-discharge outcomes can be used in antenatal, neonatal and post-discharge counseling and support of families, as well as for grant applications and department reports.

Research

A program that includes comprehensive standardized assessments, a comprehensive data base, and procedures in place for tracking families provides an opportunity for research on a number of levels including observational studies, cohort studies, and randomized control trials to examine the effects of interventions designed to improve the growth, neurologic status, developmental status, or behavior of high-risk infants. An advantage of having a structured established follow-up program in place is that it provides a mechanism to more easily implement clinical research.

Education

The follow-up program provides an excellent opportunity for education of medical students, residents, fellows, nurses, nurse practitioners, families and primary care providers regarding the care, management and outcomes of high-risk infants post discharge. All neonatal training programs in the United States currently include a requirement for fellow participation in a structured follow-up program.

Staff and Procedures of the Follow-Up Program

Basic staff would include a medical director, physicians, developmental psychologists, social worker, manager, data entry personnel, and data analyst (Table 1). Additional staff for more comprehensive evaluations or for larger programs may include nurse practitioners, occupational therapists, nutritionists, audiologist, and pulmonologists. A clinic manual with all procedures delineated, a clinic brochure, forms for all information collected, and an annual procedure for training new staff in inter-rater reliability need to be in place for all staff.

Table 1. Neonatal follow-up clinic staff.

Staff Member	Responsibilities
Medical Director	Oversees clinical, quality assurance, research and education
Physicians and Nurse Practitioners	Perform medical and neurologic assessments
Psychologists	Perform neuropsychological and behavioral testing
Social Worker	Identifies families with risk issues and facilitates needed interventions
Parent Consultant	Provides support and guidance to families
Program Manager	Supervises all aspects of day-to-day operation of the clinic
Receptionist	Schedules appointments, greets families, does billing
Data Entry	Enters data from clinic forms
Data Analyst	Manages database, completes analyses and provides reports
Nutritionist	Completes nutrition analysis and provides recommendations
Occupational Therapist	Provides therapy guidance and intervention
Pulmonologist	Manages infants with chronic lung disease
Audiologist	Provides hearing assessments

Risk Populations for Follow-Up

Infants in the following categories may be scheduled, depending on the size of the NICU, infant characteristics, and acuity level of the NICU. Premature infants weighing less than 1500 grams, 1250 grams or 1000 grams at birth, and preterm or term infants with a variety of complications including intraventricular hemorrhage, bronchopulmonary dysplasia, perinatal asphyxia, meningitis, congenital malformations and infants discharged on cardiorespiratory monitors or oxygen, may be candidates. While the majority of neonatal outcomes research has focused on the ELBW infant, more recent studies have brought attention to a long neglected population of infants, the late preterm (34–36 weeks gestation). Rates of deliveries of infants 34 and 36 weeks have increased steadily during the 1990s. Between 1990 and 2005, the rate of late preterm births increased from 7.3% to 9.1%.[3] Late preterm infants have higher rates of

Table 2. Medical risk factors.

Premature	Term
VLBW infants ≤1500; ≤1000; ≤750 grams	Perinatal Asphyxia
Preterm infants <34; ≤28; ≤27 weeks	Seizures or Meningitis
Late preterm infants 34–36 weeks	Small for gestation
Cranial Ultrasound abnormalities	Twin–twin transfusion
Necrotizing enterocolitis	Congenital Abnormalities/Birth Defects
Broncho pulmonary dysplasia	Sepsis/Meningitis
Small for Gestation	TORCH infections
Twin–twin transfusion	Hyperbilirubinemia requiring exchange
Multiples	Metabolic disorders
Sepsis/Meningitis	Other neurologic abnormalities
Congenital Abnormalities/birth defects	Other Complex Medical Morbidities
Other Complex Medical Morbidities	

mortality rates[4] and common neonatal morbidities than term infants. Table 2 lists the most common medical categories of high-risk preterm and term infants described in follow-up studies. Basic demographic data need to be collected for all outcome studies so that statistical adjustments may be made when interpreting outcomes. One of the challenges of follow-up studies which can contribute to bias in interpreting impairment rates is that poor and less educated families are less likely to return for a follow-up.[5] Other neonatal factors affecting outcome for which adjustments must be made include multiple versus singleton, inborn versus outborn, gestational age at birth and male versus female.

Assessment Schedules

Age of assessments for premature infants <34 weeks gestation in the first 30 months are standardly interpreted and based on corrected age (time since mother's expected date of delivery) rather than chronologic age (time since birth). Most, but not all studies, begin to use chronologic age at the 3-year visit. The visit schedule needs to be based on the focus of the Follow-up program. If it is primarily research, it is dependent on the outcome ages of the study protocol. The majority of recent studies have outcomes reported at 18–24 months corrected age. Many programs begin visits at 1–3 months of age with 6 month intervals between visits for the first two years of life. Because of the expense of comprehensive multi-disciplinary assessments, most programs cannot accomplish follow-up to school age. Assessments in the first 18 months to 3 years of life reliably identify major disability including mental retardation, cerebral palsy, epilepsy, blindness, and/or moderate to severe hearing impairment. These findings have historically been the outcomes of interest both to professionals and parents. Secondary to environmental influences, access to educational supports, and brain resiliency, cognitive assessment at 18 months to 3 years is not as predictive of young adult outcome as cognitive assessment at school age. Longitudinal studies of preterm children have demonstrated variability in the progression of neurologic and developmental findings and include: stability,[6] improvement,[7] and worsening[8,9] of neuropsychological findings. Limitations in the positive predictive value of early assessments may also be related to differences in follow-up rates, the inclusion or exclusion of children with major neurologic or sensory impairments, and the effects of postdischarge environment. To minimize bias in the interpretation of outcome studies, a follow-up rate of ≥90% is optimal. The validity of outcome data is further enhanced by utilization of a gender and age-matched comparison group.

Compliance for Follow-Up

For all longitudinal studies, compliance to follow-up is the greatest challenge. There are multiple barriers including language or cultural differences, lack of a phone or transportation, geographic distance from center, family stress, unemployment, poverty, and lack of a relationship between the family and program personnel. Introduction of the program prior to discharge, developing rapport with the family, obtaining contact information from multiple sources (cell phone, e-mail, home phone, work phone, relative address and phone, primary care provider and early intervention provider) are recommended. Incentives for participation include feedback to families on assessment findings including recommendations, small gifts for the child, and payment of transportation costs. Home visits by staff personnel are expensive, but indicated for families who are unable to come to the center.

Outcomes and Assessments

There are eight major categories of assessment which can be covered in early childhood in a Neonatal Follow-up Program including: growth, neurologic/neurosensory, cognitive, visual-motor/fine motor, speech and language, motor function/coordination, functional skills for daily living, and behavior.

Growth

Assessment of growth should include all birth parameters, rate of growth in the NICU and growth parameters at the time of discharge. The NICHD Neonatal Research Network uses fetal growth charts developed by Alexander *et al.*[10] which provide reference weights for infants born from 20 to 38 weeks gestation. Weight, length and head circumference should be collected routinely and longitudinally by examiners trained to reliability-using standard techniques. Measures are plotted according to gender and aged adjusted until age two, based on the National Center for Health Statistics growth charts.

Rationale for growth assessment

Preterm infants are at increased risk of small for gestation (SGA). Both SGA and appropriate for gestation (AGA) infants are at increased risk of growth restriction during their stay in the NICU. Ehrenkranz *et al.*[11] showed a clear relationship between decreasing rates of growth velocity in the NICU and both increasing rates of neonatal morbidities and subsequent rates of adverse neurodevelopmental impairment. Increased awareness of the importance of early nutrition on growth and development has resulted in significant changes in both parenteral and enteral feeding protocols of high-risk infants.

The neurologic assessment

The neurologic examination should be an integral part of every assessment of the high-risk infant. The abnormal neurologic examination and
particularly the diagnosis of moderate to severe cerebral palsy (CP) is an
important quality indicator for a NICU and a critically important diagnosis for impact on families. A diagnosis of CP is reliably obtained in
premature infants by ages 18 to 24 months corrected age by performing
a systematic neurologic examination such as the assessment developed
by Claudine Amiel Tison.[12] CP is defined as a non-progressive central
nervous system disorder with abnormal muscle tone in at least one
extremity and abnormal control of movement and posture which interfere
with age-appropriate activities.[12] CP is a challenging diagnosis to make
on infants less than one year of corrected age because of the prevalence
of hypertonicity among premature infants in the first year of life. Other
neurologic findings include hypertonicity, hypotonicity, seizure disorder,
dyspraxia, absent pincer, or facial palsy without a specific diagnosis of
CP. Moderate to severe CP is a component of neurodevelopmental
impairment (NDI), a common primary outcome. NDI has been defined as
the presence of any of the following: moderate to severe CP, blind in both
eyes, bilateral hearing impairment requiring amplification, or having a
Bayley II Mental Developmental Index or Psychomotor Developmental
Index score <70.

Rational for neurologic assessment

Extremely preterm infants have increased rates of intraventricular
hemorrhage (IVH) and periventricular leukomalacia (PVL). IVH,
ventriculomegaly at term and cystic PVL are all associated with cognitive impairment and CP.[13] Rates of CP in ELBW vary from 5% to
30%,[13-21] but are most commonly cited at 15% to 23%.[13,14,16,19,20]
While CP is the most well known and potentially most disabling motor
abnormality associated with prematurity, infants born preterm often
demonstrate other less severe differences in their neurologic development. During the first year of life, transient dystonia is a common
deviation in the motor development of VLBW infants.[22] More

recently, these transient findings have been re-described as occurring in 21% to 36% of preterm infants with a peak incidence at 7 months corrected age.[23]

Sensory

Vision abnormalities are common among former preterm infants. The standard of care within tertiary care centers determines that VLBW infants have ophthalmologic examinations for retinopathy of prematurity prior to discharge with appropriate follow-up and intervention where appropriate. This has facilitated the identification of all degrees of vision impairment. In addition, ongoing monitoring for the detection of strabismus and myopia are indicated. Bilateral blindness is included in the composite outcome of NDI.

Since NICU infants are at increased risk of all types of permanent hearing loss, including neural (auditory neuropathy/auditory dyssynchrony) hearing loss, the Joint Committee on Infant Hearing (JCIH) (2007),[24] recommended automated auditory brainstem response (ABR) screening prior to discharge for all infants that require NICU care for >5 days. Infants who fail the screen should have a comprehensive audiology assessment with diagnostic auditory brainstem response and otoacoustic emissions by 3 months of age. Children who are at least 6 months of developmental age should also have a behavioral assessment, vision reinforcement audiometry, tympanometry and otoacoustic emissions completed. Bilateral hearing loss that requires amplification is included in NDI.

Rational for sensory assessment

Rates of neurosensory disabilities are higher in ELBW infants than the general population. Unilateral or bilateral blindness occurs in 1% to 10% of ELBW infants.[21] Milder visual impairments including myopia, strabismus, and lack of stereopsis (depth perception), occur at rates of 9% to 25%.[21]

Permanent hearing loss requiring amplification with hearing aids or cochlear implants is reported in 1% to 9% of ELBW infants.[21] When transient conductive or unilateral hearing loss is included, rates of milder impairment are as high as 28%.[21]

Developmental/cognitive outcomes

The Bayley Scales of Infant Development (Bayley II)[25] has been the most commonly reported assessment of development to 36 months of age and provides a cognitive (mental developmental index (MDI)) and motor (psychomotor developmental index (PDI)) domains. A score < 70 (2 SDs below the mean) is interpreted as evidence of developmental delay. A limitation of the Bayley II was the combining of cognitive and language tasks into a single MDI and combining gross and fine motor tasks into a single PDI score. The Bayley Scales of Infant Development III (BSID-III) is currently available for assessments from 1 month to 42 months of age.[26] The BSID-III consists of three domains: the Cognitive, Language and Motor. In addition, there are subscores for receptive communication, expressive communication, fine motor and gross motor. The rationale for the development of the Bayley III was, in part, to separate the cognitive from language tasks to eliminate the bias imposed on cognitive scores for children residing in a bilingual or non–English speaking household.

The Stanford Binet Intelligence Scale — fourth edition (SB-4),[27] the Differential Ability Scales,[28] and the McCarthy Scales of Children's Abilities,[29] are tests of early cognitive/developmental ability. For studying populations of high-risk children, cognitive outcome data is best interpreted by comparison to a normal control group, a study comparison group or normative data. Many outcome studies report on overall performance in a spectrum of domains. A battery of tests is administered and may include visual perceptual skills,[30–31] speech and language skills,[32–35] cognition,[27–29,36,37] fine and gross motor function,[38–41] behavior,[42–45] functional skills and health care status.[46–48] An individual child's early test results have limited predictive validity of cognitive status and are best used to identify service needs at the time the test is administered. School age outcomes have the most validity. At school age, cognitive functioning is assessed using a variety of different measures including the Stanford Binet Intelligence Scale — fourth edition, the Wechsler Preschool and Primary Scales of Intelligence — third edition (WPPSI), the Wechsler Intelligence Scale for Children (WISC-III), the Woodcock–Johnson Psycho-Educational Battery — Revised and the

Differential Abilities Scales,[28] the McCarthy Scales of Children's Abilities.[29] Each of these assessments provides an intelligence quotient (IQ) and subtest scores that allow for a limited assessment of specific areas of strengths and weaknesses of skill attainment. The Behavior Rating Inventory of Executive Function (BRIEF)[49] is a test which taps into executive function.

Justification for cognitive assessment

The most common severe impairment seen in VLBW and ELBW infants at 18 and 30 months is cognitive impairment, defined as scores that are more than two standard deviations below the mean on standardized cognitive testing. Average score for ELBW infants at 18–22 months corrected age on the Bayley II in an NICHD cohort was 76, but varied from center to center with a range of 70 to 83.[21] In a cohort of <1000 gram infants born from 1982 to 2002, Wilson-Costello and Hack report average MDIs of 84–86 at 20-month follow-up.[18]

While cognitive functioning can by measured in infancy, it may not be predictive of cognitive functioning later in life. Hack *et al.* reported that MDI at 20 months corrected age was not predictive of cognitive functioning at 8 years of age. The positive predictive value of having a low cognitive score at 20 months (<70) was only 0.37.[50] for a low cognitive score at 8 years (<70). Ment *et al.* reported recovery of median expressive language scores from 88 to 97 and full scale IQ increased from 90 to 96 from 3 to 8 years of age among former preterm children. While environmental factors are known to impact on intelligence, differences in IQ between preterm and term controls persist after adjustment for these confounders.

At school age, former preterm children have higher rates of neuropsychological deficits and academic and poorer academic functioning. Higher prevalence, lower severity dysfunctions occur in 50–70% of children born VLBW. Children born VLBW or ELBW have relative impairments of executive functioning,[51,52] visual-motor skills and memory, especially verbal memory. Approximately 25% of VLBW infants and up to 62% of ELBW infants receive special education services and between 15% and 34% repeat a grade.[53]

Visual motor integration/fine motor skills

The third category is visual motor and fine motor skills.[30,31] The most commonly used test for visual motor skills is the Beery Developmental Test of Visual-Motor Integration fourth Ed. (Beery VMI).[30] The Beery VMI assesses the degree to which visual-perception and motor behavior is integrated. Fine motor skills can be assessed using the Peabody Developmental Motor Scales (PDMS).[39] This test presents the child with a variety of fine motor and manual dexterity tasks.

Justification for visual motor integration and fine motor assessment

Difficulties with fine motor skills, visual perception, visual motor control, hand-eye coordination, or visual-motor integration, are common in children born VLBW or ELBW. These difficulties can impact on academic performance including reading and mathematics. Fine motor difficulties have been described in as many as 70% and fine motor difficulties resulting in impairment in 23% at 5 years of age.[54–56]

Speech and language

Speech language delays are common among both preterm and term infants. The Preschool Language Scale — third edition (PLS-3)[34] is a standardized assessment which includes auditory comprehension and expressive communication subscales to assess attention, vocal development, social communication, semantics, language structure, and integrative thinking skills. The Peabody Picture Vocabulary Test (PPVT-R)[32] is a non-verbal, multiple-choice test of receptive vocabulary. The Early Language Milestone Scale — Second Edition (ELM Scale-2)[35] assesses speech and language development in three areas: auditory expressive, auditory receptive, and visual. The Sequenced Inventory of Communication Development Revised edition (SICDR)[33] is a diagnostic test that evaluates the communication abilities between 4 months and 4 years of age. It has been used successfully for children with sensory impairments and developmental retardation.

Justification for speech and language assessment

Speech and Language delays are common among former ELBW children, with delays in the acquisition of expressive language, receptive language, and articulation. Children born at or before 25 weeks gestation have significantly lower total scores on the PLS (90 vs 104) and significantly higher rates of language impairment (16% vs 2%) at 6 years of age. Scores on auditory comprehension, expressive communication and articulation subtests of the PLS are uniformly lower.[57] In addition, rates of language impairment, defined as standard scores of < 70 on language assessment, are higher. Former ELBW infants have significantly lower scores (92 vs 105) and higher rates of impairment (13% vs 4%) on the PPVT, as well as lower expressive, receptive, and total scores (85–87 vs 100–103) and higher rates of impairment (22–24% vs 3–4%) on the CELF at age 12.[56] Specific language deficits have been described including phonological short term memory and prosodic processing. At 12 years of age, children who were born <1250 grams have less pronounced differences on tests of lower level language skills (phonological processing, phonemic decoding and sight word reading) compared to term controls, but exhibit significantly more difficulty with higher level skills (syntax, semantics, verbal language memory and reading comprehension).[56]

Motor function/coordination

The Peabody Developmental Motor Scales (PDMS)[39] are a test of gross and fine motor skills of children ages birth through 83 months. The Early Screening Profiles (ESP)[40] measures motor, cognitive/language, and developmental skills in children. The ESP consists of three profiles: Motor Profile, Cognitive/Language Profile and Self-Help/Social. Another test is the Movement Assessment Battery for Children (MABC).

Justification for motor assessment

Cerebral Palsy is the most common cause of severe gross and fine motor impairment. Level of gross motor function is most commonly assessed and categorized using Palisano's Gross Motor Function Classification System

(GMFCS).[58] Scores range from 0 to 5 and increase with increasing functional impairment. In an NICHD Neonatal Network study, though 27% of a cohort of ELBW infants diagnosed with CP at 18–22 months had moderate to severe gross motor function (Level 3–5), 28% had gross motor function consistent with level 0 or 1 and were ambulatory.[13] It is important to remember that a diagnosis of CP includes a wide spectrum of motor performance.

Additional subtle motor abnormalities and coordination inefficiencies are also seen commonly in former preterm infants. In recent years, the diagnosis of developmental coordination disorder (DCD) has been used. DCD is defined as impairment in motor performance sufficient to produce functional impairment that cannot be otherwise explained by the child's age, cognitive ability, or neurologic diagnosis. Scores of less than the 5th% to 10th% on the Movement Assessment Battery for Children (MABC) are considered diagnostic. DCD is found in 31–34% of VLBW and 50% of ELBW infants.[54]

Functional measures

The eighth area of assessment includes functional measures of daily living skills. Functional assessment is the determination of the child's ability to perform tasks of daily living and to fulfill the social roles expected of a physically and emotionally healthy child of the same age and culture Four functional outcome measures are currently available.[46,48,59] The Pediatric Evaluation of Disability Inventory (PEDI) assesses developmental skills in children 6 months to 7.5 years.[59] The Vineland Adaptive Behavior Scale (VABS) measures functional skills in children birth to 18 years.[48] The Battelle Developmental Inventory (BDI) is a developmental educational assessment battery for children age 0–8 years with or without developmental delays.[47] The Battelle consists of five domains: personal-social, adaptive, motor, communicative, and cognitive. The Functional Independence Measure for Children (WeeFIM)[46] can be used in children with and without disabilities through 8 years of age.

Justification for a functional assessment

Functional outcomes are considered particularly important by parents. Children born VLBW and ELBW with and without severe impairments have higher rates of functional limitations than children who were born at term. While 93% of ELBW infants achieve sitting balance, 83% walk, and 86% feed themselves independently by 18–22 months corrected age, more subtle functional deficits become apparent later in life.[21]

Behavior

Evaluations of behavior are routinely obtained in infancy and childhood by parent, teacher, or subject interviews with standardized measures rather than by direct observation or assessment. The Child Behaviour Checklist (CBCL),[60,61] is a parent-report questionnaire designed to describe social competencies and emotional/behavioural issues of children. There are two versions: one for 1½ to 5 year olds and a second for ages 6–18. The Conners Rating Scales,[62,63] are questionnaires designed for parents or teachers to describe symptoms of inattention, hyperactivity, and oppositionality in school-age children. In addition, because of the recent increasing rates of identification of autism spectrum disorder, especially in high-risk populations, more follow-up programs are screening for this disorder. The Modified Checklist for Autism in Toddlers (M-CHAT)[64,65] and the Pervasive Developmental Disorders Screening Test II (PDDST II)[66] are screeners for autism spectrum disorder.

Justification for behavior assessment

Very low birth weight has been associated with a wide variety of behavioral and psychological diagnoses and disabilities. Two prior studies have investigated rates of autistic characteristics in children born very VLBW. Indredavik *et al.*[67] demonstrated a trend toward higher scores on the Autism Spectrum Screening Questionnaire in VLBWs at 14 years of age compared to term controls. Limperopoulos *et al.*[68] reported that 25% of VLBW infants screened positive on the M-CHAT at 18 months.

At school age (8 to 12 years old), parents and teachers of VLBW/ELBW infants report higher rates of inattention and hyperactivity.[67,69] At 12 to 14 years of age, one quarter to one half of VLBW/ELBW infants have symptoms of anxiety and/or social withdrawal, 8% to 14%

meet criteria for generalized anxiety disorder,[67] and 25% to 28% meet criteria for a psychiatric disorder.[67]

Summary

Former preterm infants and subgroups of full term infants are at increased risk of a spectrum of growth, developmental, neurologic, and behavioral sequelae. A structured follow-up program for the NICU is needed to successfully accomplish the clinical, surveillance, research and educational objectives that will ultimately result in improved outcomes for high-risk infants.

References

1. Vohr BR, Wright LL, Hack M *et al.* (2004) Follow-up care of high-risk infants. *Pediatrics Supplement* 114.
2. Broyles RS, Tyson JE, Heyne ET *et al.* (2000) Comprehensive follow-up care and life-threatening illnesses among high-risk infants: A randomized controlled trial. *JAMA* **284**: 2070–2076.
3. Engle WA, Tomashek KM, Wallman C. (2007) "Late-preterm" infants: A population at risk. *Pediatrics* **120**: 1390–1401.
4. Khashu M, Narayanan M, Bhargava S *et al.* (2009) Perinatal outcomes associated with preterm birth at 33 to 36 weeks' gestation: A population-based cohort study. *Pediatrics* **123**: 109–113.
5. Aylward GP, Hatcher RP, Stripp B *et al.* (1985) Who goes and who stays: Subject loss in a multicenter, longitudinal follow-up study. *J Dev Behav Pediatr* **6**: 3–8.
6. Rickards AL, Ryan MM, Kitchen WH. (1988) Longitudinal study of very low birthweight infants: Intelligence and aspects of school progress at 14 years of age. *Aust Paediatr J* **24**: 19–23.
7. Vohr BR, Allan WC, Westerveld M *et al.* (2003) School-age outcomes of very low birth weight infants in the indomethacin intraventricular hemorrhage prevention trial. *Pediatrics* **111**: e340–e346.
8. McCormick MC, Gortmaker SL, Sobol AM. (1990) Very low birth weight children: Behavior problems and school difficulty in a national sample. *J Pediatr* **117**: 687–693.

9. Taylor HG, Klein N, Hack M. (2000) School-age consequences of birth weight less than 750 g: A review and update. *Dev Neuropsychol* **17**: 289–321.

10. Alexander GR, Himes JH, Kaufman RB *et al.* (1996) A United States national reference for fetal growth. *Obstet Gynecol* **87**: 163–168.

11. Ehrenkranz RA, Dusick AM, Vohr BR *et al.* (2006) Growth in the neonatal intensive care unit influences neurodevelopmental and growth outcomes of extremely low birth weight infants. *Pediatrics* **117**: 1253–1261.

12. Amiel-Tison C. (1987) Neuromotor Status. In Taeusch HW, Yogman MW (Eds). *Follow-up Management of the High-Risk Infant.* Little, Brown & Company, Boston, MA.

13. Vohr BR, Msall ME, Wilson D *et al.* (2005) Spectrum of gross motor function in extremely low birth weight children with cerebral palsy at 18 months of age. *Pediatrics* **116**: 123–129.

14. Hintz SR, Kendrick DE, Vohr BR *et al.* (2005) Changes in neurodevelopmental outcomes at 18 to 22 months' corrected age among infants of less than 25 weeks' gestational age born in 1993–1999. *Pediatrics* **115**: 1645–1651.

15. Lorenz JM, Wooliever DE, Jetton JR *et al.* (1998) A quantitative review of mortality and developmental disability in extremely premature newborns. *Arch Pediatr Adolesc Med* **152**: 425–435.

16. Hack M, Wilson-Costello D, Friedman H *et al.* (2000) Neurodevelopment and predictors of outcomes of children with birth weights of less than 1000 g: 1992–1995. *Arch Pediatr Adolesc Med* **154**: 725–731.

17. Vohr BR, Wright LL, Poole WK *et al.* (2005) Neurodevelopmental outcomes of extremely low birth weight infants <32 weeks' gestation between 1993 and 1998. *Pediatrics* **116**: 635–643.

18. Wilson-Costello D, Friedman H, Minich N *et al.* (2007) Improved neurodevelopmental outcomes for extremely low birth weight infants in 2000–2002. *Pediatrics* **119**: 37–45.

19. Doyle LW, Anderson PJ. (2005) Improved neurosensory outcome at 8 years of age of extremely low birthweight children born in Victoria over three distinct eras. *Arch Dis Child Fetal Neonatal Ed* **90**: F484–F488.

20. Marlow N, Wolke D, Bracewell MA *et al.* (2005) Neurologic and developmental disability at six years of age after extremely preterm birth. *N Engl J Med* **352**: 9–19.

21. Vohr BR, Wright LL, Dusick AM *et al.* (2004) Center differences and outcomes of extremely low birth weight infants. *Pediatrics* **113**: 781–789.

22. Drillien CM. (1972) Abnormal neurologic signs in the first year of life in low-birthweight infants: Possible prognostic significance. *Dev Med Child Neurol* **14**: 575–584.

23. De Vries LS, Van Haastert IL, Rademaker KJ *et al.* (2004) Ultrasound abnormalities preceding cerebral palsy in high-risk preterm infants. *J Pediatr* **144**: 815–820.

24. Year 2007 position statement: Principles and guidelines for early hearing detection and intervention programs. *Joint Committee on Infant Hearing.*

25. Bayley N. (1993) *Bayley Scales of Infant Development-II.* Psychological Corporation, San Antonio, TX.

26. Bayley N. (2006) *Bayley Scales of Infant Development-III.* Psychological Corporation, San Antonio, TX.

27. Thorndike RI, Hagan EP, Sattler JM. (1986) *Stanford-Binet Intelligence Scale, Fourth Edition.* Riverside, Chicago, IL.

28. Elliott CD. (1990) *Differential Ability Scales. Introductory and Technical Handbook.* The Psychological Corp., New York, NY.

29. Mc Carthy DA. (1972) *Manual for the McCarthy Scales of Children's Abilities.* The Psychological Corp., New York, NY.

30. Beery K. (1997) *Developmental Test of Visual Motor Integration, Fourth Edition.* Modern Curriculum Press, Parsippany, NJ.

31. Colarusso RH, DD. (1972) *Motor-Free Visual Perception Test Manual.* Western Psychological Services, Los Angeles, CA.

32. Dunn L. (1997) *Peabody Picture Vocabulary Test-III.* American Guidance Service, Circle Pines, MN.

33. Hendrick DL, Prather M, Tobin AR. (1984) *Sequenced Inventory of Communication Development (SICD)-Revised Edition.* Pro-ed 1984, Austin, TX.

34. Zimmerman IL, Steiner V, Pond R. (1992) *Preschool Language Scale, 3rd edition.* The Psychological Corporation, San Antonio, TX.

35. Coplan J. (1993) *Early Language Milestone Scale-Second Edition.* Pro-ed, Austin, TX.

36. Wechsler D. (1989) *Manual for the Wechsler Preschool and Primary Scale of Intelligence-Revised.* Psychological Corporation, San Antonio, TX.

37. Woodcock RW, Johnson MB. (1989) *Woodcock Johnson Psycho-Educational. Battery Revised.* DLM Teaching Resources, Allen, TX.

38. Bruininks R. (1978) *Bruininks-Oseretsky Test of Motor Proficiency.* American Guidance Service, Circle Pines, MN.

39. Folio MR, Fewell RR. (1983) *Peabody Developmental Motor Scales and Activity Cards.* Developmental Learning Materials Resource, Allen, TX.

40. Harrison P, Kaufman AS, Kaufman NL *et al.* (1990) *Early Screening Profiles (ESP).* American Guidance Service.

41. Palisano RJ. (1993) Validity of goal attainment scaling in infants with motor delays. *Phys Ther* **73**: 651–658; discussion 658–660.

42. Ireton H. (1992) *Child Development Inventory.* Behavior Science Systems, Minneapolis, MN.

43. Larson SL, Vitali GJ. (1988) *Kindergarten Readiness Test (KRT).* Slosson Educational Publication, East Aura, NY.

44. Miller LJ. (1988) *Miller Assessment for Preschoolers (MAP).* The Psychological Corporation, San Antonio, TX.

45. Nehring AD, Nehring EM, Bruni JR *et al.* (1992) *Learning Accomplishment Profile — Diagnostic (LAP-D) Standardized Assessment–1992 Revision and Standardization.* Kaplan Press, Examiner's Manual, Lewisville, NC.

46. Msall ME, DiGaudio K, Duffy LC *et al.* (1994) WeeFIM. Normative sample of an instrument for tracking functional independence in children. *Clin Pediatr (Phila)* **33**: 431–438.

47. Newborg J, Jock JR, Wnek L, *et al.* (1984) *Battelle Development Inventory and recalibrated technical data and morns: Examiner's manual. DLG, LINC Associates.* Teaching Resources, Allen, TX.

48. Sparrow S, Balla D, Cicchetti D. (1984) *Vineland Adaptive Behavior Scales: Interview Edition, Survey Form Manual. A revision of the Vineland Social Maturity Scale by E.A. Doll.* American Guidance Service, Circle Pines, MN.

49. Gioia G, Isquith PK, Guy SC, Kenworthy L. (2000) *Behavior Rating Inventory of Executive Function, Professional Manual.* Psychological Assessment Resources, Inc., Odessa, FL.

50. Hack M, Taylor HG, Drotar D *et al.* (2005) Poor predictive validity of the Bayley Scales of Infant Development for cognitive function of extremely low birth weight children at school age. *Pediatrics* **116**: 333–341.

51. Anderson PJ, Doyle LW. (2004) Executive functioning in school-aged children who were born very preterm or with extremely low birth weight in the 1990s. *Pediatrics* **114**: 50–57.

52. Taylor HG, Klein N, Drotar D *et al.* (2006) Consequences and risks of <1000-g birth weight for neuropsychological skills, achievement, and adaptive functioning. *J Dev Behav Pediatr* **27**: 459–469.

53. Saigal S, den Ouden L, Wolke D *et al.* (2003) School-age outcomes in children who were extremely low birth weight from four international population-based cohorts. *Pediatrics* **112**: 943–950.

54. Foulder-Hughes LA, Cooke RW. (2003) Motor, cognitive and behavioural disorders in children born very preterm. *Dev Med Child Neurol* **45**: 97–103.

55. Goyen TA, Lui K, Woods R. (1998) Visual-motor, visual-perceptual and fine motor outcomes in very-low-birthweight children at 5 years. *Dev Med Child Neurol* **40**: 76–81.

56. Luu TM, Ment LR, Schneider KC *et al.* (2009) Lasting effects of preterm birth and neonatal brain hemorrhage at 12 years of age. *Pediatrics* **123**: 1037–1044.

57. Wolke D, Samara M, Bracewell M *et al.* (2008) Specific language difficulties and school achievement in children born at 25 weeks of gestation or less. *J Pediatr* **152**: 256–262.

58. Palisano R, Rosenbaum P, Walter S *et al.* (1997) Development and reliability of a system to classify gross motor function in children with cerebral palsy. *Dev Med Child Neurol* **39**: 214–223.

59. Haley SM, Coster WJ, Ludlow LH *et al.* (1992) *Pediatric Evaluation of Disability Inventory (PEDI), Version I, Development, standardization and administration manual.* New England Medical Center-PEDI Research Group, Boston, MA.

60. Achenbach TM. (2000) *Child Behavior Checklist 1.5–5.* ASEBA, Burlington, VT.

61. Achenbach TM. (2001) *Child Behvaior Checklist 6–18.* ASEBA, Burlington, VT.

62. Gianarris WJ, Golden CJ, Greene L. (2001) The Conners' parent rating scales: A critical review of the literature. *Clin Psychol Rev* **21**: 1061–1093.

63. Goyette GH, Conners CK, Ulrich RF. (1978) Normative data on revised Conners Parent and Teacher Rating Scales. *J Abnormal Child Psychol* **6**: 221–236.

64. Robins DL, Fein D, Barton ML *et al.* (2001) The modified checklist for autism in toddlers: An initial study investigating the early detection of autism and pervasive developmental disorders. *J Autism Dev Disord* **31**: 131–144.

65. Kleinman JM, Robins DL, Ventola PE *et al.* (2008) The modified checklist for autism in toddlers: A follow-up study investigating the early detection of autism spectrum disorders. *J Autism Dev Disord* **38**: 827–839.
66. Siegel B. (2004) *Pervasive Developmental Disorders Screening Test-II.* Psych Corp, San Antonio, TX.
67. Indredavik MS, Vik T, Heyerdahl S *et al.* (2004) Psychiatric symptoms and disorders in adolescents with low birth weight. *Arch Dis Child Fetal Neonatal Ed* **89**: F445–F450.
68. Limperopoulos C, Bassan H, Sullivan NR *et al.* (2008) Positive screening for autism in ex-preterm infants: Prevalence and risk factors. *Pediatrics* **121**: 758–765.
69. Anderson P, Doyle LW. (2003) Neurobehavioral outcomes of school-age children born extremely low birth weight or very preterm in the 1990s. *JAMA* **289**: 3264–3272.

Chapter

21

Medical Care of NICU (Neonatal Intensive Care Unit) Graduates

Bonnie E. Stephens, Leslie T. McKinley
and Betty R. Vohr

Introduction

Neonatal Intensive Care Unit (NICU) graduates are a diverse population of infants, but the most common reason for admission remains preterm birth. Advances in antenatal medicine have successfully resulted in improved survival rates of preterm infants.[1] While many preterm infant survivors ultimately thrive, they are at increased risk for medical morbidities[2] which may result in post-discharge morbidities[3–6] or special health care needs.[7–11] These infants also have increased rates of rehospitalizations within the first year of life.[12] Well-coordinated, comprehensive, multidisciplinary follow-up care is important in decreasing the severity of these morbidities.

Infants with intrauterine growth restriction (IUGR) are vulnerable to the same morbidities as preterm infants, especially if they are also preterm. Full-term infants with meconium aspiration syndrome (MAS), persistent pulmonary hypertension of the newborn (PPHN), infection, congenital diaphragmatic hernia (CDH), neonatal encephalopathy and multiple congenital anomalies also require intensive care and are at risk for health and neurodevelopmental sequelae.[13,14] However, this chapter will focus primarily on preterm infants.

Discharge Criteria

Prior to discharge, preterm infants should achieve physiologic stability, defined as the ability to feed orally in sufficient quantity to support growth, the ability to maintain euthermia, and the development of mature respiratory control. These criteria are met between 36 and 37 weeks in the majority of preterm infants, but occasionally not until 44 weeks.[15] Important exceptions include infants with incurable, terminal disorders requiring palliative care and infants who are dependent on technology such as ventilator, oxygen, apnea monitors, pulse oximetry, or tube feedings.[15,16] These will be discussed later in the chapter.

Follow-Up Care

Limited guidelines for the provision of follow-up services to NICU graduates exist, thus management differs among centers.[17] Most high-risk infants are enrolled in a NICU Follow-up Clinic staffed by specialists in neonatology and child development, who provide periodic assessments at specified times within the child's development with the goal of monitoring outcomes of NICU interventions (see also Chapter 20 "Follow-Up Assessment of High-Risk Infants").

All infants discharged from the NICU need to see a primary care physician with expertise in caring for NICU graduates within one week of NICU discharge.[15] In addition to providing well child care, anticipatory guidance, management of growth, nutrition and acute illness and illness prevention, this physician is the child's "Medical Home" or care coordinator. Pediatric subspecialists should also follow infants with continuing medical issues and/or special health care needs. Some infants require home or visiting nursing care. All should be referred for Early Intervention services.

Infants with ongoing medical problems such as chronic lung disease, seizures, or feeding difficulties and those with technological dependence should have their first follow-up visit shortly after discharge, followed by weekly to monthly visits until their condition resolves. Infants with milder conditions such as gastroesophageal reflux can be followed every few months for assessment and medication adjustment.

While the timing of follow-up varies, the goals are universal: support of nutrition and growth, prevention of infectious disease, and early detection and treatment of medical sequelae.

Corrected vs Chronologic Age

For infants born <34 weeks gestation, use corrected age (time since mother's expected date of delivery) for all assessments of growth, development and nutrition in the first 30 months of life. Use chronologic age (time since birth) thereafter. In contrast, always base immunization schedules on chronologic age regardless of gestational age at birth.

Growth, Nutrition and Feeding

Growth

The majority of very low birth weight (VLBW, ≤1500 grams) infants become growth restricted (growth parameters < 10th percentile) during NICU hospitalization.[18,19] These infants have episodes of accelerated growth, often between 4 and 12 months with growth parameters approaching the 25th to 50th percentile.[9] Head growth achieves catch-up before weight and length; it is not unusual for the head circumference to be 50th to 90th percentile with weight and length 3rd to 25th percentile in the first year of life.[20] Preterm infants with chronic lung disease, necrotizing enterocolitis, feeding difficulties are at especially high risk for growth failure. While preterm infants continue to demonstrate catch up growth throughout childhood, they continue to lag behind their normal birth weight (NBW) peers through adolescence.[21] By age 20, females born VLBW have caught up to their NBW counterparts. However males remain significantly smaller in length and weight.[21]

The ideal growth trajectory for a preterm infant remains controversial. While growth failure is associated with poor neurodevelopmental outcomes, catch-up growth may have undesirable metabolic effects, such as insulin resistance and coronary heart disease.[22] Nevertheless, growth measurements and rates remain the simplest and most well-accepted means of determining overall health.[4,23]

Perform measurement of growth at all follow-up visits.[17] Growth parameters at discharge should be made available as a baseline for calculation of growth rates. For children <2 years of age, measure weight without clothing or diaper; length in the recumbent position using a pediatric length board; maximal occipital frontal head circumference to the nearest millimeter using a standard measuring tape. After age 2, obtain standing height. Plot these measurements on standard growth charts, using corrected age prior to 30 months and chronologic age after 30–36 months.[17] Plot growth parameters at regular intervals to identify inadequate or excessive growth.

Approximate growth rates for girls and boys at the 50th percentile of the WHO Growth Standards (www.cdc.gov/growthcharts/who; accessed October 12, 2010):

	Weight	Length
Birth to 3 months	31 g/d	0.9 cm/wk
3 to 6 months	17 g/d	0.5 cm/wk
6 to 9 months	10 g/d	0.3 cm/wk
9 to 12 months	8 g/d	0.3 cm/wk

During the catch-up phase, premature infants may gain at greater rates. High nutritional intakes accompany rapid growth. Weight and length should be less than two percentile rankings apart. Weight and length are in proportion when the age-independent measure of weight-for-length falls between the 25th and the 75th percentile.

Nutrition

While evidence for post-discharge feeding recommendations is sparse, it is accepted that because of high rates of growth failure, preterm infants require nutrient enriched feedings, either nutrient enhanced formulas ("transitional formulas") or fortified human milk, for some period postdischarge.[36,37,47,48]

There is unequivocal evidence that breast milk is the optimal source of nutrition for all neonates. Most importantly, higher cognitive scores at 18 and 30 months follow-up are associated with higher intake of breast milk.[24,25] Infants and mothers should receive adequate breastfeeding support during neonatal hospitalization and after discharge. Mothers who supply all feedings as breast milk by hospital discharge have a better chance of success at breastfeeding after discharge.

Unsupplemented human milk provides inadequate protein, calcium, phosphorus, vitamins and minerals to support growth and prevent osteopenia in the preterm infant.[26,27] Current recommendations for preterm infants fed exclusively human milk is fortification of expressed breast milk and supplementation with a multivitamin with iron and vitamin D.[26,27] Expressed human milk is most commonly fortified with a human milk fortifier during neonatal hospitalization and with transitional formula powder following discharge. Fortified expressed breast milk or supplemental transitional formula is no longer needed when breastfeeding alone produces adequate growth (Table 1).

For healthy, preterm infants, 110–130 Kcal/kg/day are recommended, but 130–150 Kcal/kg/day may be needed for infants with chronic lung disease. At NICU discharge, many preterm infants consume 165–200 mL/kg/d of transitional formula concentrated to a calorie level that will support adequate weight gain. Transitional formulas come ready-to-use (22 Kcal/oz) and as powder. While the standard dilution is 22 Kcal/oz, transitional formula powder can be mixed to concentrations of 24, 27 or 30 Kcal/oz.

How long an infant should remain on transitional formula is unclear. Taking parental stature into account, length, weight and head circumference should show evidence of catch-up to at least the 25–50th percentiles. When an infant maintains these percentiles and can consume ~26 oz/d of formula, it is appropriate to change to term formula. Preterm infants may benefit from transitional formula until 6–9 months corrected age.

Table 1. Directions for preparing breast milk to different caloric densities.

20 kcal/oz = HM20
22 kcal/oz = 45 mL HM20 + ¼ tsp Trans formula powder
24 kcal/oz = 45 mL HM20 + ½ tsp Trans formula powder
27 kcal/oz = 30 mL HM20 + ½ tsp Trans formula powder
30 kcal/oz = 30 mL HM20 + ½ tsp Trans formula powder + 0.45 mL corn oil

Errors in mixing instructions are common. At each follow-up visit, ask the caregiver to state the recipe that she/he is using to verify appropriate caloric density. Make modifications as necessary.

AAP recommendations for starting solid foods for preterm infants are comparable to those for term infants, using corrected age, but developmental readiness for solid foods may appear later for premature infants. Solid foods are generally less nutrient dense than breast milk or formula, thus introduction of solids prior to 4–6 months corrected age may compromise nutritional intake.

Compromised nutrition may also result if caregivers start cow's milk or fruit juices too soon. It is recommended that fruit juice begin after 6–8 months corrected age and whole cow's milk no sooner than one year corrected age. Children over one year of age who continue to have poor growth may need a supplemental pediatric formula. These formulas are generally 30 Kcal/oz and come in a ready-to-use form.

At each follow-up visit, obtain a 24-hour food recall and complete nutritional assessment. If intake is inadequate, unbalanced, or excessive, provide nutrition counseling. Refer infants with ongoing growth or nutritional issues to a pediatric Registered Dietitian. Nutrition support is also available from the Early Intervention and the Women Infant and Children (WIC) Programs.

Iron therapy and anemia

Up to 85% of preterm infants develop iron deficiency. Iron is accumulated during the third trimester of pregnancy so the smaller, more preterm infants are at greatest risk. Unless a preterm infant receives external sources of iron, their endogenous iron stores meet their needs for only 2–3 months. Iron deficiency can lead to poor growth, gastrointestinal disturbances, thyroid dysfunction, altered immunity, temperature instability, anemia and motor deficits.[28]

Daily iron requirements for the preterm infant are 5–6 mg/kg/day. The iron content of human breast milk is 0.5 mg/L. Transitional formula provides 13 mg iron/L. Current recommendations are to provide supplemental iron at a dose of 2 mg/kg/day for infants exclusively breastfed and 1 mg/kg/day for formula fed infants, for the first 12 months of life.[28]

Screen preterm infants for iron deficiency with a hemoglobin and hematocrit at 4 months, 6 months and 9–12 months of age. Iron deficiency will result in a low hemoglobin, low serum ferritin and low transferrin. Infants found to be iron deficient should receive 3–6 mg/kg/day of elemental iron for 3 months.[28]

Vitamin D deficiency and osteopenia

While the incidence of osteopenia in low birth weight infants has decreased with improvements in neonatal nutrition, preterm infants remain at elevated risk for osteopenia and bone fractures. Premature infants receiving prolonged parenteral nutrition or unsupplemented enteral feedings during neonatal hospitalization are at highest risk.

The AAP recommends all infants receive 400 IU of vitamin D daily. Most multivitamin preparations for infants contain 400 IU of vitamin D per 1 mL.[29] To assure adequate intake, exclusively breastfed infants should receive 400 IU of supplemental vitamin D per day. Formula fed infants should receive 400 IU of vitamin D per day from formula and supplements combined.

Feeding

Persistent oromotor dysfunction or suck-swallow incoordination can occur in some extremely preterm infants, infants with perinatal asphyxia, or infants with congenital anomalies of the head and neck such as cleft lip, cleft palate and micrognathia. Severe oromotor dysfunction can result in aspiration, which can lead to inflammatory pneumonitis.

Preterm infants, especially those with lung disease, are often "slow feeders." This may be due to oromotor dysfunction and to the increased energy expenditure required for feeding. These infants are at risk for growth failure due to inadequate dietary intake or increased energy expenditure required for prolonged feeding.

Oral aversion occurs most frequently in extremely preterm infants with a history of prolonged intubation and mechanical ventilation. It may also be a presentation of gastroesophageal reflux. Oral aversion can result in inadequate oral intake for growth.

For infants with severe feeding difficulties, placement of a gastrostomy tube may be necessary. Unless contraindicated due to aspiration or other swallowing dysfunction, oral feedings should continue to be encouraged along with tube feedings. Involvement with an occupational and/or speech therapist is helpful in working through feeding difficulties. Referral to a comprehensive, multidisciplinary feeding team may also be necessary.

Apnea of Prematurity

Apnea of prematurity is defined as cessation of breathing for ≥20 seconds or periodic breathing (3 or more respiratory pauses >3 seconds with <20 seconds of respiration between) associated with bradycardia (<60–80 beats per minute), oxygen desaturation (<80–85%) and/or cyanosis in an infant <37 weeks gestation.[30] Infants born <28 weeks gestation have 100% incidence of periodic breathing. Up to 85% of infants <34 weeks have apnea. Pathologic apneas cease in 92% of infants by 37 weeks. However, apneas may persist until up to 43 weeks, especially in infants born <28 weeks.[30]

Apneas may be central, obstructive or mixed. Central apnea occurs with absence of brainstem stimulus to breathe, resulting in absence of breathing effort. Obstructive apnea occurs with central effort to breathe, but air flow is blocked by mucous or airway collapse. Mixed apneas contain both central and obstructive components. The role of gastro-esophageal reflux in apnea of prematurity is controversial. Further studies are needed to assess this relationship.

The significance of apnea in preterm infants is unclear, but it is thought that infants with more frequent or severe events are at higher risk of cognitive impairment. Thus, most infants with central apnea are treated with methylxanthines (caffeine) to decrease the frequency and severity of apneas. While the majority of infants no longer have severe apnea at the time of discharge, a small number of infants remain on caffeine. All infants discharged with persistent events should have a home apnea monitor and parents should receive instruction in cardiopulmonary resuscitation (CPR) and use of the monitor prior to discharge.

Parents of infants on a home monitor should keep a daily record of alarms and events and report any events or concerns to their pediatrician. Parents are advised to avoid smoking in the home, fireplace smoke, high altitudes, airplane flights and exposure to anyone with a respiratory infection.

Infants discharged on caffeine and/or apnea monitors should be seen at least every 4 weeks. Allow infants on caffeine to outgrow the dose naturally; if no events occur as the dose is outgrown, discontinue the caffeine; if events occur, increase the dose for weight gain. Once off caffeine, infants should remain on a monitor until event free for 4 weeks.

Preterm infants are at increased risk for SIDS. However, studies have failed to show a reduction in SIDS with home monitoring.[31]

Bronchopulmonary Dysplasia/Chronic Lung Disease

Chronic lung disease (CLD, oxygen requirement at 36 weeks in a preterm infant) is a common sequelae of prematurity and can result in considerable morbidity even after NICU discharge. Infants with CLD are often discharged later than those without, due to prolonged oxygen and/or ventilatory requirements. While VLBW infants with and without CLD are at increased risk of symptomatic pulmonary disease and rehospitalizations after discharge, infants with CLD remain at higher risk of growth failure, feeding problems due to oral defensiveness or oromotor dysfunction, gastroesophageal reflux, infection, respiratory illness, rehospitalizations, prolonged apnea of prematurity and neurodevelopmental impairment.[32] Systemic and pulmonary hypertension are more common in infants with CLD. These infants may also develop tracheomalacia and/or bronchomalacia.

Infants with moderate to severe CLD are often discharged on supplemental oxygen, monitors, diuretics and bronchodilators. Providing home oxygen results in earlier discharge in infants who are otherwise stable and ready for discharge. Adequate oxygenation with supplemental oxygen to keep saturations ≥93–95% decreases the incidence of SIDS, results in improved weight gain and catch-up growth, decreases pulmonary artery pressure resulting in improvement in pulmonary hypertension, improves lung compliance, airway resistance and work of breathing, decreases incidence of central and obstructive apnea and improves sleep architecture in preterm infants with CLD.[33,34] Continue oxygen therapy until the infant consistently demonstrates normal oxygen saturations, good growth velocity and "sufficient stamina for a full range of activity"[15] and pulmonary hypertension has resolved.

Evidence for treatment of CLD with long-term diuretic therapy is sparse and its use is controversial.[32] For infants discharged on diuretics, wean and discontinue oxygen first. Once stable off oxygen, wean diuretics unless the infant has outgrown the dose, in which case they may be stopped. Infants receiving diuretic therapy should be monitored closely for electrolyte disturbances.[32]

There is no evidence for long-term use of bronchodilators in CLD. Albuterol is rarely used as maintenance therapy, but can be beneficial during acute respiratory illness.

Survivors of CLD often demonstrate airway hyper-reactivity, obstruction, hyperinflation and decreased pulmonary function into adolescence and adulthood. A gradual improvement in lung function over time has been documented.[31,32]

The incidence of neurodevelopmental impairment increases significantly with the severity of CLD, reaching 62% among those with severe CLD.[35]

Gastroesophageal Reflux

Gastroesophageal reflux (GER) is seen in higher rates at lower gestational ages and in infants with neurologic impairment. GER occurs secondary to transient relaxation of the lower esophageal sphincter in combination with horizontal positioning and a relatively large volume of milk intake. Delayed gastric emptying has been shown not to contribute.[36]

Diagnosis of GER disease (GERD) is often made based on clinical suspicion. Many symptoms have been attributed to GERD; however, there is a lack of practical, valid diagnostic methods, especially in the outpatient setting. Ph-probe only diagnoses acidic reflux, while the pH of infants' gastric contents is >4 the majority of the time.[36] Multiple intraluminal impedence is more valid, but time consuming to perform and interpret.[36,37]

Though rare, GERD can result in complications including recurrent aspiration pneumonia and failure-to-thrive due to odynophagia, parents' reluctance to feed an infant who vomits after feeding, or caloric loss from repeated vomiting.

Conservative treatment for reflux includes keeping the infant upright for 20 minutes after feeding and keeping the head of the infant's bed elevated to 15–45 degrees, smaller more frequent feedings and thickening feedings with cereal or commercial thickener.[37] If these treatments are unsuccessful, consider pharmacologic therapy with an H2Blocker or a proton pump inhibitor. Duration of treatment is individualized but the majority of infants outgrow GER by 6–12 months of age. Monitor for symptoms of GERD as an infant outgrows their dose; if they occur, increase dosages for weight. If maximum pharmacologic support does not alleviate symptoms, a pediatric surgery consult is warranted to evaluate the need for fundoplication.

Inguinal Hernias and Hydroceles

Because preterm infants are born prior to closure of the processus vaginalis, indirect inguinal hernias are common. Lower birth weight, male gender, and prolonged mechanical ventilation increase the risk. Bilateral inguinal hernias occur more commonly than unilateral.[38]

Peak incidence of hernias in preterm infants is at term equivalent, so while many are diagnosed and surgically repaired prior to discharge, many are diagnosed in the outpatient setting. Incarceration is more common than in term infants, but recurrence rate is low.[31,38]

Check for hernias at each follow-up physical exam; if a hernia is diagnosed, surgical repair should be scheduled.[38]

Neurologic and Neurosensory Sequelae

Seizures

Infants in the NICU have seizures for a variety of reasons including hypoxic-ischemic encephalopathy, cerebral hemorrhage or infarction, meningitis, sepsis, CNS malformations, metabolic disorders, congenital infection and idiopathic reasons.

Due to the lack of evidence, treatment of neonatal seizures varies widely. Infants discharged from the NICU after a seizure should be followed closely by a neurologist who can make decisions about the need for seizure prophylaxis. While there are no published prospective trials, available data does not support the use of Phenobarbital after hospital discharge for the treatment of isolated neonatal seizures.[39]

Sequelae of intraventricular hemorrhage and periventricular leukomalacia

Grade 3–4 intraventricular hemorrhage (IVH) is associated with a 2–6 fold increased risk of cerebral palsy (CP).[40,41] A 3–10 fold increased risk of CP is associated with cystic periventricular leukomalacia (PVL).[40,41] Posthemorrhagic hydrocephalus may increase the risk of CP by 12 times[42] and the presence of PVL and hydrocephalus by 15 times.[41]

Perform a thorough neurologic exam to assess for signs of CP and a head circumference, looking for rapidly increasing head circumference at each follow-up visit. A rapidly increasing head circumference or fontanel size or a tense or pulsating fontanel suggests the development of late onset hydrocephalus, requiring further evaluation.

Visual disturbances

Retinopathy of prematurity (ROP) is a disorder of the developing retina that occurs only in preterm infants and can result in retinal detachment and blindness. Infants born <32 weeks or 32–35 weeks with an unstable clinical course are at risk for ROP as their retina are not fully vascularized at birth.[43]

All infants at risk for ROP should be screened in the NICU.[43] Infants whose ROP has not resolved prior to discharge need outpatient ophthalmology follow-up every 1–3 weeks. Infants with treated or resolved ROP remain at risk for late retinal detachment and other visual disturbances and need follow-up by an ophthalmologist every 3–6 months. Even infants without ROP are at elevated risk for strabismus and refractive errors and need ophthalmologic follow-up every 6–12 months.

Hearing loss

While infants in the NICU for prematurity, congenital or acquired infection, respiratory failure requiring mechanical ventilation, hypoxic ischemic encephalopathy, or certain genetic syndromes are at elevated risk for congenital hearing loss, all infants regardless of risk should be screened. Refer all infants who fail the initial newborn screen for comprehensive audiology diagnostic assessment with an audiologist experienced in evaluating infants, followed by referral to early intervention services. Infants who pass the neonatal screen, but have a risk factor for hearing loss, should be referred for an audiology diagnostic assessment by 24–30 months of age, or sooner if there are clinical signs of hearing loss of language delay.

Other Complications

Torticollis and plagiocephaly

The "Back to Sleep" campaign has resulted in an increase in positional torticollis and deformational plagiocephaly. Deformational plagiocephaly is a skull deformity with asymmetric flattening of the occiput resulting from prolonged supine positioning. Positional torticollis is a stiff neck with contraction of neck muscles and rotation of the head to one side which is often associated with deformational plagiocephaly.[44]

Preterm infants are at higher risk for torticollis and plagiocephaly as they spend many more months supine than term infants. Counsel parents at discharge and early follow-up visits to alternate head position during supine positioning for sleep, have frequent "tummy time" while awake, and spend minimal time in a car safety seat when not a passenger in a vehicle.[44]

At each follow-up visit look at the infant not only from the front, back and sides, but also down at the top of the head. From this view point, plagiocephaly will appear as a parallelogram-shaped skull. Imaging studies are usually not required for diagnosis.[44]

Treatment involves parental education, positioning with the rounded side of the occiput down, supervised "tummy time" as frequently as possible, gentle stretching exercise of the neck with each diaper change, and referral to a physical therapist.

Plagiocephaly that is unresponsive to 2–3 months of conservative management requires the use of a skull-molding helmet. The best results from a helmet occur between 4 and 12 months of age while the skull is still malleable. Surgery is rarely required unless plagiocephaly is resistant to all non-surgical measures or associated with craniosynostosis.[44]

Cholestasis

Preterm infants are at risk for feeding intolerance requiring prolonged parenteral nutrition. This may result in cholestasis with elevated direct bilirubin levels. Once enteral feedings are established, it can take weeks to months for cholestasis to resolve. Monitor bilirubin and liver enzyme levels on a regular basis until resolution is seen. For direct bilirubin levels >2 mg/dL, medications that increase biliary flow such as ursodiol or phenobarbital are prescribed. Discontinued these once direct bilirubin levels decrease to <2 mg/dL. Infants with cholestasis requiring pharmacologic treatment should be followed by a Pediatric Gastroenterologist.

Short bowel syndrome

Short bowel syndrome is defined as insufficient bowel length to digest and absorb adequate nutrients for growth. Necrotizing enterocolitis requiring intestinal resection is the most common cause, though intestinal atresias, gastroschisis and volvulus can all result in short bowel. Short bowel syndrome is associated with dehydration, malnutrition, poor growth, infection and neurodevelopmental impairment.[45]

Physicians of infants with short bowel syndrome need to work closely with their pediatric surgeon and gastroenterologist as enteral feeding is gradually advanced and parenteral nutrition slowly weaned. Monitor growth and symptoms of malabsorption closely.[46] Infants with short bowel syndrome are more likely to require prolonged parenteral nutrition, gastrostomy tube feedings, elemental infant formulas, long NICU stays, and readmissions after NICU discharge. Some infants with short bowel will require bowel transplantation.

Health Maintenance

Back to sleep

Preterm infants are at increased risk of SIDS.[47] Parents should be counseled regarding SIDS prevention. All infants should be placed supine for sleeping.[15] Supine sleeping position has led to an increase in rates of positional skull deformities, discussed earlier in this chapter.

Car safety seats

Prior to hospital discharge, all infants born <37 weeks should undergo a car safety seat observation to ensure that they do not develop apnea, bradycardia or desaturation in their car safety seat. The AAP recommendations for infant car seat safety should be followed for all NICU graduates with the following considerations[48]:

1. Most rear-facing car safety seats are designed for infants weighing at least 4–5 pounds. Low birth weight infants have relative hypotonia and risk for airway obstruction.
2. For infants with apnea, bradycardia and/or desaturation in a car seat, a car bed may be indicated. A similar observation in the car bed prior to discharge is important as some infants have apneas, bradycardias and desaturations in a car bed.
3. Preterm infants should only be placed in a car safety seat for travel. Placement in car safety seat can worsen reflux and plagiocephaly in addition to placing the infant at risk for apnea.
4. Some infants are discharged from the NICU requiring medical equipment such as oxygen, ventilators and monitors. Portable devices are available, but are heavy and could cause injury if they hit a child during a sudden stop or crash. This equipment should be secured to the vehicle floor or underneath a seat to prevent injury.[49]

Infants with a tracheostomy should be placed in a car seat with a three-point or five-point harness, never in a seat with a harness-tray/shield combination or an armrest due to the risk of falling forward and causing airway injury. Toddlers with hypotonia and poor head control should be placed in a convertible car seat with lateral support, a rolled towel between the legs and crotch strap. Infants with hypertonia may need a roll placed under their knees.[49]

Immunizations/infection control

Preterm infants are at increased risk of morbidity from vaccine-preventable diseases. They are, however, less likely than term infants to receive immunizations on time. With the exception of hepatitis B, medically stable preterm infants should receive all recommended childhood vaccines at the same chronologic age as full-term infants. Immunizations of preterm infants frequently are started in the NICU. A complete immunization record should be provided to the medical home at discharge. Vaccine dosages are the same as those given to term infants. Intramuscular vaccines should be administered in the anterolateral thigh.

Hepatitis B should be given to all infants born >2000 grams at birth. Infants born ≤2000 grams should only receive hepatitis B vaccine at birth if maternal hepatitis B status is positive or unknown. In these cases, hepatitis B vaccine and hepatitis B immune globulin should be given within 12 hours of birth. In preterm infants whose maternal hepatitis B status is negative, the first hepatitis B vaccine should be given at 30 days or hospital discharge if <30 days.

Palivizumab is licensed for the prevention of serious morbidity from respiratory syncytial virus (RSV) in infants at high risk for these complications. It is recommended for all eligible infants during the RSV season (typically November through March) and is given as an intramuscular injection every 30 days during this season. Eligible infants include:

1. Infants born <28 weeks gestation who are <12 months at the start of RSV season (eligible for 5 doses)
2. Infants born <32 weeks gestation who are <6 months at the start of RSV season (eligible for 5 doses)
3. Infants born 32–35 weeks who attend daycare or live with another child <5 years of age (eligible for 3 doses)
4. Infants ≤12 months with congenital abnormalities of the airway or neuromuscular disease (eligible for 5 doses)

5. Infants ≤24 months with cyanotic congenital heart disease, moderate to severe pulmonary hypertension, or congestive heart failure requiring pharmacologic management (eligible for 5 doses per year).
6. Infants ≤24 months with CLD requiring medical management (oxygen, etc.) within 6 months of the RSV season (eligible for 5 doses per year).

Technology Dependence

While for many infants, the dependence on technological support is self-limited and resolved by NICU discharge, a subgroup require technological support post-discharge.[15,16]

Home oxygen

Home oxygen allows infants with chronic lung disease and residual oxygen requirement to achieve early discharge and avoids the risks that inadequate oxygenation poses, such as poor growth and cor pulmonale.[15] Infants discharged on oxygen should also be discharged on an apnea monitor or pulse oximeter.[15]

Infants discharged on oxygen should receive monthly follow-up until off of oxygen. Oxygen therapy should be continued until the infant consistently demonstrates normal oxygen saturations, good growth velocity and "sufficient stamina for a full range of activity,"[15] and pulmonary hypertension has resolved. It should then be gradually weaned to keep saturations ≥93–95%.

Home monitors

The indications for home monitoring with a cardiac apnea monitor are not well established, thus use of home monitoring varies widely. Home apnea monitors are not indicated for the prevention of sudden infant death syndrome (SIDS)[15,16]; they should not replace the need for development of mature respiratory control and should not be used to justify the discharge of infants who continue to have central or obstructive apneas.[15] Most NICUs recommend home apnea monitoring for infants with prolonged apnea of prematurity requiring methylxanthine therapy and those with chronic lung disease requiring home oxygen and/or mechanical ventilation.[16]

Monitor settings at discharge are usually: Apnea $\geq$20 seconds; Bradycardia $\leq$80 beats/minute; Tachycardia $\geq$220 beats/minute. To avoid false-positive bradycardia alarms, the bradycardia setting should be lowered as follows: <38 weeks: 100 beats/minute; 38–44 weeks: 80 beats/minute; 1–3 months: 70 beats/minute; 3–12 months: 60 beats/minute. Apnea monitor alarms are known to cause additional stress for the family; careful assessment of the infant's respiratory status is indicated to ensure that the monitor is discontinued as soon as the infant is medically stable.

Home ventilation

Home ventilation requires multidisciplinary care coordination, in-depth parental education with demonstration of mastery of the specific skills needed, and close follow-up and support in the outpatient and in-home setting.[15] Arrangement of home nursing care is crucial. In some areas, respite care for the parents is also available.

Gastrostomy tube (G-tube) feeding

Preterm infants are at high risk for feeding difficulties. It is best to learn this skill in the hospital with nursing and occupational or speech therapy support. However, if unable to acquire these skills due to significant oral aversion, abnormal mental status, or aspiration, G-tube should be surgically placed and parents should be taught how to administer tube feedings and care for the G-tube site. It is recommended that feeding volumes be adjusted at least once per week, based on weight gain, to maintain adequate growth. Oral feeding should be continued with tube feeding unless the infant's ability to protect their own airway is compromised due to a swallowing abnormality or abnormal neurologic status.[15]

Intravenous nutrition

Home intravenous nutrition is rarely required, usually in the setting of short-bowel syndrome where enteral feedings are not adequately absorbed.[15]

This necessitates central venous access in the form of a percutaneous central venous catheter or surgically placed central line.

Palliative Care

For infants with incurable, terminal illness families often prefer to spend the last few days or weeks of the infant's life at home.[15,16] In these cases, palliative care is provided by both the family and home nursing staff with a goal of preventing physical pain and suffering and optimizing quality of life for both the infant and their family, in combination with curative therapies or as part of a hospice program where life-prolonging therapies are not provided.[16] In rare instances, withdrawal of assisted ventilation can occur at home.[15]

In preparation for discharge to palliative care in the home setting, medical follow-up, home nursing, delivery and education of parent regarding home equipment and supplies, bereavement support services, and respite care resources should be provided.[15] Decisions should be made regarding resuscitation status and family preference about rehospitalization versus continued home care in the case of worsening medical status. Resuscitation status should be clearly documented.

Conclusions

The medical needs of the NICU graduate are variable and diverse and should be managed by careful coordination between pediatrician and an established NICU follow-up program.

References

1. Fanaroff AA, Hack M, Walsh MC. (2003) The NICHD neonatal research network: Changes in practice and outcomes during the first 15 years. *Semin Perinatol* **27**(4): 281–287.
2. Lemons JA, Bauer CR, Oh W *et al.* (2001) Very low birth weight outcomes of the National Institute of Child health and human development neonatal research network, January 1995 through December 1996. NICHD Neonatal Research Network. *Pediatrics* **107**(1): E1.

3. Blakely ML, Lally KP, McDonald S *et al.* (2005) Postoperative outcomes of extremely low birth weight infants with necrotizing enterocolitis or isolated intestinal perforation: A prospective cohort study by the NICHD Neonatal Research Network. *Ann Surg* **241**(6): 984–989; discussion 989–994.

4. Ehrenkranz RA, Dusick AM, Vohr BR *et al.* (2006) Growth in the neonatal intensive care unit influences neurodevelopmental and growth outcomes of extremely low birth weight infants. *Pediatrics* **117**(4): 1253–1261.

5. Laptook AR, O'Shea TM, Shankaran S *et al.* (2005) Adverse neurodevelopmental outcomes among extremely low birth weight infants with a normal head ultrasound: Prevalence and antecedents. *Pediatrics* **115**(3): 673–680.

6. Schmidt B, Asztalos EV, Roberts RS *et al.* (2003) Impact of bronchopulmonary dysplasia, brain injury, and severe retinopathy on the outcome of extremely low birth weight infants at 18 months: Results from the trial of indomethacin prophylaxis in preterms. *JAMA* **289**(9): 1124–1129.

7. Blaymore–Bier J, Pezzullo J, Kim E *et al.* (1994) Outcome of extremely low birth weight infants: 1980–1990. *Acta Paediatr* **83**(12): 1244–1248.

8. Costeloe K, Hennessy E, Gibson AT *et al.* (2000) The EPI Cure study: Outcomes to discharge from hospital for infants born at the threshold of viability. *Pediatrics* **106**(4): 659–671.

9. Hack M, Fanaroff AA. (2000) Outcomes of children of extremely low birth weight and gestational age in the 1990s. *Semin Neonatol* **5**(2): 89–106.

10. Sauve RS, Robertson C, Etches P *et al.* (1998) Before viability: A geographically-based outcome study of infants weighing 500 grams or less at birth. *Pediatrics* **101**(3 Pt 1): 438–445.

11. Wood NS, Marlow N. (1999) Non-neurological morbidity among extremely preterm children at two and a half years. *Proceedings of the Royal College of Paediatrics and Child Health* A40: G98.

12. Chien YH, Tsao PN, Chou HC *et al.* (2002) Rehospitalization of extremely low birth weight infants in first 2 years of life. *Early Hum Dev* **66**(1): 33–40.

13. Chiu P, Hedrick HL. (2008) Postnatal management and long-term outcome for survivors with congenital diaphragmatic hernia. *Prenat Diagn* **28**(7): 592–603.

14. Rees CM, Pierro A, Eaton S. (2007) Neurodevelopmental outcomes of neonates with medically and surgically treated necrotizing enterocolitis. *Arch Dis Child Fetal Neonatal Ed* **92**(3): F193–F198.

15. Hospital discharge of the high-risk neonate. (2008) *Pediatrics* **122**(5): 1119–1126.

16. Hummel P, Cronin J. (2004) Home care of the high-risk infant. *Adv Neonatal Care* **4**(6): 354–364.

17. Follow-up care of high-risk infants. (2004) *Pediatrics* **114**(5): 1377–1397.

18. Ehrenkranz RA. Growth outcomes of very low-birth weight infants in the newborn intensive care unit. *Clin Perinatol* **27**(2): 325–345.

19. Ehrenkranz RA, Younes N, Lemons JA *et al.* (1999) Longitudinal growth of hospitalized very low birth weight infants. *Pediatrics* **104**(2 Pt 1): 280–289.

20. Hack M, Merkatz IR, McGrath SK *et al.* (1984) Catch-up growth in very low birth weight infants. Clinical correlates. *Am J Dis Child* **138**(4): 370–375.

21. Hack M, Schluchter M, Cartar L *et al.* (2003) Growth of Very Low Birth Weight Infants to Age 20 Years. *Pediatrics* **112**(1): e30–e38.

22. Saigal S, Stoskopf B, Streiner D *et al.* (2006) Growth trajectories of extremely low birth weight infants from birth to young adulthood: A longitudinal, population-based study. *Pediatr Res* **60**(6): 751–758.

23. Georgieff MK, Hoffman JS, Pereira GR *et al.* (1985) Effect of neonatal caloric deprivation on head growth and 1-year developmental status in preterm infants. *J Pediatr* **107**(4): 581–587.

24. Vohr BR, Poindexter BB, Dusick AM *et al.* (2007) Persistent beneficial effects of breast milk ingested in the neonatal intensive care unit on outcomes of extremely low birth weight infants at 30 months of age. *Pediatrics* **120**(4): e953–e959.

25. Vohr BR, Poindexter BB, Dusick AM *et al.* (2006) Beneficial effects of breast milk in the neonatal intensive care unit on the developmental outcome of extremely low birth weight infants at 18 months of age. *Pediatrics* **118**(1): e115–e123.

26. Griffin IJ, Cooke RJ. (2007) Nutrition of preterm infants after hospital discharge. J *Pediatr Gastroenterol Nutr* **45** (Suppl 3): S195–S203.

27. Klein CJ. (2002) Nutrient requirements for preterm infant formulas. *J Nutr* **132**(6 Suppl 1): 1395S–1577S.

28. Rao R, Georgieff MK. (2009) Iron therapy for preterm infants. *Clin Perinatol* **36**(1): 27–42.

29. Wagner CL, Greer FR. (2008) Prevention of rickets and vitamin D deficiency in infants, children, and adolescents. *Pediatrics* **122**(5): 1142–1152.

510   *B. E. Stephens, L. T. McKinley and B. R. Vohr*

30. Apnea, sudden infant death syndrome and home monitoring. *Pediatrics* **111**(4 Pt 1): 914–917.

31. Verma RP, Sridhar S, Spitzer AR. (2003) Continuing care of NICU graduates. *Clin Pediatr* (Phila) **42**(4): 299–315.

32. Shah PS. (2003) Current perspectives on the prevention and management of chronic lung disease in preterm infants. *Paediatr Drugs* **5**(7): 463–480.

33. Kotecha S, Allen J. (2002) Oxygen therapy for infants with chronic lung disease. *Arch Dis Child Fetal Neonatal Ed* **87**(1): F11–F14.

34. Poets CF. (1998) When do infants need additional inspired oxygen? A review of the current literature. *Pediatr Pulmonol* **26**(6): 424–428.

35. Ehrenkranz RA, Walsh MC, Vohr BR *et al.* (2005) Validation of the National Institutes of Health consensus definition of bronchopulmonary dysplasia. *Pediatrics* **116**(6): 1353–1360.

36. Poets CF. (2004) Gastroesophageal reflux: A critical review of its role in preterm infants. *Pediatrics* **113**(2): e128–e132.

37. Birch JL, Newell SJ. (2009) Gastrooesophageal reflux disease in preterm infants: Current management and diagnostic dilemmas. *Arch Dis Child Fetal Neonatal Ed* **94**(5): F379–F383.

38. DeCou JM, Gauderer MW. (2000) Inguinal hernia in infants with very low birth weight. *Semin Pediatr Surg* **9**(2): 84–87.

39. Guillet R, Kwon J. (2007) Seizure recurrence and developmental disabilities after neonatal seizures: Outcomes are unrelated to use of phenobarbital prophylaxis. *J Child Neurol* **22**(4): 389–395.

40. Vohr BR, Wright LL, Poole WK *et al.* (2005) Neurodevelopmental outcomes of extremely low birth weight infants <32 weeks' gestation between 1993 and 1998. *Pediatrics* **116**(3): 635–643.

41. Ment LR, Bada HS, Barnes P *et al.* (2002) Practice parameter: Neuroimaging of the neonate: Report of the Quality Standards Subcommittee of the American Academy of Neurology and the Practice Committee of the Child Neurology Society. *Neurology* **58**(12): 1726–1738.

42. Msall ME, Buck GM, Rogers BT *et al.* (1991) Risk factors for major neurodevelopmental impairments and need for special education resources in extremely premature infants. *J Pediatr* **119**(4): 606–614.

43. Screening examination of premature infants for retinopathy of prematurity. *Pediatrics* **117**(2): 572–576.

44. Persing J, James H, Swanson J *et al.* (2003) Prevention and management of positional skull deformities in infants. American Academy of Pediatrics Committee on Practice and Ambulatory Medicine, Section on Plastic Surgery and Section on Neurological Surgery. *Pediatrics* **112**(1 Pt 1): 199–202.

45. Cole CR, Hansen NI, Higgins RD *et al.* (2008) Very low birth weight preterm infants with surgical short bowel syndrome: Incidence, morbidity and mortality and growth outcomes at 18 to 22 months. *Pediatrics* **122**(3): e573–e582.

46. Wessel JJ, Kocoshis SA. (2007) Nutritional management of infants with short bowel syndrome. *Semin Perinatol* **31**(2): 104–111.

47. Thompson JM, Mitchell EA. (2006) Are the risk factors for SIDS different for preterm and term infants? *Arch Dis Child* **91**(2): 107–111.

48. Bull MJ, Engle WA. (2009) Safe transportation of preterm and low birth weight infants at hospital discharge. *Pediatrics* **123**(5): 1424–1429.

49. Bull M, Agran P, Laraque D *et al.* (1999) American Academy of Pediatrics. Committee on Injury and Poison Prevention. Transporting children with special health care needs. *Pediatrics* **104**(4 Pt 1): 988–992.

Index